Geriatric Mental Health Disaster and Emergency Preparedness

John A. Toner, EdD, PhD, is associate professor of Medical Psychology, director of Residency/Fellowship Programs, and co-director of the Statewide Geriatric Psychiatry Residency/Fellowship Program at the Columbia University Stroud Center and Department of Psychiatry. He is a senior research scientist at the New York State Psychiatric Institute and holds interdepartmental and interuniversity appointments in the Mailman School of Public Health, where he has been a recipient of the Calderone Prize for Faculty Research, and the State University of New York, Upstate Medical University, where he is a director of the Center for Aging Research, Education, and Services. He is the director of the Columbia–New York Geriatric Education Center of the Consortium of New York Geriatric Education Centers and the Rural Geriatric Mental Health Initiative (POISE). Trained in gerontology and geriatric neuropsychology, Dr. Toner has devoted over 20 years to educating and recruiting medical doctors and other health care professionals to work in medically underserved areas. He is an editorial board member and fellow of numerous scientific journals and professional societies.

Therese M. Mierswa, MSW, is a Fordham University Andrus Scholar Geriatric Social Worker currently serving as the coordinator for assisted living in the Maryknoll Fathers and Brothers Retirement Community in Ossining, New York. Prior to this position, she was the program coordinator for the Columbia University Statewide Geriatric Psychiatry Residency Program. Ms. Mierswa has a Certificate of Training from the AMA and National Disaster Life Support Foundation in Basic Disaster Life Support, a certificate in Geriatric Mental Health and Emergency Preparedness from the Consortium of New York Geriatric Centers (CNYGEC), and CMI Education Institute credits in crisis debriefing for survivors of trauma and violence.

Judith L. Howe, PhD, is associate professor in the Brookdale Department of Geriatrics and Palliative Medicine, Mount Sinai School of Medicine; associate director/education and evaluation, Geriatric Research, Education, and Clinical Center (GRECC) at the James J. Peters VA Medical Center; and director, Consortium of New York Geriatric Education Centers. She is a board member of the Association for Gerontology in Higher Education (AGHE) and president of the National Association of Geriatric Education Centers. Dr. Howe is the Editor designate of the *Gerontology and Geriatric Education Journal*. Dr. Howe is a fellow of the New York Academy of Medicine, AGHE, and the Gerontological Society of America.

Geriatric Mental Health Disaster and Emergency Preparedness

JOHN A. TONER, EdD, PhD, EDITOR

THERESE M. MIERSWA, MSW, ASSOCIATE EDITOR

JUDITH L. HOWE, PhD, ASSOCIATE EDITOR

SPRINGER PUBLISHING COMPANY
New York

Springer Publishing Company, LLC
11 West 42nd Street
New York, NY 10036
www.springerpub.com

Acquisitions Editor: Sheri W. Sussman
Senior Editor: Rose Mary Piscitelli
Cover design: David Levy
Composition: Laura Stewart, Apex CoVantage, LLC
Ebook ISBN: 978-0-8261-2222-3

10 11 12/ 5 4 3 2 1

The author and the publisher of this Work have made every effort to use sources believed
to be reliable to provide information that is accurate and compatible with the standards
generally accepted at the time of publication. The author and publisher shall not be
liable for any special, consequential, or exemplary damages resulting, in whole or in part,
from the readers' use of, or reliance on, the information contained in this book. The
publisher has no responsibility for the persistence or accuracy of URLs for external or
third-party Internet Web sites referred to in this publication and does not guarantee
that any content on such Web sites is, or will remain, accurate or appropriate.

Library of Congress Cataloging-in-Publication Data

Geriatric mental health disaster and emergency preparedness / John A. Toner,
editor ; Therese M. Mierswa, associate editor, Judith L. Howe, associate editor.
    p. ; cm.
  Includes bibliographical references and index.
  ISBN 978-0-8261-2221-6 (alk. paper)
1. Geriatric psychiatry. 2. Older people—Mental health services. I. Toner,
John A. II. Mierswa, Therese M. III. Howe, Judith L.
  [DNLM: 1. Disaster Medicine—methods. 2. Mental Health Services.
3. Aged. 4. Geriatric Psychiatry—methods. 5. Stress Disorders,
Post-Traumatic. WT 145 G232 2010]
  RC451.4.A5G4653 2010
  618.97'689—dc22   2010000409

Printed in the United States of America by Hamilton Printing

Dedicated to Flo Aaroe,
who personifies what it means to
take the high road,
and to the countless number of
invisible and silent survivor-victims of disasters;
to Rev. James J. Dineen, SJ,
who brought spiritual support
to victims' families and workers at Ground Zero;
and to Flo's son,
Bruce E. Simmons,
August 13, 1960–September 11, 2001.

What though the radiance which was once so bright
Be now for ever taken from my sight,
Though nothing can bring back the hour
Of splendour in the grass, of glory in the flower;
We will grieve not, rather find
Strength in what remains behind;
In the primal sympathy
Which having been must ever be;
In the soothing thoughts that spring
Out of human suffering;
In the faith that looks through death,
In years that bring the philosophic mind
—William Wordsworth

Contents

PART I: INTRODUCTION

PART II: COMMUNITY RESPONSE TO THE NEEDS OF OLDER PERSONS IN DISASTERS

PART III: CLINICAL RESPONSE TO THE NEEDS OF OLDER PERSONS DURING DISASTERS

PART IV: IDENTIFYING AND CLASSIFYING MENTAL AND RELATED HEALTH PROBLEMS

Contributors

Othmane Alami, MD
Acting Medical Director
Mental Health PSL Community Outreach Team
Minneapolis, Minnesota
Adjunct Clinical Assistant Professor
University of Minnesota at Minneapolis

Lynda Atack, RN, PhD
Professor
Baccalaureate Nursing Program
School of Community and Health Sciences
Centennial College
Toronto, Canada

Annette M. Atanous, MSSW
Education Specialist
U.S. Department of Veterans Affairs
James J. Peters VA Medical Center
Geriatric Research, Education, and Clinical Center (GRECC)
Bronx, New York

D. Peter Birkett, MD
Director
Statewide Geriatric Psychiatry Residency/ Fellowship Program
Associate Research Scientist
Columbia University Stroud Center
New York, New York

Trish Dryden, RMT, MEd
Director
Applied Research and Innovation
Centennial College
Toronto, Canada

Michael B. Friedman, LMSW
Director
Center for Policy, Advocacy, and Education
Geriatric Mental Health Alliance of New York
New York, New York

Terry Fulmer, PhD, RN, FAAN
Erline Perkins McGriff Professor
Dean
New York University College of Nursing
New York, New York

William Grant, EdD
Executive Director
Center for Emergency Preparedness
SUNY Upstate Medical University
Syracuse, New York

Neil Hall, MD, MBA
Attending Physician
Associate Research Scientist
Columbia University Stroud Center
New York, New York

Judith L. Howe, PhD
Associate Professor
Brookdale Department of Geriatrics and Palliative Medicine
Mount Sinai School of Medicine
New York, New York
Associate Director/Education and Evaluation
VISN 3 Geriatrics Research, Education, and Clinical Center Program (GRECC)
    at James J. Peters VA Medical Center
Bronx, New York
Director
Consortium of New York Geriatric Education Centers
Director
VA Interprofessional Palliative Care Fellowship Program

Joanne Izzo, MDiv, LCSW-R
Social Worker
Posttraumatic Stress Disorder Outpatient
Department of Veterans Affairs
Brooklyn Campus, New York Harbor Healthcare Medical Center
Brooklyn, New York

Beth A. Kallmyer, LCSW
Director
Client Services
Alzheimer's Association
Chicago, Illinois

Jed A. Levine, MA
Executive Vice President
Director of Programs and Services
New York City Chapter of the Alzheimer's Association
New York, New York

Richard Mandelbaum, RH, AHG
Registered Herbalist
Forestburgh, New York

Lucia McBee, LCSW, MPH, CYI
Social Work Supervisor
Jewish Home Lifecare
Adjunct Lecturer
Columbia University School of Social Work
New York, New York

Evelyn S. Meyer, MA, LMSW
Artist and Freelance Author
Los Angeles, California

Therese M. Mierswa, MSW
Coordinator
Assisted Living
Maryknoll Fathers and Brothers
Ossining, New York

Mark R. Nathanson, MD
Director
Psychiatric Emergency Services
Elmhurst Hospital and Medical Center
Elmhurst, New York
Assistant Clinical Professor
Columbia University Department of Psychiatry
Attending Physician
New York Presbyterian Hospital
New York, New York

Nora O'Brien-Suric, MA
Senior Program Officer
The John A. Hartford Foundation
New York, New York

Ian Portelli, PhD, MMS, CRA
Director
Emergency Medicine Research
New York University School of Medicine
Department of Emergency Medicine
NYU Center for Catastrophe, Preparedness, and Response
New York, New York

Jenny Riddell, MA
Lecturer and Psychotherapist
Department of Interdisciplinary Studies in Professional Practice
School of Community and Health Sciences
City University, London, UK

Douglas M. Sanders, PhD
Deputy Clinical Director and Licensed Clinical Psychologist
Rockland Psychiatric Center (Middletown Campus)
Cognitive Remediation Program
Middletown, New York

Andrea Sherman, PhD
President
Transitional Keys
Master Trainer
National Center for Creative Aging
Washington, DC

Philippa Sully, MSc, RN
Visiting Lecturer in Reflective Practice
Department of Interdisciplinary Studies in Professional Practice
School of Community and Health Sciences
City University, London, UK

Concetta M. Tomaino, DA, MT-BC, LCAT
Executive Director/Co-Founder
Institute for Music and Neurologic Function
Senior Vice President
Music Therapy Services
Beth Abraham Family of Health Services
Bronx, New York

John A. Toner, EdD, PhD
Director
Geriatric Residency and Fellowship Programs
Co-Director
Columbia University Statewide Geriatric Psychiatry Residency/
    Fellowship Program
Director
Columbia–New York Geriatric Education Center of the Consortium of New York
    Geriatric Education Centers (CNYGEC)
Associate Clinical Professor and Senior Research Scientist
Columbia University Stroud Center in the Faculty of Medicine and New York State
    Psychiatric Institute
New York, New York

Nina Tumosa, PhD
Professor
Saint Louis University
Health Education Officer
VISN 15 GRECC
Co-Director
Gateway Geriatric Education Center of Missouri and Illinois
St. Louis, Missouri

Andrea Villanti, MPH, CHES
Senior Education Coordinator
Department of Epidemiology
Johns Hopkins Bloomberg School of Public Health
Baltimore, Maryland

Malcolm T. Wandrag, MSc
Lecturer
Civil Emergency Management
City University
London, UK

Kimberly A. Williams, LCSW
Director
The Geriatric Mental Health Alliance of New York
The Center for Policy, Advocacy, and Education
Mental Health Association of New York City
New York, New York

Foreword

With the increase in the number and complexity of disaster events, there is one factor that remains constant in determining the effectiveness of disaster mental health response and recovery—that is, preparedness. Evidence shows that disaster mental health programs for older persons are most effective when there is an existing plan for the rapid mobilization, response, and service implementation of mental health providers. However, this is rarely the case. Older victims of disasters are often neglected and left alone in their despair, as was the case in the aftermaths of September 11, 2001, and Hurricane Katrina. *Ageism,* a term I first coined in 1969, refers to the denial on a societal level of the special needs of a large segment of the population. This is particularly true regarding the emotional/mental health needs of older persons during times of crises, such as disasters.

After the September 11 World Trade Center attacks, many older persons and people with disabilities living near the disaster area were left stranded in their homes without assistance. In response, the International Longevity Center-USA, of which I am president and chief executive officer, contacted local and citywide organizations that serve older people to find out how they had dealt with the emergency and to discover what resources were available to aid these vulnerable sectors of the city in the event of a future emergency. We were frankly shocked to find an overwhelming lack of plans and systems to care for vulnerable populations such as the elderly and impaired. In particular, we noted the critical shortage of mental health practitioners experienced in working with older clients and a lack of general knowledge about how mental health problems are manifested in older persons. With better awareness of the symptoms, practitioners can intervene more quickly and appropriately to sustain the best possible quality of life for the older person during and subsequent to a disaster or emergency.

This volume provides the first-ever comprehensive overview of the essential information everyone working with older persons should know about the mental health effects of disasters on the elderly. It emphasizes the essential role that choice and choosing play in maintaining quality of life for older persons affected by disasters and emergencies. It also gives key evidence-based and interdisciplinary approaches for identifying and classifying mental health disorders, such as PTSD, depression, and substance abuse, to which older persons are particularly vulnerable. This is a must-read book for clinicians, service providers, policy makers, program planners, and teachers in the fields of mental health, aging, and emergency preparedness.

Robert N. Butler, MD

Preface

The rage you feel does more damage to the vessel in which it is stored than to the object on which it is poured. Give it up girl.

—Anonymous

Here is the copy of the verse you wanted, John. I found this on the sidewalk as I was going into my lawyer's office! Good advice—wherever you are! Stay well—my best to the kids. See you in May! Love, Flo xx.

—Flora Aaroe, March 22, 2009

On September 11, 2001, life, as most of us had come to know it in America, changed. The physically, emotionally, and socially numbing catastrophe of the tragic attacks on the World Trade Center (WTC) in New York City and the Pentagon in Washington, DC, have left a void in the American psyche. Yet as a society we have moved on. And we have done so because of our collective wisdom, which guides us in the direction of hope, rebirth, and redemption, with an ever-present awareness that our individual and societal *vessels* are better served by doing so.

Flo Aaroe is the 72-year-old mother of a WTC victim. Within the 12-month period leading up to September 11, her husband of many years fell victim to a lingering terminal illness and died, her son-in-law was killed in a motorcycle accident, she was forced to move from her home, and most tragic of all, her son, Bruce, was killed in the terrorist attack on Tower II of the WTC. In the emotional abyss of her life at the time, Flo saw hope where there seemed to be only hopelessness. She found peace where around her fermented rage. Out of the abyss—and primarily due to a supportive network of family and friends (and excellent mental health interventions)—Flo came to know herself as never before . . . she became whole. In 2009, Flo reflected on the past 8 years as she recounted the experiences of her first deep dive in Cancun, Mexico, and her hot air balloon safari in eastern Pennsylvania. Up, up, and away! You go, girl!

Flo is representative of the thousands of *invisible and silent survivor-victims* of the September 11 events and the many other man-made and natural disasters of our time. The visible survivor-victims of these disasters, such as the grieving young widows and their infant/toddlers or adolescent children, the homeless young families, and so forth, receive most of the attention from the government, the media, and society at large. But the older, invisible, and silent survivor-victims of disaster are often left alone in their despair. These are the older disaster survivors themselves, and also the parents, the grandparents, the siblings, and the friends of younger victims lost in disasters. This book is about them and their needs . . . and particularly about their mental health needs, which are most often neglected either because they do not seek help—the *stiff upper lip* mentality—or because they are bypassed by first responders and follow-up mental health providers.

The primary purpose of this book is to provide a comprehensive overview of the essential information everyone working or hoping to work in the field of aging should know about disasters, emergencies, and their effects on the mental health and well-being of older persons. Another purpose of the book is to efficiently provide the reader with evidence-based approaches for identifying and classifying mental health problems, such as posttraumatic stress disorder (PTSD), depression, and substance use, that may occur in older adults during and post disasters/emergencies. Additionally, the book provides state-of-the-art resources related to clinical, individual, and community responses to the mental health needs of older people in disasters. Specifically, in addition to providing evidence-based approaches to assessment and diagnosis of mental health problems, the book helps define the special needs and approaches to the care of *at-risk* groups of older persons such as veterans and holocaust survivors; older adults who are isolated, dependent, have mobility problems or communication deficits, are cognitively impaired, or have other comorbidities; elders who use Meals on Wheels, vital medications, or home care; or older persons who are in senior centers, nursing homes, or assisted living settings. This book utilizes quality of life as its unifying theme and emphasizes the work of Barry Gurland and associates at the Columbia University Stroud Center for Quality of Life in establishing the critical role that choices and choosing have in promoting good quality of life, particularly during disasters, emergencies, and other crises in older persons' lives. The general aims of the book are to (1) increase understanding of the mental health issues in older adults; (2) provide tools that can foster resiliency and recovery at the community, group, and individual levels;

and (3) influence the development of positive responses to disasters—
that is, responses that have the potential to minimize adverse mental and
physical outcomes in older persons and maximize individual and group
recovery in the context of quality of life.

The burgeoning older population in the United States, particularly
the rapid increase in numbers of those over the age of 85, calls for resources to prepare a workforce to serve this population. The U.S. Census
Bureau projection for the year 2025 is that 18.2% of the national population will be 65 years or older, and by 2050 the proportion of those over the
age of 65 will more than double. Moreover, in certain disaster-prone areas of the country such as the southeastern coastal areas, older adults
are significantly more heavily represented. Therefore, it is imperative to
prepare those in the workforce involved in natural and/or man-made disasters and disaster preparedness with the skills and knowledge to work
with this rapidly growing population, as they are likely to interface with
older persons during disasters and emergencies.

Recent studies of PTSD in older persons have challenged popular
stereotypes and revealed the substantial proportions of older persons who
develop PTSD and the high proportion who continue to suffer chronic
mental health and associated physical conditions post-disaster. Some
studies provide evidence that medical and social impacts on older persons
and their caregivers can be comparable or worse than for younger persons. Paradoxically, there is evidence that older adults have greater resilience to the effects of disasters than younger persons. Regardless, this
book provides disaster preparedness strategies for reducing disaster-
related impacts on older persons and their caregivers and building upon
their natural resilience.

Emerging evidence from disasters such as the 2001 World Trade
Center disaster, the 2004 Sumatra tsunami and earthquake, and 2005's
Hurricane Katrina suggests that the affected communities, disaster responders, and health care professionals can greatly benefit from systematic disaster preparedness such as that provided by this book.

This book lays the foundation upon which clinicians, policy makers,
program planners, teachers, and researchers can build. The primary target audience of this book is case managers and other specialists in services to older persons, such as social workers, nurses, psychologists, nurse
practitioners, psychiatrists, primary care physicians, clergy, and elder care
attorneys. It will also be a resource to older people themselves and their
family caregivers as well as other formal and informal care providers
such as friends and neighbors. Finally, the book will be a useful resource

to public welfare agencies, educational institutions, health care facilities, community outreach providers such as Meals on Wheels programs, transportation services for older persons, visiting nurse associations, and other mental health associations.

The eighteen chapters that comprise the book are organized into the following five sections: Introduction, Community Response to the Needs of Older Persons in Disasters, Clinical Response to the Needs of Older Persons During Disasters, Identifying and Classifying Mental and Related Health Problems, and Special Populations. The first three chapters form the Introduction. Chapter 1 sets the stage for our discussion of disaster and emergency preparedness and provides an overview of the essentials of disaster-related mental health in older persons. Chapter 1 also describes the strictly circumscribed criteria for evidence as adopted from, among others, the Cochrane Review for Effective Practice and begins the discussion of evidence-based care practices in the context of quality of life and the choice and choosing model. Quality of life, and more specifically the choice and choosing model of quality of life, serves as a unifying theme for the book. This theme links the five parts of the book into a cohesive whole. Chapter 2 demonstrates the overlapping mental and physical health issues related to older persons and disasters and provides useful tips to clinicians and nonclinicians alike about how mental health particularly affects physical health and vice versa in this age group. Chapter 3 provides an overview of the national Geriatric Emergency Preparedness and Response (GEPR) network and captures the progress that has been made to focus national attention on older people, the heretofore invisible and silent survivor-victims.

Chapter 4 is the lead chapter in the Community Response section. The authors point out that nearly half of all U.S. states do not have official plans that specifically address disaster preparedness for older persons. Furthermore, it is clear from the authors' research that there are no consistent national or state emergency preparedness plans that detail how to provide services to older persons during disasters. Chapters 5 and 6 provide descriptions of two cross-national models of geriatric mental health disaster preparedness programs. The first is a Canadian model that draws on evidence-based literature and the results of key informant interviews conducted by the authors to describe governmental, community-based, and academic geriatric mental health disaster initiatives under way in Canada. Chapter 6 describes a national and cross-national mental health services model originating in England with broad applicability internationally. The chapter focuses on the use of facilitated reflective practice as key to the preparation for and delivery of interdisciplinary services to older persons in disasters. Chapters 7, 8, and 9 complete the section by providing public health guidelines for developing community mental health disaster preparedness plans. Each chapter presents examples of self-help programs that have been used successfully to promote optimal health, promote quality of life, assess the likelihood of recurrence of disease, and manage disease (an explanation of these programs is contained in chapter 7). These tools, as outlined in chapter 8, are designed to help individuals better control fear levels, minimize disruption in their quality of life, increase personal safety, provide peace of mind, deliver culturally and ethnically appropriate information, and improve coping with post-traumatic stress. Chapter 9 concludes that first responders cannot meet the overwhelming demands subsequent to catastrophic events, so it is incumbent on community leaders to develop disaster preparedness plans that involve volunteers, including older persons themselves.

The three subsequent chapters comprise the Clinical Response section and focus on state-of-the-art evidence-based clinical practices relevant to treating the mental health needs of older persons during disasters. Chapter 10 examines psychosocial and pharmacological interventions for older persons during disasters with a special focus on the major domains of mental health symptoms experienced by older persons in disasters and the identification of mediating and buffering factors that promote resilience and quality of life. The authors also specify interventions that integrate and are sensitive to both common symptoms as well as idiosyncratic responses to disaster. Chapter 11 provides an overview of the important role of case management in assisting older persons with mental disorders or troubling emotional reactions in the aftermath of a disaster. The authors point out, however, that while there has been considerable research about the effectiveness of case management with older adults, the literature related to the effectiveness of case management with older persons experiencing mental, emotional, or substance abuse issues in the aftermath of a disaster is extremely limited. Chapter 12 reviews a number of complementary and alternative medicine (CAM) interventions, which are designed to enhance the ability of older persons and their caregivers to respond to the mental and physical stressors of disaster. The chapter describes the general reasons that CAM might be effective for older persons and describes in detail several specific treatments, applications, and recommendations that promote quality of life.

Three additional chapters expand upon the scope of the Clinical Response section and comprise the section titled Identifying and Classifying

Mental and Related Health Problems. Chapter 13 examines the inter-disciplinary treatment team as a resource for identifying and classifying mental health and related problems in older persons during disasters and describes evidence-based interdisciplinary teamwork methods that have been incorporated into a model interdisciplinary team training program and applied to geriatric mental health disaster preparedness. This chapter also describes strategies for team training in geriatric mental health and disaster preparedness and applications of the choice and choosing model of quality of life to interdisciplinary teamwork. Chapter 14 uses a case study approach to emphasize the risk factors for psychological distress in older persons including the nature and severity of the disaster, the vulnerability of the older patient/client before and during the disaster, threat to life, previous history of psychological disturbances, past treatment efficacy, and current access to mental health services. The authors provide an in-depth review of evidence-based geriatric assessment for the recognition and differential diagnosis of mental health problems, including the systematic assessment of quality of life. The concluding chapter in this section probes the normal versus pathological aspects of bereavement and grief. The author introduces strategies for determining if the symptoms of grief—agitation and weeping, disbelief, hallucinations, panic attacks, phobias, anger, and depression—are *normal* or part of a mental health disease process such as PTSD, for example.

The final section of the book, Special Populations, is devoted to three chapters that address the special needs of specific subgroups of older persons who are particularly vulnerable to developing new mental health symptoms and/or experiencing exacerbation of existing mental health problems. These three groups are the following: veterans (chapter 16), older persons suffering from Alzheimer's disease and related disorders (chapter 17), and older persons who are mistreated and/or abused during disasters and emergencies (chapter 18).

John A. Toner, EdD, PhD

Acknowledgments

In connection with this book project, the editors have incurred several substantial debts of gratitude. Dr. Hugh Barr gave generously of his time and constructive thinking and was instrumental in facilitating the recruitment of our cross-national collaborators.

Sheri W. Sussman deserves special thanks for her crucial assistance in many aspects of this book and for her consistent encouragement and support throughout the course of the project. Without her intuitive knowledge of the importance of this project and her support in overcoming numerous seemingly insurmountable obstacles, this volume might never have been realized.

Dr. Barry Gurland, scholar, mentor, director of the Columbia University Stroud Center, and co-director of the Consortium of New York Geriatric Centers (CNYGEC), provided encouragement and critical administrative support for this project. He gave tirelessly and willingly of his time and advice.

We thank our spouses: Nancy Knight Toner, Robert Harangozo, and the late Thomas J. Skeffington, whose personal sacrifices, untiring patience, love, and intermittent interest have made it all possible. We are especially appreciative of our children—Clark, Catherine, and Andrew; Caroline; and Michael and Peter—and the sacrifices they, too, have made for this book project. Our wish for them is that they always be prepared for the unexpected.

A note of gratitude to Mark A. Fionda, Jr., for his technical assistance in the preparation of the tables in this book.

Introduction

A Primer for Disaster and Emergency Preparedness and Evidence-Based Care Practices in Geriatric Mental Health

JOHN A. TONER AND OTHMANE ALAMI

Older persons represent the fastest growing segment of the American population. The U.S. Census Bureau projects that 18.2% of the U.S. population will be over the age of 65 by 2025, and by 2050 the population of older persons will more than double (Himes, 2007). This dramatic growth in the population of older persons in the United States is even more pronounced in certain disaster-prone regions such as Florida and the Gulf coast. Yet relatively little is known about the mental health impacts of disasters on older persons (Busuttil, 2004; Yehuda & Hyman, 2005) and even less about effective interventions for older persons who have been exposed to disasters (Owens, Baker, Kasckow, Ciesla, & Mohamed, 2005). Large-scale epidemiological studies of disaster-related mental health have been conducted with samples of older persons but these have focused on PTSD in older persons (van Zelst, de Beurs, Beekman, Deeg, & van Dyck, 2003). These studies have found high prevalence rates of PTSD in cohorts of older people, who often develop PTSD in the acute phase following a disaster (Neal, Hill, Hughes, Middleton, & Busuttil, 1995; Rauch, Morales, Zubritsky, Knott, & Oslin, 2006). Many older persons who initially develop acute symptoms of PTSD eventually suffer chronicity of symptoms (Elklit & O'Connor, 2005; Livingston, Livingston, & Fell, 2008). Some studies have shown that impacts on older persons can be comparable (Chung, Dennis, Easthope, Farmer, & Werrett, 2005; Kohn, Levav, Garcia, Machuca, & Tamashiro, 2005)

3

or worse (Adams & Boscarino, 2006) than for younger subjects, depending on the circumstances and other corollary risk factors.

Pioneering work has begun to expand the field of study of the consequences of disasters on the mental health of older persons. Predictors of acute (Mecocci, et al., 2000; Yazgan, Dedeoglu, & Yazgan, 2006) and chronic (Goenjian, et al., 1994; Goenjian, et al., 2008; Marshall, et al., 2006) PTSD in older persons are being identified and related to or distinguished from predictors in younger age groups (Chung, et al., 2005; Livingston, Livingston, Brooks, & McKinley, 1992). Groups of older persons at high risk for developing symptoms of PTSD are being characterized (Chung, 2007; Elklit & O'Connor, 2005). This growing number of findings may lead to more rational and effective interventions (Marshall, et al.; Yazgan, et al.). Some studies have found that older subjects have greater resilience than younger subjects, both after disasters (Phifer, 1990; Seplaki, Goldman, Weinstein, & Lin, 2006) and in recovery (Kato, Asukai, Miyake, Minakawa, & Nishiyama, 2007). Published reports have suggested interventions that may facilitate successful coping on the part of older persons during and after disasters and have provided information that expands our understanding of the biological pathways for stress reactions (Goenjian, et al., 2008). Additional studies have focused on methods of recruiting and sustaining the involvement of older persons in community resilience efforts (Acierno, Ruggiero, Kilpatrick, Resnick, & Galea, 2004; Norris & Murrell, 1988). Factors that are protective for older persons may account for the relative resilience of some in the face of disaster (Bramsen, VanDer Ploeg, & Boers, 2006; Lin, et al., 2002; Norris & Murrell). Several studies have focused on other impacts, in addition to PTSD, on the mental health of older persons (Neupert, Almeida, Mroczek, & Spiro, 2006; Spiro, Hankin, Mansell, & Kazis, 2006; Yazgan, et al.). These studies have noted special subgroups of older persons that are of additional concern, particularly those who are isolated, dependent, have mobility problems or communication deficits, are cognitively impaired, or have other comorbidities; use Meals on Wheels, vital medications, or home care; or are in senior centers, nursing homes, or assisted living settings.

OVERVIEW OF DISASTER AND EMERGENCY PREPAREDNESS

The purpose of this chapter is to provide an overview of the mental health consequences of disasters and emergencies, including acts of terrorism and natural disasters. The chapter also provides a review of evidence-based care practices and criteria for determining the extent to which care practices are evidence based. With this in mind, evidence-based care practices should be evaluated in the context of the extent to which they promote good and/or improved quality of life. Barry Gurland and his associates at the Columbia University Stroud Center for Studies of Quality of Life in Health and Aging have completed groundbreaking work in this area. Several recent papers have critically reviewed and proposed criteria for judging current quality of life models and measures (Gurland & Gurland, 2008a). They have also described a new model of quality of life in older persons based on the processes of facilitating choices and choosing that are matched to these criteria (Gurland & Gurland, 2008b) and examined the potential of the choices and choosing model for advancing the scientific base for the field of study related to promoting quality of life in health care generally (Gurland, Gurland, Mitty, & Toner, 2009) and mental health specifically (Gurland & Katz, 2006). Recognizing the importance of quality of life, and more specifically the choices and choosing model of quality of life, we feel that the foundation has been established for developing and adapting evidence-based care practices related to the mental health consequences of disasters and emergencies, using the choices and choosing model to promote quality of life in older persons in the aftermath of disasters and emergencies.

Older persons, particularly those who are frail, face extraordinary physical and mental health challenges in the days and months that follow a disaster. In addition, a system of emergency preparedness is generally not in place for those caring and responsible for older persons—both in the informal and formal sectors of care. For instance, following the attacks on the World Trade Center and also Hurricane Katrina, older persons and people with disabilities living in the hardest-hit areas were trapped for days before being rescued (O'Brien, 2003).

Several studies have informed our conceptualization of the mental health consequences of various types of disasters. Some have focused on direct victims and rescue workers. Others have focused on the mental health consequences of terrorist-based disasters on individuals, communities, and entire populations within and beyond disaster zones (Vlahov, 2002, p. 295). Disasters and emergencies are concurrently psychological and physiological regardless of whether the disaster is physical, biological, or chemical. Although most public health efforts have concentrated on individual treatment and prevention, the social and political imperative exists to develop evidence-based interventions and effective educational programs and resources for health care professionals and paraprofessionals. The goal is to promote the healing of individuals and communities by incorporating community-based public information and training and utilizing individual- and community-centered educational methods.

Mental health and social service providers in a variety of settings have reported a growing sense of anxiety among their older clients in the aftermath of recent disasters and particularly in response to the wars in Iraq and Afghanistan (Yehuda & Hyman, 2005). These concerns are even more marked for certain older cohorts such as holocaust survivors and veterans for whom television reports and talk of war may reawaken anxieties in those already coping with PTSD. Gullette (2006) found subsequent to the Hurricane Katrina disaster in New Orleans that those who were most vulnerable to the effects of the disaster were older, poor, female, African American, and disabled.

Definition of Terms

Disaster

According to the American Red Cross, a disaster is defined as an event that involves 10 or more deaths and involves 100 or more persons. Disasters involve an appeal for assistance (International Federation of Red Cross and Red Crescent Societies, 1999). The Federal Emergency Management Agency (FEMA) expands this definition in terms of the severity of the event that warrants governmental response and defines a disaster as "an occurrence of severity and magnitude that normally results in deaths, injuries, and property damage and that cannot be managed through the routine procedures and resources of government. It requires immediate, coordinated, and effective response by multiple government and private sector organizations to meet human needs and speed recovery" (Center for Mental Health Services, 1999, p. 6).

Emergency

FEMA defines an emergency in the terms used in the Robert T. Stafford Disaster Relief and Emergency Assistance Act of 1988. An emergency refers to "any occasion or instance for which, in the determination of the President, Federal assistance is needed to supplement State and local efforts and capabilities to save lives and to protect property and public health and safety, or to lessen or avert the threat of a catastrophe in any part of the United States" (Robert T. Stafford Disaster Relief and Emergency Assistance Act, 1988). Emergencies are sudden occurrences and may be due to epidemics, technological catastrophes, or strife from natural or man-made causes, including terrorism. Emergencies are distinguished from disasters in that, although emergencies and disasters both require a rapid reallocation of resources, emergencies can be handled by allocating existing agency resources. Disasters require additional resources from other outside agencies.

Preparedness

Veenema (2007, p. 612) defines preparedness as the following: "All measures and policies taken before an event occurs that allow for prevention, mitigation, and readiness. Preparedness includes designing warning systems, planning for evacuation and relocation, storing food and water, building temporary shelter, devising management strategies, and holding disaster drills." For the purpose of this book, preparedness also includes all mental health measures, such as assessment and screening, to determine risks for the onset of mental health problems.

Response

Response is "the phase in a disaster when relief, recovery and rehabilitation occur; also includes the delivery of services, the management of activities and programs designed to address the immediate and short-term effects of an emergency or disaster" (Veenema, 2007, p. 613).

Types and Characteristics of Disasters

According to DeWolfe (2000), there are four major types of disasters: natural disasters such as fires, floods, earthquakes, hurricanes, and tornados; technological disasters such as blackouts and computer/electronic malfunctions; health disasters such as epidemics; and social disasters such as riots and genocides.

Disasters are unpredictable, varied events with mental health implications for older persons and the communities in which they live. The severity of mental health impacts on older people is determined by the characteristics of the disaster itself. DeWolfe emphasizes that the following characteristics of disasters determine impacts: natural versus human causation, degree of personal impact, size and scope of the disaster, visible impact/low point, and the probability of recurrence.

Natural Versus Human Causation

Recent studies have provided conflicting results regarding the mental health impacts of natural versus human-caused disasters; however, there are distinct psychological effects associated with each. Human-caused disasters, such as terrorist attacks, airline crashes, and so forth, result in the survivors' struggle to reconcile the loss of life with the reality of violence and human error and the belief that the loss was unnecessary and preventable. On the other hand, natural disasters are most often seen as acts of God, which are beyond human control and without evil intent. In the disaster following Hurricane Katrina, natural and human-caused factors collided to yield a natural disaster that was made worse through human error and neglect (Gullette, 2006).

Degree of Personal Impact

Studies have demonstrated that the more personal the survivors' exposure to the disaster, the more severe the post-disaster effects (Vlahov, 2002). Such factors as witnessing the death of a victim, the death of a family member, or the destruction of one's home are high-impact factors, which result in more anxiety, depression, PTSD, somatic symptoms, and addictions.

Size and Scope of the Disaster

As with the degree of personal impact, a relationship exists between the size and scope of the devastation and the mental health impacts. The devastating loss of an entire community removes everything that is familiar to the survivor. Most survivors become disoriented at the most basic levels (Adams & Boscarino, 2006; Chung, et al., 2005; Kohn, et al., 2005). This disorientation can be life-threatening in older persons, particularly those who are isolated, have communication deficits, or are otherwise members of special subgroups of vulnerable older persons (Neupert, et al., 2006; Spiro, et al., 2006; Yazgan, et al., 2006).

Visible Impact/Low Point

Most disasters have a corresponding recovery period that begins at a clearly defined end/low point. In natural disasters, the end point of a devastating flood, earthquake, or hurricane signals the recovery and rebuilding process.

Although this recovery and rebuilding process may be delayed in the case of earthquake aftershocks and the secondary effects of floods, eventually the disaster ends and the healing begins. Human-caused disasters are altogether different. Technological events—for example, nuclear accidents—may not exhibit high visible impact or an observable end/low point, yet the prolonged threat of health consequences can result in chronic stress and anxiety due to the continuous threat (Rahu, 2003; Sumner, 2007).

Probability of Recurrence

Mental health consequences of disasters are exacerbated when there is a perceived immediate or long-term risk of recurrence.

EVIDENCE-BASED CARE (EBC) PRACTICES

Introduction and Definition of EBC

Testing medical interventions for efficacy has existed since the time of Avicenna's The Canon of Medicine in the 11th century. However, it was only in the 20th century that this effort evolved to affect almost all fields of health care and policy. In 1972, professor Archie Cochrane, a Scottish epidemiologist, published a book entitled *Effectiveness and Efficiency: Random Reflections on Health Services* (Cochrane, 1972). His book, which was reprinted in 1999, as well as his subsequent advocacy, led to increasing acceptance of the concepts behind EBC practices. EBC is the application of tested and proven guidelines to the care of patients in clinical settings in order to ensure the best prediction of medical treatment outcomes. EBC uses systemic methods to support the application of evidence from valid clinical research to clinical practice, thus reducing variability of care. It is designed to optimize the effectiveness of care by linking research and practice with clinical education and the decision-making process (Gambrill, 1999). While many aspects of care depend on individual factors that are only partially subject to scientific methods, EBC can help clarify those parts of clinical practice that are, in principle, subject to scientific methods and apply these methods. Health care professionals, allied health care providers, and health care institutions can use EBC as a tool to help them measure their performance and identify areas for further study and improvement (Torpy, 2009).

Criteria for Determining Whether a Care Practice Is Evidence Based

While past clinical guidelines were based mostly on the clinical wisdom of experts, EBC uses a hierarchy of evidence to guide clinical decision making and to classify the level of evidence that supports an intervention free from the various biases that beset clinical research. EBC uses techniques such as meta-analysis of the scientific literature, risk-benefit analysis, and randomized controlled trials (RCTs). EBC seeks internally valid evidence that is externally valid for clinical practice. Since no individual study can include full clinical reality, meta-analyses of various diagnostic and therapeutic studies including various relevant subgroups, such as older patients or those with comorbidity, are indispensable. To support individual decision making, these meta-analyses should evaluate effect modification between subgroups rather than seeking overall effect measures adjusted for subgroup differences. A rigorous meta-analysis of multiple studies has the advantage of using quantitative methods to provide a single best estimate of the effect of an intervention (Guyatt & Rennie, 2002). The systematic review of published research studies is a major method for evaluating particular treatments. The Cochrane Collaboration is one of the most well-known and well-respected examples of systematic reviews. A 2007 analysis of 1,016 systematic reviews from all 50 Cochrane Collaboration Review Groups found that 44% of the reviews concluded the intervention was likely to be beneficial, 7% concluded the intervention was likely to be harmful, and 49% concluded the evidence did not support either benefit or harm. Of these reviews, 96% recommended further research (El Dib, Atallah, & Andriolo, 2007). In contrast, patient testimonials, case reports, and even expert opinion have little value as proof because of the placebo effect, the biases inherent in the observation and reporting of cases, difficulties in ascertaining who is an expert, and more.

Reviewing the strength of evidence for a clinical practice requires evaluating the quality, including minimizing of bias; quantity, including magnitude of effect and sample size; and consistency, such as similar findings reported using similar and different experimental designs. All these elements help to characterize the level of confidence that can be assigned to a body of knowledge (West, et al., 2002). Systems to stratify evidence by quality have been developed, including one by the U.S. Preventive Services Task Force for ranking evidence about the effectiveness of treatments or screening (Barton, 2007):

- Level I: Evidence obtained from at least one properly designed randomized controlled trial
- Level II-1: Evidence obtained from well-designed controlled trials without randomization
- Level II-2: Evidence obtained from well-designed cohort or case-control analytic studies, preferably from more than one center or research group
- Level II-3: Evidence obtained from multiple time series with or without the intervention; dramatic results in uncontrolled trials might also be regarded as this type of evidence
- Level III: Opinions of respected authorities based on clinical experience, descriptive studies, or reports of expert committees

Gray offered a different hierarchical classification of evidence for the effectiveness of research studies (Gray, 1997):

1. A meta-analysis or systematic review of well-designed randomized controlled trials
2. A single, properly designed randomized controlled trial
3. Studies without randomization
4. Other quasi-experimental studies from more than one center or research group
5. Expert reports and authorities' recommendations based on descriptive studies or clinic evidence

Problems With and the Need for Evidence-Based Geriatric Psychiatry

The field of mental health, especially geriatric psychiatry, seems to be lagging behind in using evidence-based strategies. Conventional drug trials typically exclude people over 65 years of age, and even when they do include older persons, they commonly select individuals who are healthy or have few physical disabilities to minimize reports of adverse events and withdrawal from pharmaceutical trials (Banerjee & Dickinson, 1997). Psychotherapies and psychosocial interventions are a special challenge since they are difficult to deliver in a uniform way. This contrasts with pharmacological trials in which the intervention and control condition are clearly identified and measured. Older patients tend to take multiple medications, have multiple comorbidities, be more sensitive to drug-drug interaction, and have issues that could impair their adherence to treatment. They are also more sensitive to medication side effects, and they respond to psychotherapy according to their level of cognitive impairment (Banerjee & Dickinson). To make matters worse, there is a lack of empirical evidence that can guide the clinician because a majority of clinical trials for psychotropic medications are based on young individuals. This unfortunate combination has made older persons with mental disorders at a higher risk for poorer quality care (Bartels, et al., 2002). While in geriatric psychiatry the empirical research base is limited, the principles of evidence-based decision making can still be applied and hopefully will lead to a significant improvement in quality of care.

OVERVIEW OF PSYCHOPHARMACOLOGICAL AND NONPSYCHOPHARMACOLOGICAL TREATMENTS

This section provides a brief overview of the major psychopharmacological medications and nonpsychopharmacological treatments, such as psychosocial and behavioral strategies, commonly used with older persons suffering from mental health problems. For a thorough, in-depth discussion of these treatments, please see chapter 10 and chapter 14.

Medication management in the field of geriatric mental health is a real and constant challenge. Older persons tend to take multiple medications, have multiple comorbidities, have issues that can impair their adherence to treatment, and be more sensitive to side effects. In fact, medications for mental health problems, also known as psychotropics, are among the most common medications associated with preventable adverse drug events in older persons (Gurwitz, et al., 2003). To make matters worse, there is a lack of empirical evidence to guide the health care provider because a majority of clinical trials for psychotropic medications use young individuals. These elements make the decision to start psychotropic treatment of an older patient a challenge because the clinician has to assess the risk-benefit ratio.

PSYCHOPHARMACOLOGICAL TREATMENTS

Antidepressants

Selective Serotonin Reuptake Inhibitors (SSRIs)

SSRIs are considered first-line agents for the treatment of depression based on their safety and side effects profiles rather than their efficacy. In fact, randomized controlled trials support that SSRIs and tricyclics have the same efficacy (Anderson, 2000) and are superior to placebo (Wilson, Mottram, Sivananthan, & Nightingale, 2005). The safety profiles of SSRIs give them a clear advantage over other antidepressants. They are relatively benign in overdose (Barbey & Roose, 1998), and, unlike tricyclics, they have a relatively benign cardiovascular profile (Glassman, 1993). The most common side effects of SSRIs are gastrointestinal. Both hyponatremia and syndrome of inappropriate antidiuretic hormone (SIADH) have been associated with the use of SSRIs in older patients. The incidence of SIADH in older persons treated with SSRIs may be as high as 12% (Fabian, et al., 2004).

Tricyclic Antidepressants (TCAs)

The clinical utility of classical TCAs in the geriatric population is limited by their side effect and safety profiles despite their robust effectiveness. TCAs have anticholinergic side effects and lead to anticholinergic-induced urinary retention and confusion. The major safety problem with TCAs is their cardiovascular side effects (Glassman, 1993). They are lethal in overdose, and as little as three times the daily dose can result in death from heart block or arrhythmia. Given the prevalence of occult and manifest ischemic heart conditions in the older population, TCAs should be avoided. Unlike the classical TCAs, newer TCA-related antidepressants have better side effect profiles and offer the clinician and patient an acceptable alternative in situations where SSRIs are not acceptable (Mottram, Wilson, & Strobl, 2006).

Monoamine Oxidase Inhibitors (MAOIs)

MAOIs are rarely used in the older population because of their side effect profiles as well as the requirement for dietary and medications restriction, a serious challenge in older persons whose memory can be impaired. However, the FDA quite recently approved a transdermal patch of selegeline that may not require dietary restrictions. The risk of orthostasis, a serious risk factor for falls, limits their use.

Benzodiazepines

Benzodiazepines are avoided in older patients because of their numerous side effects. Benzodiazepines can cause impairment of information acquisition, impairment of consolidation and storage of memory, or both (Greenblatt, 1992). Among patients with dementia, the use of benzodiazepines can exacerbate cognitive deficits in multiple domains. Even in patients without dementia, chronic use of benzodiazepines also may be associated with deficits in sustained attention and visuospatial impairment that are insidious and not recognized by the patient (Ashton, 1995; Ayd, 1994). Amnestic effects may be more marked in heavy alcohol drinkers (Ashton).

Antipsychotics

When atypical antipsychotics were introduced, there was a clear resurgence in antipsychotic prescribing for older patients (Briesacher, et al., 2005). Older patients started receiving atypicals for various conditions, but this changed when atypicals were found to increase the risk of stroke, metabolic syndrome, and death in older persons with dementia (Schneider, Dagerman, & Insel, 2005). The view that atypicals were superior to conventional antipsychotic was seriously challenged by the findings of the Clinical Antipsychotic Trials in Intervention Effectiveness (CATIE) schizophrenia study. Aside from olanzapine, the atypical antipsychotics were no more effective than the conventional antipsychotic pherphenazine (Lieberman, et al., 2005). To make matters worse, a study found that conventional antipsychotics were as likely to increase the risk of death in older patients as atypical drugs (Wang, et al., 2005). Today, antipsychotics are used with caution in the geriatric population not only because of newly recognized stroke and mortality risks but also because of well-known side effects. Antipsychotics can cause hypotension as well as orthostatic hypotension, both associated with falls, myocardial infarction, and stroke. Many antipsychotics can cause QTC prolongations that can evolve into torsades de pointes, which may result in dizziness or syncope or may progress to ventricular fibrillation and sudden death (Taylor, 2003). They can also cause stroke via different mechanisms, including thromboembolic effects, orthostasis, and cardiac dysrhythmia, among others. The FDA has issued a warning regarding the risk of stroke among older patients with dementia and psychosis or other behavioral disturbances. In two large population-based retrospective cohort studies, comparing atypicals to conventional antipsychotics showed no increase in risk of stroke with atypical agents (Gill, et al., 2005). The extrapyramidal symptoms in older persons are also of concern: while the risk of drug-induced parkinsonism increases in the older population on antipsychotics, the risk of akathisia and acute dystonia decreases with age (Wirshing, 2001). Tardive dyskinesia is also of concern: antipsychotic-induced tardive dyskinesia is five to six times more prevalent in older persons than in younger patients (Jeste, 1999).

Medications for Dementia

Cholinesterase inhibitors are the mainstay of dementia treatment. The drugs have slightly different pharmacological properties, but they all work by inhibiting the breakdown of acetylcholine—an important neurotransmitter associated with memory—by blocking the enzyme acetylcholinesterase. Compared with placebo, cholinesterase inhibitors have a beneficial effect on cognitive function and measures of global clinical state at 6 months or more, and there is also evidence that they may improve behavioral disturbances and stabilize daily functions (Birks, 2006). There is some suggestion that these drugs may also exert neuroprotective effects (Krishnan, 2003). Memantine is a low-affinity antagonist to glutamate N-methyl d-aspartate (NMDA) receptors that may prevent excitatory neurotoxicity in dementia. It was approved in 2003 by the FDA for the treatment of moderate to severe Alzheimer's disease. Memantine has a slight beneficial, clinically detectable effect on cognitive function and functional decline measured at 6 months in patients with moderate to severe Alzheimer's disease (McShane, Areosa Sastre, & Minakaran, 2006).

NONPHARMACOLOGIC APPROACHES

Psychotherapy

Psychotherapy can be used as both a primary and an adjunctive therapy. While it was once thought that psychotherapy was of limited use in older persons because of the potential for cognitive impairment, there is now evidence that any type of psychotherapy can be as effective for older persons as for younger populations (Thompson, Gallagher-Thompson, & Breckenridge, 1987). Age itself cannot be used as an indication or contraindication of a specific therapy. Older persons can be reluctant to undergo therapy because of negative beliefs toward psychotherapy. When dealing with an older person, the therapist is expected to be flexible and to adjust his therapy to the many life changes that older persons potentially face. When using cognitive behavioral therapy (CBT), some of the more important adaptations include emphasizing behavioral techniques, particularly earlier in therapy, and frequently repeating information using different sensory modalities (Grant & Casey, 1995). Psychodynamic therapies may require an understanding of physical illness and the implications of approaching the end of life (Shiller, 1992). Reminiscence therapy, which involves the discussion of past activities, events, and experiences with another person or a group of people, is one of the most popular psychosocial interventions in dementia care and is highly rated by staff and participants. There is some evidence that reminiscence therapy can lead to improvement in a patient's mood, cognition, and functional ability. It can also alleviate the strain on caregivers (Woods, Spector, Jones, Orrell, & Davies, 2005).

Electroconvulsive Therapy (ECT)

ECT involves the application of an electric current to the head with the aim of inducing a controlled tonic-clonic convulsion and is usually carried out at intervals of days. Some reports suggest ECT is particularly effective in late-life depression (Flint & Rifat, 1998) as well as in therapy-resistant depressive older people with extensive white matter hyperintensities (Coffey, et al., 1988). Currently there is no evidence to suggest ECT causes any kind of brain damage, although temporary cognitive impairment is frequently reported (Devanand, Dwork, Hutchinson, Bolwig, & Sackeim, 1994; Scott, 1995). ECT seems to be a safe procedure even in older persons with cardiovascular disorders (Rice, Sombrotto, Markowit, & Leon, 1994). ECT is used more frequently to treat depressed older persons and its use is declining less rapidly than in the general population (Glen & Scott, 1999).

TREATMENT OF SOME OF THE MOST COMMON MENTAL HEALTH CONDITIONS IN OLDER PERSONS

Anxiety Disorders

Anxiety symptoms are quite common in the older population. The prevalence rate of anxiety disorders among older persons living in the community has been estimated between 10% and 15% (Beekman, et al., 1998; Kessler, et al, 2005b). However, primary anxiety disorders in later life are rare, as most patients develop anxiety symptoms secondary to a medical condition or in the context of a depressive disorder (Flint, 2005). The impact of anxiety disorders in later life can be significant: They can impair quality of life by having a negative impact on functioning and well-being and are associated with increased health care utilization (de Beurs, et al., 1999). Moreover, patients suffering from anxiety disorders have an increased risk of depression (Beekman, et al., 2000); left untreated, anxiety disorders tend to become chronic (Larkin, Copeland, & Dewney, 1992). In two large cohort studies, anxiety disorders in later life were prospectively associated with an increased mortality rate (Brenes, et al., 2007). Because of the potential for serious complications, anxiety disorders should be treated early and aggressively. A recent review concluded that SSRIs are efficacious for late-life anxiety disorders whereas the effect of benzodiazepines and tricyclic agents was not significant, which might be explained by a lack of statistical power (Pinquart & Duberstein, 2007).

Generalized Anxiety Disorder (GAD)

SSRI are the first line of treatment for GAD for most older patients, regardless of whether depression is present. Benzodiazepines have a more limited role for the treatment of GAD in older patients, and when they are used, lorazepam and oxazepam are preferred (Flint, 2005). Buspirone and pregabalin can also be used (Feltner, et al., 2003). Buspirone appears to have little amnestic effect (Lawlor, et al., 1992). When symptoms of GAD occur secondary to a medical condition or medications, treatment needs to be directed toward the underlying cause. CBT is well established as an effective mode of treatment for anxiety disorders. It may be used in conjunction with certain medications, such as antidepressants, but there is some suggestion that co-treatment with benzodiazepines reduces its efficacy (Van Balkom, et al., 1996). There is also some evidence that CBT is not as effective in the treatment of GAD in older patients as it is in younger patients (Mohlman, 2004).

Panic Disorder

Panic disorder can be secondary to a general medical condition or medications, or it can be primary. The recommended pharmacologic treatment for panic disorder in older patients is an SSRI antidepressant. The potential for an antidepressant to induce a panic attack or anxiety symptoms imposes a low starting dose and a slow titration. A benzodiazepine may be needed as adjunctive therapy during the initial weeks of treatment (Flint & Gagnon, 2003), but the frequent association of panic disorder with alcohol dependence complicates this use. CBT can be helpful in the treatment of panic disorder.

Posttraumatic Stress Disorder

PTSD with onset in earlier life can become symptomatic again in late life (Murray, 2005) or can result from a different trauma in old age, such as a serious fall. Older patients with PTSD have more somatic symptoms than do younger patients (Owens, et al., 2005). In older as in younger patients, the treatment of choice for PTSD is CBT, and the first-line pharmacologic treatment is an SSRI antidepressant (Asnis, et al., 2004)

Depression

Depression is a relatively common condition in the older population, with a higher prevalence in demented patients, patients in nursing homes, and patients with chronic or debilitating medical conditions. Comorbid depression adversely affects the outcome of several medical conditions and has been documented for ischemic heart disease. Depressed patients with un-stable angina, postmyocardial infarction, or congestive heart failure have a higher cardiac mortality rate than do medically comparable patients who are not depressed (Musselman, Evans, & Nemeroff, 1998). Suicide is a particular concern in older persons, especially those with severe or psychotic depression, comorbid alcoholism, recent loss or bereavement, a new disability, or sedative-hypnotic abuse. Treating depression has been shown to reduce the risk of suicide in at-risk older persons (Barak, et al., 2005). The majority of older persons with depression are treated by their primary care physician (PCP), but a significant portion are treated with doses that are not optimal (Wang, et al., 2005). Medications can help but may not be enough, and psychosocial support may be needed (Roose & Schatzberg, 2005). The majority of depressed older persons will eventually respond to aggressive treatment for depression (Flint & Rifat, 1996). Older persons are at chronic risk of undertreatment because of low expectations regarding recovery and fears about aggressive pharmacotherapy and ECT (Heeren, Derksen, van Heycop Ten Ham, & van Gent, 1997). While all classes of antidepressant medications have the same efficacy, SSRIs have been considered first-line agents for the treatment of geriatric depression mainly because of their better side effect profiles. The belief that older persons do not respond well to antidepressants and require a longer duration of treatment has led to the rule that the minimum duration necessary for an adequate antidepressant trial is 12 weeks. New data analyses of 12-week antidepressant treatment trials in late-life depression focused on time to response and the early identification of nonresponders (Sackeim, Roose, & Burt, 2005). Neither the overall response or remission rates nor the time to achieve sustained remission support the belief that older persons are less responsive to antidepressants or take longer to respond. A significant number of older persons with depression have memory issues that can make strict adherence to their antidepressant problematic, exposing them to the risk of withdrawal. In such case, using fluoxetine, an SSRI with a long half-life, can be a good choice.

Dementia

Cholinesterase inhibitors are the mainstay of dementia treatment. In Alzheimer disease, cholinesterase inhibitors can have some benefits, albeit modest ones: cognitive improvement, stabilization of daily function, and some delay of disease progression. There is some suggestion that these drugs may also exert neuroprotective effects (Krishnan, 2003). Memantine, an NMDA antagonist, was introduced in 2003 and was specifically labeled for the treatment of dementia at moderate to severe levels. Combining an anticholinesterase inhibitor with memantine can be beneficial; results from a randomized controlled study suggest that such combination was well tolerated and could positively affect cognition, activities of daily living, global outcome, and behavior in patients with moderate to severe dementia (Areosa Sastre, Sherriff, & McShane, 2006). Vitamin E, selegiline, secretase inhibitors, Ginkgo biloba, statin drugs, estrogen, and nonsteroidal anti-inflammatory drugs (NSAIDs) have been used for the treatment of cognitive disorders, including dementia, but the evidence to support their use is weak. There is also some evidence that psychotherapy can improve the mood, cognition, and functional ability of patients with dementia (Woods, et al., 2005).

Agitation in Dementia

Antipsychotics remain the treatment of choice for behavioral complications of dementia (Street, et al., 2000). Studies have shown that antipsychotics are used in 30%–50% of older institutionalized patients (Giron, et al., 2001). While no antipsychotic has been approved by the FDA for the treatment of psychosis and agitation in demented older persons, placebo-controlled studies consistently show comparable advantage for antipsychotics over placebo for symptoms of both psychosis and behavioral dyscontrol (Devanand, Sackeim, Brown, & Mayeux, 1989). Benzodiazepines should be used in low doses and restricted to short-term crisis management of agitated and anxious behaviors if antipsychotics or other medications are ineffective.

Delirium

Short-term antipsychotic administration is a standard treatment strategy in patients with delirium, particularly antipsychotic medications with low anticholinergic properties such as haloperidol (Tune, 2002). Atypical antipsychotics are useful in the management of delirium. In geriatric medical practice, it is always better to minimize the number and dosage of medications, especially those that are prone to cause delirium. When a patient develops delirium, treating the underlying cause is of extreme importance. If the patient exhibits the hypoactive form of delirium, he can be managed safely using nursing intervention, such as avoiding excessive sensory stimulation, providing orientation cues such as a calendar or clock, encouraging family presence for reassurance, and other such strategies. Using physical restraints should be limited to patients who are at serious risk of falling or pulling IV lines or urinary catheters. Patients with the agitated form of delirium may end up requiring pharmacological interventions. Antipsychotics with low anticholinergic activity, like haloperidol or risperidone, are preferred. If the delirium is caused by alcohol withdrawal, benzodiazepines can reduce withdrawal severity, the incidence of delirium, and seizures (Mayo-Smith, 1997)

Insomnia

Prevalence rates of insomnia in people aged 65 and older range between 12% and 40% (Morin, et al., 1999). Older adults primarily report difficulty in maintaining sleep, and, while not all sleep changes are pathological in later life (Bliwise, 1993; Morin & Gramling, 1989), severe sleep disturbances may lead to depression and cognitive impairments (Ford & Kamerow, 1989). Night waking produces significant stresses for carers and is a common cause for demands for institutional living arrangements (Pollak, Perlick, Linsner, Wenston, & Hsieh, 1990). The sleep deprivation of insomnia may result in excessive daytime sleepiness, fatigue, irritability, impairment of concentration, and an increased risk of involvement in a traffic accident. Insomniacs report lower quality of life scores than good sleepers (Leger, Scheuermaier, Philip, Paillard, & Guilleminault, 2001), and continued unresolved insomnia may be associated with significant psychiatric morbidity, predominantly depression (Millman, Fogel, McNamara, & Carlisle, 1989; Roth, 2001). Furthermore, sleep deprivation has been associated with a reduced tolerance to pain (Johnson, 1969) and may reduce immune function (Moldofsky, Lue, Davidson, & Gorezynski, 1989). Bringing back a normal sleep pattern is of extreme importance. The most common treatments for sleep disorders are pharmacological, particularly for insomnia (Hohagen, et al., 1994; Kupfer & Reynolds, 1997; Morin, et al., 1999). Two consensus conferences sponsored by the National Institute of Health (National Institute of Health [NIH], 1983, 1990) concluded that short-term use of hypnotic medications might be useful for acute and situational insomnia across all age groups but that long-term use remains controversial because of the potential risk of tolerance and dependency. The same NIH studies indicate that the drug of choice for the symptomatic treatment of insomnia is a benzodiazepine receptor agonist.

EVIDENCE-BASED APPROACHES TO SPECIFIC MENTAL HEALTH ISSUES DURING DISASTERS

Bereavement

Older people may go through many losses during a disaster: loss of relatives, pets, neighbors, friends, and so forth. Psychotherapy alone or coupled with psychopharmacology may be necessary in patients going through severe bereavement. Older adults who go through a loss during a disaster are more likely to suffer severe bereavement because of the absence of perceived or actual social support, the suddenness of the loss, and the presence of multiple concurrent stressful life events (Windholz, Marmar, & Horowitz, 1985).

PTSD

Because of an exposure to a situation where their life as well as their physical integrity is threatened, older persons can develop posttraumatic stress disorder. In older as in younger patients, the treatment of choice for PTSD is CBT, and the first-line pharmacologic treatment is an SSRI antidepressant (Asnis, et al., 2004).

Delirium

In a disaster area, the risk for older persons to develop delirium increases. Delirium is characterized by an acute change in cognition and attention, although the symptoms may be subtle and usually fluctuate throughout the day. This heterogeneous syndrome requires prompt recognition and evaluation because the underlying medical condition may be life-threatening. The risk of developing delirium can be reduced by preventing and correcting dehydration, minimizing unnecessary noise and stimuli, promoting good sleep hygiene, and repeated reorientation (Miller, 2008). The treatment of delirium centers on the identification and management of the medical condition that triggered the delirious state. Antipsychotic agents may be needed when the cause is nonspecific and other interventions do not sufficiently control symptoms such as severe agitation or psychosis. Also, a patient who develops delirium can become agitated and aggressive. Using haloperidol in agitated patients with dementia can decrease the degree of aggression (Lonergan, Luxenberg, Colford, & Birks, 2002).

Insomnia

In a disaster zone, older persons may end up in a noisy and overcrowded shelter where sleep may be difficult. As such, they may develop insomnia, which can affect their well-being in a negative way. Bringing back a normal sleep pattern is of extreme importance. The simplest approach is adherence to some basic rules of sleep hygiene: avoiding daytime napping, maintaining adequate nighttime pain relief; addressing environmental conditions; avoiding alcohol and caffeine late at night; and minimizing noise, light, and excessive heat during the sleep period. However, the chaos and disorganization caused by a disaster can make it difficult to implement these basic rules. CBT can have a mild positive impact on different aspects of insomnia in older adults (Montgomery & Dennis, 2003). Several pharmacological treatments are also available for the symptoms of insomnia, and the most commonly prescribed group of sleep-promoting drugs are benzodiazepines. Short-acting benzodiazepines such as temazepam and triazolam are favored to reduce impaired functioning the next day. Benzodiazepines with a longer half-life are avoided since they can have serious hangover effects, including drowsiness, confusion, and unsteady gait.

CONCLUSION

The importance of the mental health consequences of disasters on older persons is underlined by these early findings. However, the large gaps and uncertainties in our knowledge base present major challenges to professionals and caregivers in the face of disasters and emergencies. This book aims to address these public health and clinical challenges and fill in some of these gaps by providing the reader with evidence-based support for best practices.

REFERENCES

Acierno, R., Ruggiero, K., Kilpatrick, D., Resnick, H., & Galea, S. (2004). Risk and protective factors for psychopathology among older versus younger adults after the 2004 Florida hurricanes. *American Journal of Geriatric Psychiatry, 14,* 1051–1059.

Adams, R., & Boscarino, J. (2006). Predictors of PTSD and delayed PTSD after the World Trade Center disaster: The impact of exposure and psychosocial resources [Original articles]. *The Journal of Nervous and Mental Disease, 194*(7), 485–493.

Anderson, I. M. (2000). Selective serotonin reuptake inhibitors versus tricyclic antidepressants: A meta-analysis of efficacy and tolerability. *Journal of Affective Disorders, 58,* 19–36.

Areosa Sastre, A., Sherriff, F., & McShane, R. (2006). Memantine for dementia. In Cochrane Dementia and Cognitive Improvement Group, *Cochrane Database of Systematic Reviews:* CD003154. PMID 15495043.

Ashton, H. (1995). Toxicity and adverse consequences of benzodiazepine use. *Psychiatric Annals, 25,* 158–165.

Asnis, G. M., Kohn, S. R., Henderson, M., & Brown, N. L. (2004). SSRIs versus non-SSRIs in posttraumatic stress disorder: An update with recommendations. *Drugs, 64,* 383–404.

Ayd, F. J. (1994). Prescribing anxiolytics and hypnotics for the elderly. *Psychiatric Annals, 24,* 91–97.

Banerjee, S., & Dickinson, E. (1997). Evidence based healthcare in old age psychiatry. *International Journal of Psychiatry in Medicine, 27,* 283–292.

Barak, Y., Aizenberg, D., Szor, H., Swartz, M., Maor, R., & Knobler, H. (2005). Increased risk of attempted suicide among aging Holocaust survivors. *American Journal of Geriatric Psychiatry, 13*(8), 701–704.

Barbey, J. T., & Roose, S. P. (1998). SSRI safety in overdose. *Journal of Clinical Psychiatry, 59*(Suppl. 15), 42–48.

Bartels, S. J., Dums, A. R., Oxman, T. E., Schneider, L. S., Arean, P. A., Alexopoulos, G. S., et al. (2002). Evidence-based practices in geriatric mental health care. *Psychiatric Services, 53,* 1419–1431.

Barton, M. B. (2007). How to read the new recommendation statement: Methods update from the U.S. Preventive Services Task Force. *Annals of Internal Medicine, 147*(2), 123–127.

Beekman. A. T., de Beurs, B. E., van Balkom, A. J., Deeg, J. H., van Dyck, R., & van Tilburg, W. (2000). Anxiety and depression in later life: Co-occurrence and communality of risk factors. *American Journal of Psychiatry, 157,* 89–95.

Birks, J. (2006). Cholinesterase inhibitors for Alzheimer's disease. *Cochrane Database of Systematic Reviews, 1.* (Art. No. CD005593. DOI No. 10.1002/14651858.CD005593).

Bliwise, D. L. (1993). Sleep in normal aging and dementia. *Sleep, 16*(1), 40–81.

Bramsen, I., Van Der Ploeg, H. M., & Boers, M. (2006). Posttraumatic stress in aging World War II survivors after a fireworks disaster: A controlled prospective study. *Journal of Traumatic Stress, 19*(2), 291–300.

Brenes, G. A., Kritchevsky, S. B., Mehta, K. M., Yaffe, K., Simonsick, E. M., & Ayonayon, H. N. (2007). Scared to death: Results from the health, aging, and body composition study. *American Journal of Geriatric Psychiatry, 15,* 262–265.

Briesacher, B. A., Limcangco, M. R., Simoni-Wastila, L., Doshi, J. A., Levens, S. R., Shea, D. G., et al. (2005). The quality of antipsychotic drug prescribing in nursing homes. *Archives of Internal Medicine, 165,* 1280–1285.

Busuttil, W. (2004). Presentations and management of posttraumatic stress disorder and the elderly: A need for investigation. *International Journal of Geriatric Psychiatry, 19,* 429–439.

Center for Mental Health Services. (1999). *Psychosocial issues for older adults in disasters* (Publication No. ESDRB SMA 99–3323). Washington, DC: U.S. Department of Health and Human Services.

Chung, M. C. (2007) Post-traumatic stress disorder in older people. *Aging Health, 3*(6), 743–749.

Chung, M. C., Dennis, I., Easthope, Y., Farmer, S., & Werrett, J. (2005). Prevalence, risk factors, and aging vulnerability for psychopathology following a natural disaster in a developing country: Differentiating posttraumatic stress between elderly and younger residents. *Psychiatry: Interpersonal and Biological Processes, 68*(2), 164–173.

Cochrane, A. L. (1972). *Effectiveness and efficiency: Random reflections on health services.* London: Royal Society of Medicine Press.

Coffey, C. E., Figiel, G. S., Djang, W. T., Cress, M., Saunders, W. B., & Weiner, R. D. (1988). Leukoencephalopathy in elderly depressed patients referred for ECT. *Biological Psychiatry, 24*(2), 143–161.

de Beurs, E., Beekman, A. T., van Balkom, A. J., et al. (1999). Consequences of anxiety in older persons: Its effect on disability, well-being, and use of health services. *Psychological Medicine, 29,* 583–593.

Devanand, D. P., Dwork, A. J., Hutchinson, E. R., Bolwig, T. G., & Sackeim, H. A. (1994). Does ECT alter brain structure? *American Journal of Psychiatry, 151*(7), 957–970.

Devanand, D. P., Sackeim, H. A., Brown, R. P., & Mayeux, R. (1989). A pilot study of haloperidol treatment of psychosis and behavioral disturbance in Alzheimer's disease. *Archives of Neurology, 46*(8), 854–857.

DeWolfe, D. (2000). *Training manual for mental health and human service workers in major disasters* (2nd ed.) (Publication No. ADM 90-538). Washington, DC: Substance Abuse and Mental Health Services.

El Dib, R. P., Atallah, A. N., & Andriolo, R. B. (2007). Mapping the Cochrane evidence for decision making in health care. *Journal of Evaluation of Clinical Practice, 13*(4), 689–692.

Elklit, A., & O'Connor, M. (2005). Post-traumatic stress disorder in a Danish population of elderly bereaved. *Scandinavian Journal of Psychology, 46,* 439–445.

Fabian, T. J., Amico, J. A., Kroboth, P. D., Mulsant, B., Corey, S., Begley, A., et al. (2004) Paroxetine-induced hyponatremia in older adults: A 12-week prospective study. *Archives of Internal Medicine, 164,* 327–333.

Feltner, D. E., Crockatt, J. G., Dubovsky, S. J., Cohn, C. K., Shrivastava, R. K., Targum, S. D., et al. (2003). A randomized, double blind, placebo-controlled, fixed-dose, multicenter study of Pregabalin in patients with generalized anxiety disorder. *Journal of Clinical Psychopharmacology, 23,* 240–249.

Flint, A. J. (2005). Generalized anxiety disorder in elderly patients: Epidemiology, diagnosis, and treatment options. *Drugs & Aging, 22,* 101–114.

Flint, A. J., & Gagnon, N. (2003). Diagnosis and management of panic disorder in older patients. *Drugs & Aging, 20,* 881–891.

Flint, A. J., & Rifat, S. L. (1996). The effects of sequential antidepressant treatment on geriatric depression. *Journal of Affective Disorders, 36,* 95–105.

Flint, A. J., & Rifat, S. L. (1998). The treatment of psychotic depression in later life: A comparison of pharmacotherapy and ECT. *International Journal of Geriatric Psychiatry, 13*(1), 23–28.

Ford, D. E., & Kamerow, D. B. (1989). Epidemiologic study of sleep disturbances and psychiatric disorders. *Journal of the American Medical Association, 262,* 1479–1484.

Gambrill, E. (1999). Evidence-based clinical behavior analysis, evidence-based medicine, and the Cochrane collaboration. *Journal of Behavioral Therapy and Experimental Psychiatry, 30,* 1–14.

Gill, S. S., Rochon, P. A., Hermann, N., Lee, P. E., Sykora, K., Gunraj, N., et al. (2005). Atypical antipsychotic drugs and risk of ischemic stroke: Population-based retrospective cohort study. *British Medical Journal, 330,* 445.

Giron, M.S.T., Wang, H. X., Bernsten, C., Thorsdlund, M., Winblad, B., & Fastbom, J. (2001). The appropriateness of drug use in an older nondemented and demented population. *Journal of the American Geriatrics Society, 49,* 277–283.

Glassman, A. (1993). The safety of tricyclic antidepressants in cardiac patients: Risk-benefit reconsidered. *Journal of the American Medical Association, 269,* 2673–2675.

Glen, T., & Scott, A. (1999). Rates of electroconvulsive therapy use in Edinburgh 1992–1997. *Journal of Affective Disorders, 54*(1–2), 81–85.

Goenjian, A. K., Najarian, L. M., Pynoos, R. S., Steinberg, A. M., Manoukian, G., Tavosian, A., et al. (1994). Posttraumatic stress disorder in elderly and younger adults after the 1988 earthquake in Armenia. *American Journal of Psychiatry, 151*(6), 895–901.

Goenjian, A., Noble, E., Walling, D., Goenjian, H., Karayan, I., Ritchie, T., et al. (2008). Heritabilities of symptoms of posttraumatic stress disorder, anxiety, and depression in earthquake exposed Armenian families. *Psychiatric Genetics, 18*(6), 261–266.

Grant, R., & Casey, D. (1995). Adapting cognitive behavioural therapies for the frail elderly. *International Psychogeriatrics, 7*(4), 561–571.

Gray, J. A. M. (1997). *Evidence-based health care: How to make health policy and management decisions.* New York: Churchill Livingston.

Greenblatt, D. J. (1992). Pharmacology of benzodiazepine hypnotics. *Journal of Clinical Psychiatry, 53*(Suppl. 6), 7–13.

Gullette, M. (2006). Katrina and the politics of later life. In C. Hartman & G. Squires (Eds.), *There is no such thing as a natural disaster: Race, class, and Hurricane Katrina* (pp. 103–120). New York: Taylor and Francis Group.

Gurland, B. J., & Gurland, R. V. (2008a). The choices, choosing model of quality of life: Description and rationale. *International Journal of Geriatric Psychiatry, 24,* 90–95.

Gurland, B. J., & Gurland, R. V. (2008b). The choices, choosing model of quality of life: Linkages to a science base. *International Journal of Geriatric Psychiatry, 24,* 84–89.

Gurland, B. J., Gurland, R. V., Mitty, E., & Toner, J. A. (2009). The choices, choosing model of quality of life: Clinical evaluation and intervention. *Journal of Interprofessional Care, 23*(2), 110–120.

Gurland, B., & Katz, S. (2006). Quality of life in Alzheimer's and related dementias. In H. Katschnig, H. Freeman, & N. Sartorius (Eds.), *Quality of life in mental disorders* (2nd ed., pp. 179–198). New York: John Wiley & Sons.

Gurwitz, J., Field, T., Harrold, L., Rothschild, J., Debellis, K., Seger, A., et al. (2003). Incidence of preventability of adverse drug effects among older persons in the ambulatory setting. *Journal of the American Medical Association, 289*(9), 1107–1116.

Guyatt, G., & Rennie, D. (2002). *Users' guides to the medical literature: A manual for evidence-based clinical practice/the evidence-based medicine working group.* Chicago: American Medical Association Press.

Heeren, T. J., Derksen, P., van Heycop Ten Ham, B. F., & van Gent, P. P. (1997). Treatment outcome and predictors of response in elderly depressed inpatients. *British Journal of Psychiatry, 170,* 436–440.

Himes, C. (2007). Elderly Americans. In H. Cox (Ed.), *Aging* (19th ed., pp. 3–7). Dubuque, IA: McGraw-Hill Contemporary Learning Series.

Hohagen, F., Kaeppler, C., Schramm, E., Rink, K., Weyerer, S., Riemann, D., et al. (1994). Prevalence of insomnia in elderly general practice attenders and the current treatment modalities. *Acta Psychiatrica Scandinavica, 90*(2), 102–108.

International Federation of Red Cross and Red Crescent Societies. (1999). *World Disasters Report.* Dordrecht, The Netherlands: Martinus Nijhoff.

Jeste, D. (1999). Incidence of tardive dyskinesia in early stages of low-dose treatment with typical neuroleptics in older patients. *American Journal of Psychiatry, 156,* 309–311.

Johnson, L. C. (1969). Psychological and physiological changes following total sleep deprivation. In A. Kales (Ed.), *Sleep: Physiology and pathology* (pp. 206–220). Philadelphia, PA: Lippincott.

Kato, H., Asukai, N., Miyake, Y., Minakawa, K., & Nishiyama, A. (2007). Post- traumatic symptoms among younger and elderly evacuees in the early stages following the 1995 Hanshin-Awaji earthquake in Japan. *Acta Psychiatrica Scandinavica, 93*(6), 477–481.

Kessler, R. C., Berglund, P., Demler, O., Jin, R., Merikangas, K. R., & Walters, E. E. (2005b). Lifetime prevalence and age of onset distributions of DSM-IV disorders in the National Comorbidity Survey Replication. *Archives of General Psychiatry, 62,* 593–660.

Kohn, R., Levav, I., Garcia, I. D., Machuca, M. E., & Tamashiro, R. (2005). Prevalence risk factors and aging vulnerability for psychopathology following a natural disaster in a developing country. *International Journal of Geriatric Psychiatry, 20*(9), 835–841.

Krishnan, R. (2003). Randomized, placebo-controlled trial of the effects of donepezil on neuronal markers and hippocampal volumes in Alzheimer's disease. *American Journal of Psychiatry, 160,* 2003–2011.

Kupfer, D. J., & Reynolds III, C. F. (1997). Management of insomnia. *New England Journal of Medicine, 336*(5), 341–346.

Larkin, B. A., Copeland, J. R., & Dewey, M. E. (1992). The natural history of neurotic disorders in an elderly urban population. *British Journal of Psychiatry, 160,* 81–86.

Lawlor, B. A., Hill, J. L., Radcliffe, J. L., Minichiello, M., Molchan, S. E., & Sunderland, T. (1992). A single oral dose challenge of buspirone doesn't affect the memory process in older volunteers. *Biological Psychiatry, 32,* 101–103.

Leger, D., Scheuermaier, K., Philip, P., Paillard, M., & Guilleminault, C. (2001). SF-36: Evaluation of quality of life in severe and mild insomniacs compared with good sleepers. *Psychosomatic Medicine, 63*(1), 49–55.

Lieberman, J. A., Stroup, T. S., McEvoy, J. P., Swartz, M. S., Rosenheck, R. A., Perkins D. O., et al. (2005). Effectiveness of antipsychotic drugs in patients with chronic schizophrenia. *New England Journal of Medicine, 353,* 1209–1223.

Lin, M. R., Huang, W., Huang, C., Hwang, H. F., Tsai, L. W., & Chiu, Y. N. (2002). The impact of the Chi-Chi earthquake on quality of life among elderly survivors in Taiwan—A before and after study. *Quality of Life Research, 11*(4), 379–388.

Livingston, H., Livingston, M., & Fell, S. (2008).The Lockerbie disaster: A 3-year follow-up of elderly victims. *International Journal of Geriatric Psychiatry, 9,* 989–994.

Livingston, H., Livingston, M., Brooks, D., & McKinley, W. (1992). Elderly survivors of the Lockerbie Air Disaster. *International Journal of Geriatric Psychiatry, 7,* 725–729.

Lonergan, E., Luxenberg, J., Colford, J. M., & Birks, J. (2002). Haloperidol for agitation in dementia. *Cochrane Database of Systematic Reviews, 2.* (Art. No. CD002852. DOI No. 10.1002/14651858.CD002852).

Marshall, R., Turner, J., Lewis-Fernandez, R., Koenan, K., Neria, Y., & Dohrenwend, B. (2006). Symptom patterns associated with chronic PTSD in male veterans: New findings from the National Vietnam Veterans Readjustment Study. *The Journal of Nervous and Mental Disease, 194*(4), 275–278.

Mayo-Smith, M. F. (1997). Pharmacological management of alcohol withdrawal: A meta-analysis and evidence-based practice guideline. *Journal of the American Medical Association, 278,* 144–151.

McShane, R., Areosa Sastre, A., & Minakaran, N. (2006). Memantine for dementia. *Cochrane Database of Systematic Reviews, 2.* (Art. No. CD003154. DOI No. 10.1002/14651858. CD003154.pub5).

Mecocci, P., Di Iorio, A. D., Pezzuto, S., Rinaldi, P., Simonelli, G., & Maggio, D. (2000). Impact of the earthquake of September 26, 1997, in Umbria, Italy, on the socioenvironmental and psychophysical conditions of an elderly population. *Aging* (Milano), *12*(4), 281–286.

Miller, M. (2008). Evaluation and management of delirium in hospitalized older patients. *American Family Physician, 78*(11), 1265–1270.

Millman, R. P., Fogel, B. S., McNamara, M. E., & Carlisle, C. C. (1989). Depression as a manifestation of obstructive sleep apnea: Reversal with nasal continuous positive airway pressure. *Journal of Clinical Psychiatry, 50*(9), 348–351.

Mohlman, J. (2004). Psychosocial treatment of late life generalized anxiety disorder: Current status and future directions. *Clinical Psychology Review, 24,* 149–169.

Moldofsky, H., Lue, F. A., Davidson, J. R., & Gorezynski, R. (1989). Effects of sleep deprivation on immune function. *Federation of American Societies for Experimental Biology Journal, 3,* 1972–1977.

Montgomery, P., & Dennis, J. A. (2003). Cognitive behavioural interventions for sleep problems in adults aged 60+. *Cochrane Database of Systematic Reviews, 1.* (Art. No. CD003161. DOI No. 10.1002/14651858.CD003161).

Morin, C. M., & Gramling, S. E. (1989). Sleep patterns and aging: Comparison of older adults with and without insomnia complaints. *Psychology and Aging, 4*(3), 290–294.

Morin, C. M., Hauri, P. J., Espie, C. A., Spielman, A. J., Buysse, D. J., & Bootzin, R. R. (1999). Nonpharmacologic treatment of chronic insomnia. *Sleep, 22*(8), 1134–1156.

Mottram, P. G., Wilson, K., & Strobl, J. J. (2006). Antidepressants for depressed elderly. *Cochrane Database of Systematic Reviews, 1.* (Art. No. CD003491. DOI No. 10.1002/14651858.CD003491.pub2).

Murray, A. (2005). Recurrence of post traumatic stress disorder. *Nursing Older People, 17,* 24–30.

Musselman, D., Evans, D. L., & Nemeroff, C. B. (1998). The relationship of depression to cardiovascular disease: Epidemiology, biology, and treatment. *Archives of General Psychiatry, 55,* 580–592.

National Institute of Health. (1990, March). The treatment of sleep disorders of older people. *NIH Consensus Statement, 8*(3), 1–22. Retrieved September 5, 2009, from http://www.ncbi.nlm.nih.gov/books/bv.fcgi?rid=hstat4.chapter.6897

National Institute of Health. (1983, November). Health, drugs, and insomnia: The use of medications to promote sleep. *NIH Consensus Statement, 4*(10), 1–14. Retrieved September 5, 2009, from http://consensus.nih.gov/1983/1983InsomniaDrugs039html.htm

Neal, L. A., Hill, N., Hughes, J., Middleton, A., & Busuttil, W. (1995). Convergent validity of measures of PTSD in a population of former prisoners of war. *International Journal of Geriatric Psychiatry, 10,* 617–622.

Neupert, S. D., Almeida, D. M., Mroczek, D. K., & Spiro, A. (2006). The effects of the Columbia shuttle disaster on the daily lives of older adults: Findings from the VA Normative Aging Study. *Aging & Mental Health, 10*(3), 272–281.

Norris, F. H., & Murrell, S. A. (1988). Prior experience as a moderator of disaster impact on anxiety symptoms in older adults. *American Journal of Community Psychiatry, 16*(5), 665–683.

O'Brien, N. (2003, January–February). *Emergency preparedness for older people* (Issue Brief) (pp. 1–5). New York: International Longevity Center-USA.

Owens, G., Baker, D., Kasckow, J., Ciesla, J., & Mohamed, S. (2005). Review of assessment and treatment of PTSD among elderly American armed forces veterans. *International Journal of Geriatric Psychiatry, 20,* 1118–1130.

Phifer, J. F. (1990). Psychological distress and somatic symptoms after natural disaster: Differential vulnerability among older adults. *Psychology and Aging, 5*(3), 412–420.

Pinquart, M., & Duberstein, P. R. (2007). Treatment of anxiety disorders in older adults: A meta-analytic comparison of behavioral and pharmacological interventions. *American Journal of Geriatric Psychiatry, 111,* 639–651.

Pollak, C. P., Perlick, D., Linsner, J. P., Wenston, J., & Hsieh, F. (1990). Sleep problems in the community elderly as predictors of death and nursing home placement. *Journal of Community Health, 15,* 123–135.

Rahu, M. (2003). Health effects of the Chernobyl accident: Fears, rumors, and the truth. *European Journal of Cancer, 39*(3), 295–299.

Rauch, S., Morales, K., Zubritsky, C., Knott, K., & Oslin, D. (2006). Posttraumatic stress, depression, and health among older adults in primary care. *American Journal of Geriatric Psychiatry, 14,* 316–324.

Rice, E. H., Sombrotto, L. S., Markowit, J. C., & Leon, A. C. (1994). Cardiovascular morbidity in high-risk patients during ECT. *American Journal of Psychiatry, 151*(11), 1637–1641.

Robert T. Stafford Disaster Relief and Emergency Assistance Act. (1988). Pub. L. No. 93-288,§102. Washington, DC: Federal Emergency Management Agency.

Roose, S., & Schatzberg, A. (2005). The efficacy of antidepressants in the treatment of late-life depression. *Journal of Clinical Psychopharmacology, 25*(4), S1–S7.

Roth, T. (2001). The relationship between psychiatric disease and insomnia. *International Journal of Clinical Practice, 116*(Suppl.), 3–8.

Sackeim, H. A., Roose, S. P., & Burt, T. (2005). Optimal length of antidepressant trials in late-life depression. *Journal of Clinical Psychopharmacology, 25*(Suppl. 1), S34–S37.

Schneider, L. S., Dagerman, K. S., & Insel, P. (2005). Risk of death with atypicals: Antipsychotic drug treatment for dementia. *Journal of the American Medical Association, 294,* 1934–1943.

Scott, A. L. (1995). Does ECT alter brain structure. *American Journal of Psychiatry, 152*(9), 1403.

Seplaki, C. L., Goldman, N., Weinstein, M., & Lin, Y. H. (2006). Before and after the 1999 Chi-Chi earthquake: Traumatic events and depressive symptoms in an older population. *Social Science and Medicine, 62*(12), 3121–3132.

Shiller, A. (1992). Psychotherapy with elderly patients: Experiences from a psychiatric psychotherapeutic consultation service. *Psychosomatics, Medicine, and Psychoanalysis, 38*(4), 371–380.

Spiro, A., Hankin, C., Mansell, D., & Kazis, L. (2006). Posttraumatic stress disorder and health status: The Veterans Health Study. *Journal of Ambulatory Care Management, 29*(1), 71–86.

Street, J. S., Clark, W. S., Gannon, K. S., Cummings, J. L., Bymaster, F. P., Tamura, R. N., et al. (2000). Olanzapine treatment of psychotic and behavioral symptoms in patients with Alzheimer disease in nursing care facilities: A double-blind, randomized, placebo-controlled trial. The HGEU Study Group. *Archives of General Psychiatry, 57,* 968–976.

Sumner, D. (2007). Health effects resulting from the Chernobyl accident. *Journal of Medicine, Conflict, and Survival, 23*(1), 31–45.

Taylor, D. M. (2003). Antipsychotics and QT prolongation. *Acta Psychiatrica Scandinavica, 10,* 85–95.

Thompson, L. W., Gallagher-Thompson, D., & Breckenridge, J. S. (1987). Comparative effectiveness of psychotherapies for depressed elders. *Journal of Consulting and Clinical Psychology, 55,* 385–390.

Torpy, J. (2009). Evidence based medicine. *Journal of the American Medical Association, 301*(8), 1145–1158.

Tune, L. (2002). The role of antipsychotics in treating delirium. *Current Psychiatry Reports, 4*(3), 209–212.

Van Balkom, A. J., de Beurs, E., Koele, P., Lange, A., & van Dyck, R. (1996). Long term benzodiazepine use is associated with smaller treatment gain in panic disorder with agoraphobia. *Journal of Nervous and Mental Disease, 184,* 133–135.

van Zelst, W. H., de Beurs, E., Beekman, A. T. F., Deeg, D. J. H., van Dyck, R. (2003). Prevalence and risk factors of posttraumatic stress disorder in older adults. *Psychotherapy & Psychosomatics, 72*(6), 333–343.

Veenema, T. (Ed.). (2007). *Disaster nursing and emergency preparedness for chemical, biological, and radiological terrorism and other hazards.* New York: Springer Publishing Company, LLC.

Vlahov, D. (2002). Urban disaster: A population perspective. *Journal of Urban Health, 79*(3), 295–297.

Wang, P. S., Schneeweiss, S., Avorn, J., Fischer, M. A., Mogun, H., Solomon, D. H., et al. (2005). Risk of death in elderly users of conventional vs. atypical antipsychotic medications. *New England Journal of Medicine, 353,* 2335–2341.

West, S., King, V., Carey, T. S., Lohr, K. N., McKoy, N., Sutton, S. F., et al. (2002, April). *Systems to rate the strength of scientific evidence. Evidence report/technology assessment*

No. 47 (AHRQ publication 02-E016). Rockville, MD: U.S. Department of Health and Human Services. Retrieved September 5, 2009, from http://www.ncbi.nlm.nih.gov/books/bv.fcgi?rid=hstat1.chapter.70996

Wilson, K., Mottram, P., Sivananthan, A., & Nightingale, A. (2005). Antidepressants versus placebo for the depressed elderly. *Cochrane Review. The Cochrane Library, 2.*

Windholz, M. J., Marmar, C. R., & Horowitz, M. J. (1985). A review of the research on conjugal bereavement: Impact on health and efficacy of intervention. *Comprehensive Psychiatry, 26,* 433–477.

Wirshing, W. C. (2001). Movement disorders associated with neuroleptic treatment. *Journal of Clinical Psychiatry, 62*(Suppl. 21), 15–18.

Woods, B., Spector, A. E., Jones, C. A., Orrell, M., & Davies, S. P. (2005). Reminiscence therapy for dementia. *Cochrane Database of Systematic Reviews, 2.* (Art. No. CD001120. DOI No. 10.1002/14651858.CD001120.pub2).

Yazgan, C., Dedeoglu, C., & Yazgan, Y. (2006). Disability and post-traumatic psychopathology in Turkish elderly after a major earthquake. *International Psychogeriatrics, 18*(1), 184–187.

Yehuda, R., & Hyman, S. (2005). The impact of terrorism on brain and behavior: What we know and what we need to know. *Neuropsychopharmacology, 30,* 1773–1780.

2

Older Persons in Disasters and Emergencies: The Overlapping Mental and Physical Health Issues

NEIL HALL

This chapter discusses the interactions of acute and chronic mental and physical conditions in disaster situations. It focuses on the key aspects of aging and resultant frailty that make disasters particularly problematic for older persons. Its purpose is to help health care providers understand the unique aspects of older persons and to assist them in successfully planning and providing care for the elderly during disasters.

First, it is important to define whom we are talking about when we say *older persons.* Most people think of an age, namely 65, as the criterion for being old. This arbitrary point, unrelated to any physiologic criteria, exists mainly because of its original connection with eligibility for social security and Medicare.

Many envision an older person as a bent, thin, white-haired woman walking slowly with a cane or driving under the speed limit on the highway. But *gerontologists*[1] and *geriatricians*[2] have long recognized that most people in their late 60s and early 70s are quite healthy and active, even vigorous, which is inconsistent with the typical image. From a physiologic standpoint, it is reasonable to think of people aged 65–74 as late middle aged, those past age 75 as old, and those over 85 as frail.

FUNCTION AND FRAILTY

The concept of *function*[3] is central to understanding the care of the older person. The word *function*, as used in gerontology, means the ability to do the things needed to maintain one's body and household in adequate condition. This definition focuses mostly on physical and cognitive abilities, rather than on the occupational, social, and psychological concept of function used in the discipline of psychiatry and in the *DSM-IV*. But the maintenance of function requires physical, cognitive, and emotional capacities to perform the required activities.

Function is divided into two main categories: activities of daily living (ADLs) and instrumental activities of daily living (IADLs). ADLs are the simple activities required to maintain one's body in a condition acceptable in social situations—bathing, dressing, toileting, mobility (usually walking), maintaining continence of urine and stool (or controlling external manifestations of incontinence), and feeding oneself (Katz, Downs, Cash, & Grotz, 1970).

IADLs are activities requiring a higher level of cognition and emotional function that are needed to maintain one's living situation. These include managing finances, shopping, preparing meals, cleaning, managing transportation, keeping a schedule, using a telephone, self-administering medications, and similar endeavors (Lawton & Brody, 1969).

Frailty is much more relevant than age in disaster situations. The concept of frailty refers to more than just weakness or physical fragility. It broadly encompasses the inability of the individual to maintain function in the face of significant challenges—infection, injury, environmental changes, nutritional deficiency, and so forth—to normal equilibrium (Campbell & Buchner, 1996). Disease can make one frail at any age, and complications of medical problems such as heart disease, diabetes, and chronic lung disease become increasingly common as people age. By age 85, the normal and unrelenting effects of aging have reduced virtually everyone to the point of frailty even without any major disease.

The body and mind constantly respond to external and internal events and conditions that may put the individual at risk. Some of these include environmental issues such as high or low ambient temperature, a slippery floor, or poor air quality; internal situations such as infections, metabolic disturbances, and disease processes; and emotional factors, such as anxiety, depression, and others. Each of us has an innate capacity to deal with these stressors, a capacity that may be overwhelmed if an event is powerful enough. As individuals age, their physical capacity to overcome these stressors wanes. When this capacity becomes sufficiently low that relatively small stressors overwhelm the individual's ability to cope, that person is *frail.*

Most persons aged 65–75, unless they have had major toxic effects such as cigarettes and alcohol or disease effects, especially diabetes mellitus and heart disease, will be able to cope about as well as persons in their 50s and early 60s and should not be considered at unusual risk in disasters. But virtually all persons aged 85 and over are physically frail, as are a proportion, increasing with age, of those between 75 and 85.

STRENGTHS AND WEAKNESSES OF OLDER PERSONS

Emotional Strengths and Weaknesses

Many older persons will be able to cope with disasters as well as, or perhaps better than, younger persons (Foster, 1997). The emotional response to catastrophe is often as problematic as the physical consequences. But older persons are often more emotionally tolerant of stresses than their children. This may be related to the fact that they have survived through more traumas in their lives. And perhaps those who have shown more resilience with psychological coping are more likely to have survived to older age (Tugade, Fredrickson, & Barrett, 2004).

Although older persons may exhibit greater emotional strength and reserve, they also may have greater concerns in disaster situations. In addition to normal worries, they often worry about their physical health, especially if they have significant diseases. Those less healthy and robust will naturally have more concern about their ability to cope physically with the disaster, therefore increasing the risk of anxiety.

Healthy Older Persons as a Resource

Contrary to the perception of older persons as merely receivers of assistance in disasters, we need to recognize that they also can contribute. Their wisdom and experience may help them modulate fearful reactions that may be harmful; their examples may be helpful to others in meeting the challenges. Many older persons have already served as caregivers to frail family members, and most have cared for children. They have lived lives with careers and experiences that may be very useful in dealing with disasters.

Because of their relative health and experience, persons in the 65- to 75-year-old age group have the potential to be of tremendous assistance in crises. Persons between 75 and 85 who are in good health also may be of help in ways that do not require many physical demands. These *healthy older persons* should be considered a resource in disasters, able to help others both physically and emotionally. Even frail older persons usually have preserved cognitive capacity and can contribute. Of course, persons of any age who focus on doing something to contribute to the well-being of others tend to cope better in a disaster.

Physical Changes With Aging and Resultant Weaknesses

The key consideration for older persons in disasters is their physical frailty. If there are threats to the body, the decreased resistance and resilience of older bodies means they may require more support from others to prevent distress or death. In medicine, this relates mainly to the physiologic ability to maintain bodily processes, including brain activities, in the face of disease, injury, environmental stressors, or other causes of potential physiologic disequilibrium.

The normal aging process that results in frailty for virtually everyone over age 85 includes changes in every body system. Table 2.1 shows the major changes and their implications regarding health and disease. Persons caring for older persons in disasters will need to consider these changes when designing programs to improve outcomes for the most vulnerable. Most significant problems of older persons are caused by disease, not by normal aging. If there is loss of function, assume there is underlying disease that potentially can be treated.

In addition to the normal changes of aging, of course, older persons have more disease processes. Particularly common and problematic diseases include atherosclerotic heart disease, congestive heart failure, chronic lung disease, diabetes mellitus, and chronic kidney disease. This chapter, of course, cannot discuss the details of managing these diseases, but key needs that may be helpful to consider when planning for caring for older persons during disasters are expressed in Table 2.2. Medical management and preparation for disasters need to be arranged with trained personnel.

Medications and Risk in Disasters

No discussion of the care of older persons, especially frail older persons, can omit medications. Certain medical problems, particularly reduced

Table 2.1

NORMAL CHANGES WITH AGING

ORGANS/SYSTEM	NORMAL CHANGES	COMMENTS
General	Decreased physiologic reserve (ability to compensate for changes in internal environment that often are caused by changes in or threats from the external environment—such as temperature changes or infectious agents—or because of something ingested or not ingested, such as medicine, food, and water).	Greater chance of dangerous disequilibrium. Might not be able to overcome something that a younger person could shake off, particularly from things done or prescribed by a clinician (iatrogenesis).
Nervous System	Slower to learn new information and to recall already learned information. Slowed reflexes. Change in sleep patterns (longer to get to sleep, less deep sleep, more frequent awakenings, but not decreased need for sleep).	A nuisance to the patient but no clinical significance. Major memory loss, or dementia, is not normal. Increased risk of falls and auto accidents. Problems with sleep may lead to decreased quality of life and increased use of sleep aids, which may cause side effects.
Skin	Thinner and dryer.	More easily injured. Itching from dry skin.
Vision	Decreased transmission of light to the retina because of smaller pupil, less transparent lens, increased glare from light source, decreased ability to track a moving object and to differentiate an object from its background, decreased ability to adapt to dark environment.	Increased risk of falls and auto accidents.
Hearing	Loss of high-frequency hearing. Hard to determine how much loss is from normal aging, how much from disease or noise exposure.	Any hearing loss results in missed information, reduced socialization.
Smell and Taste	Significant loss of smell; slight loss of taste.	Loss of flavor leading to decreased enjoyment of food, which may contribute to malnutrition. Potential to increase salt application to improve taste.

(Continued)

Table 2.1

NORMAL CHANGES WITH AGING (*Continued*)

ORGANS/SYSTEM	NORMAL CHANGES	COMMENTS
Respiration	Decreased ability to exchange oxygen. Less vigorous cough.	More at risk for inadequate oxygen supply when a medical problem (such as pneumonia) is added. Increased risk of pneumonia.
Heart and Blood Vessels	Decreased maximum heart rate. Decreased elasticity of blood vessels.	Decreased maximal work. Increased blood pressure.
Stomach	Questionable slight decrease in acid production; minimally slowed emptying of stomach.	Not clinically significant.
Small Intestine	Minimal decrease in absorption.	Usually not clinically significant, but may contribute to nutrition problems caused by decreased intake.
Large Intestine	Slowed movement of contents.	Tendency to constipation.
Liver	Decreased blood flow to liver and decreased liver function.	Usually not clinically significant.
Kidney	Decreased ability to excrete wastes and drugs, to preserve water, and to get rid of excess water. One of the most predictable changes with aging.	Increased risk of excess drug accumulation. Greater risk of dehydration and fluid overload. This is one of the most clinically significant changes with aging. Requires careful management.
Musculo-skeletal	Decreased muscle strength; decreased bone strength.	Increased risk of weakness that reduces functional abilities, particularly the ability to walk. Physical activity, especially walking, is one of the most important methods of delaying dependence. Bed rest is a tremendous curse for the elderly. Increased risk of fractures, but walking increases bone strength.
Genito-urinary	Increased urine production at night. Decreased bladder capacity. Increased prostate size.	More frequent nighttime urination, disturbing sleep. Decreased urine flow and higher risk of urinary retention and infection in men.

Immune Function	Decrease in white cell function, but not in numbers. Various "barrier defenses" decreased, particularly in lung and urinary tract.	Increased risk of infections. Often exacerbated by malnutrition, which also reduces immunity.
Laboratory Tests	Most are not different. Postprandial blood sugar rises; erythrocyte sedimentation rate (ESR) rises; possible slight decrease in hemoglobin/hematocrit (debated).	Generally not clinically significant. If a lab test is abnormal, look for a cause other than aging. (However, don't worry about an ESR less than 50 mm/hr.)
Emotional Function	Not significantly changed. If anything, elders are more able to withstand problems that cause emotional reactions.	If an elderly person has an emotional symptom (particularly depression), don't consider it a normal, "understandable" finding. Evaluate and treat it!

renal function, are much more common as people age, and these problems often require low doses of medication to avoid complications. Other diseases, such as congestive heart failure, coronary artery disease, diabetes mellitus, chronic lung disease, and hypertension, also are more common and create medication dependency.

The frequency and severity of adverse reactions to medications tend to be greater in older people. Kidney function is predictably reduced as people age. Any drug or active drug metabolite that is cleared by the kidney should be prescribed in a lower dose in persons over age 85 or in younger older persons with hypertension and/or diabetes mellitus, which also worsen kidney function. Using normal doses may result in excess drug accumulation and adverse effects. The old adage of start low, go slow—which pertains to initial dose and dose increases—is useful for these types of drugs.

Probably the main reason older persons are at much greater risk of adverse drug reactions is the fact that they take more medications. Any added medicine has not only its own risks, but also the risks of interactions with drugs already taken. New medicines, including and perhaps especially psychotropic medications, should be given only after careful consideration. Because medical providers want to help people, we sometimes turn to medications when the need for them is questionable in the hope they might help. A helpful adage when considering whether or not

Table 2.2

COMMON MEDICAL PROBLEMS AND DISASTERS

DISEASE	KEY CONCERNS IN DISASTERS	CONSIDERATIONS FOR MANAGEMENT
Coronary Artery Disease	Angina or myocardial infarction brought on by emotional or physical stress or absent medications.	Continue heart medications. Watch for coronary artery symptoms (chest pain, shortness of breath, fainting, sweating, nausea). Have emergency medications available.
Congestive Heart Failure (CHF)	Worsened heart function secondary to stress or stopping medications, possibly from eating foods with excess salt.	Continue CHF medications. Have others available for urgent treatment. Watch for increased shortness of breath, particularly with exercise. Avoid high-salt foods (most canned foods and prepared meals unless labeled "low salt" or "healthy").
Diabetes Mellitus	Excessively low or high blood sugar. Diabetics prone to coronary artery disease often have no chest pain, even with myocardial infarction.	Continue diabetes medications, but if food is substantially reduced, may need to reduce dosage. Watch for and be ready to treat changes with low blood sugar—sweating, pallor, shaking, confusion, coma. Assure plenty of fluids (generally at least 1/2 ounce per pound of weight per day).
Chronic Lung Disease	Worsening if poor air quality, infectious diseases, or absence of medications. Anxiety may also cause shortness of breath.	Continue medications; have emergency medications and oxygen available. Surgical-type masks can reduce particulate inhalation or infectious disease.
Chronic Kidney Disease (Renal Insufficiency)	If on dialysis, will need to continue or patient may die. Dehydration will rapidly worsen condition for any kidney patient. Much greater risk of adverse drug reactions.	Provide fluids as noted in "Diabetes Mellitus." Severe renal disease may require fluid restrictions. If patient is on dialysis but no dialysis is available, focus on comfort measures.

to prescribe in the older person is when in doubt, don't. Exceptions to this are depression and pain, which usually warrant a trial of medications.

In a major disaster that disrupts the delivery of medical supplies, the key problem may be the absence of medicines for those diseases that not much else can help. Persons with common life-threatening problems, including congestive heart failure, chronic lung disease, diabetes mellitus, and coronary artery disease, may suffer severe and potentially fatal exacerbations of their conditions without their medicines, for which there are no readily available substitutes. The major psychiatric problems, particularly anxiety disorders and schizophrenia, usually need continued medications to prevent rapid relapse. Depression tends to relapse more slowly without medications, but it also may become much worse if untreated for days or weeks.

Short of stockpiling crucial medications, there appears to be little possibility of preventing the consequences of the absence of medications. However, sometimes older patients get better when some of their meds are stopped, so some patients might get better if they couldn't get their usual meds![4]

Inevitability of Higher Losses Among Older Persons

Given the high level of medical support needed to sustain the lives of many frail elders and their reduced capacity to withstand physical stresses in general, in severe disaster situations it is inevitable there will be high losses in this population. This has been demonstrated in extreme heat situations, in which older persons die in disproportionate numbers (Vandentorren & Empereur-Bissonnet, 2006).

Persons working in disaster relief must be prepared for this possibility, and programs to assist in dealing with these losses should be available. Although not frequently discussed, the potential of facing hard decisions about who will receive scarce resources to support life and who will be allowed to die because of not receiving them must be considered when training leaders of disaster relief efforts. Our country's recent weather disaster, Hurricane Katrina, unfortunately created such a dilemma, and the unfortunate results reflected the lack of training and guidance (Fink, 2009).

OVERLAP OF THE PHYSICAL AND EMOTIONAL ISSUES

Interplay of Emotional Experiences (Past and Present) and Physical Experience, Including Neuro-Endocrine-Physiologic Connections

The connection between mental processes and the body has tremendous implications in disasters. The obvious tie is between emotional responses and actions influenced by fear, depression, and anger. But there also are internal physiologic responses developed through eons of evolution to help preserve life. These responses are mediated through the nervous and endocrine systems. In limited application, they can be lifesaving. But they take their toll on the individual when they are extensive in scope or duration. And while they may be helpful to a healthy body, they may harm those with underlying severe illness. A brief description of these processes follows.

The sympathetic nervous system responds to perceived acute danger by setting off the *fight-or-flight response.* In addition to general heightened mental alertness, this response includes the release of epinephrine and norepinephrine from the adrenal glands, located just above the kidneys. Environmental, and sometimes just mental, stimuli perceived as threatening cause the cerebral cortex to signal the brain stem (locus ceruleus), which in turn stimulates the adrenal glands via the sympathetic nerves. The adrenals then release the hormones epinephrine and norepinephrine into the bloodstream. Transported throughout the body,

Table 2.3

POTENTIAL HARMS OF THE FIGHT-OR-FLIGHT RESPONSE		
BODILY CHANGE	**POTENTIAL HELP**	**POTENTIAL HARM IN DISEASE**
Increased heart rate.	Assist in physical activity needed for survival.	In heart failure, may reduce the heart's pumping effectiveness. In coronary artery disease, may precipitate chest pain.
Increased respiratory rate.	Assist in physical activity needed for survival.	May precipitate hyperventilation syndrome, causing dizziness, chest pain, inability to function physically.
Blood flow shunted away from some organs (especially gastrointestinal tract and kidney) and heart, brain, muscles.	Improve muscle function.	In persons with reduced renal function, further reduces this function. In persons with poor circulation to intestines, may precipitate pain.
Increased production of glucose, raising blood sugar.	Increase fuel supply for muscles and brain.	In diabetes, raises blood sugar further.

these hormones produce widespread and sometimes extreme physiologic changes in body organs and function. In persons with certain diseases these changes may be harmful instead of helpful. Examples of the physiologic processes and potential harmful effects in diseases common in older persons are shown in Table 2.3. Other complex stress response processes increase blood coagulation, perhaps especially in older persons, which may increase the chance of acute obstruction of coronary arteries leading to myocardial infarction (Wirtz, et al., 2008).

In addition to this acute response, the brain under stress stimulates the release of another adrenal gland hormone that works more slowly. Acting through the hypothalamus, stress causes the release of corticotropin (ACTH) from the pituitary gland into the bloodstream. ACTH stimulates the release of cortisol from the adrenal glands. Cortisol, normally present in relatively low amounts, has diffuse bodily effects. With increases over a short time span it generally is protective of the organism, reducing excess inflammation and bolstering the physiologic systems that aid survival. But over weeks to months, elevated cortisol may produce significant problems. Indeed, chronically very high levels of cortisol, caused either by the intake of oral cortisol-like drugs or by tumors, results in a disease called Cushing's syndrome, which dramatically shortens life if untreated. Some of the adverse effects of excess cortisol include the following: elevated blood sugar, reduction of muscle mass, thinning of the skin, increased central body fat, thinning of the bones, water retention, and elevated blood pressure (McEwen, 1998). Perhaps the most significant adverse effect for older persons is a reduced ability to fight infections, to which they already are more susceptible for multiple reasons. Cortisol also affects the brain and can lead to confusion, sleep disturbance, and depression (Varghese & Brown, 2001). The connection between abnormalities of cortisol and cortisol regulation and depression is strong (Barden, 2004).

Physical Effects of Emotions/Mental Disease

Established emotional problems may produce behavioral and physical changes with substantial consequences in disaster situations. Depression blunts a person's ability to respond to situations in an energetic manner and, thus, may put the person at increased risk. It also may lessen appetite and nutritional intake with resultant physical weakening. In the frail older person particularly, undernutrition may result in a reduced ability to fight infections and will generally weaken all the body's functions. Specific nutrient deficiencies will also affect other diseases, especially those of the heart and brain. Depression also affects the sensation of pain and is a major factor in chronic pain syndromes, both producing and aggravating them. As noted earlier, the pituitary-adrenal connection and response is affected by depression and may be a factor in reducing resistance to infection in chronically depressed individuals.

Anxiety frequently accompanies depression, but it is also extremely common by itself. The brain often responds to anxious feelings by setting off the fight-or-flight reaction, although sometimes at a lower intensity. In acute situations, anxiety may precipitate the physical problems caused by the release of adrenal hormones as noted earlier. Panic attacks, part of the spectrum of anxiety disorders, may result in multiple physical symptoms, including heart palpitations, chest pain, shortness of breath, dizziness, numbness of the extremities, and even muscle spasms affecting the hands. They are very distressing and may initially be difficult to differentiate from life-threatening problems such as myocardial infarction or pulmonary embolus, especially in older people, who are more prone to these severe problems.

Psychotic disorders, particularly paranoia, may cause people to avoid others, including the support system that may be necessary for their survival. The acute worsening of schizophrenia induced by disaster stresses may produce a complete inability to attend to personal physical needs, particularly shelter and food.

Emotional Effects of Physical Experiences

Being in a disaster situation, perhaps seeing significant loss or injury of family and friends and possibly suffering personal physical harm, produces major emotional responses. Immediate losses or threats of loss and physical distress produce anxiety and sadness, which may be severe. Persons with underlying psychiatric illness have a much greater chance of relapsing into uncontrolled psychiatric states precipitated by these stressors. Those with past trauma, especially PTSD, may suffer flashbacks or more severe reactions to their current situation. Longer duration stress may cause depression in anyone, perhaps in part because of the cortisol excess noted earlier; those already prone to the disease succumb sooner or more severely. There is the potential for early interventions to reduce the severity of acute and chronic emotional problems caused by disasters

(Anand, 2009). Older persons with intact cognition should be able to benefit from these same interventions.

The Importance of Social Interactions on Physical and Emotional Problems

Humans need interaction in all situations, but in disasters the need may be particularly acute. The comforting presence of others produces emotional support in dealing with disasters and losses, and the presence of others may induce better behavior in individuals under stress. Aside from the reassurance that one is not alone in facing problems, social interaction also can produce better outcomes by stimulating thoughts on how to address problems and using the strength of the group to overcome difficulties. Social support has been demonstrated as a factor in improving emotional outcomes of disasters (Cook & Bickman, 1990; Forbes & Roger, 1999).

Some older people are already grouped in living situations, and many others living in individual settings may belong to groups, such as churches and community organizations. These can set the foundation for group interactions; reaching isolated individuals can sometimes be accomplished through these groupings. The potential for healthy older persons to reach out to other older persons and to assist them in group settings may be particularly useful. But even persons who are physically frail may benefit the group through their wealth of experience or emotional stability.

The U.S. Department of Veterans Affairs, National Center for PTSD is a good resource for further information about psychosocial support in disasters. Also, the International Federation of Red Cross and Red Crescent Societies Reference Center for Psychosocial Support has extensive information, including a free handbook and training kit.

CONCLUSION

Older persons are a diverse group who require extra support in any disaster situation but who also may be of tremendous assistance to others. The key to preparing for and implementing disaster activities to support frail older persons is the recognition of their reduced ability to maintain physical and cognitive function and their high need for medicines and sustaining treatments. Disaster relief workers and leaders must be prepared for the possibility of higher death tolls in older persons, and leaders should be trained in making difficult decisions of rationing if resources are inadequate.

Contrasting with their increased physical susceptibilities, older persons may be more resilient in dealing with the emotional stresses of disasters. But the effects of acute and chronic emotional and physical stress, with their consequent hormonal and diffuse physiologic changes, have greater potential to negatively affect those with weaker cardiovascular and other organ systems—symptoms markedly more common in older persons. Accordingly, older persons should be included in any programs designed to reduce emotional reactions to disasters.

Despite concerns about their frailty, a large proportion of older persons, especially those under 75, will be able to contribute positively and significantly to relief efforts. Although with reduced strength and stamina, they are often still relatively robust physically and can do lighter but important physical tasks. They also have a wealth of knowledge and experience from work and life in general. Even very old persons often have wisdom and emotional strength that can be of great assistance to younger people facing a disaster. Planners and managers of disaster relief programs should include this great resource in their plans and activities.

NOTES

1. Experts in the study of aging and older persons in society.
2. Physicians specializing in elderly medical care.
3. *Function* may also be used to describe the status of various organs and capacities—e.g., cardiac function or cognitive function—but the broader definition is used here.
4. Those wishing to learn more about potentially harmful medicines for the elderly should consult *The Beers List* (Fick et al., 2003).

REFERENCES

Anand, P. (2009). Adult disaster psychiatry: Clinical synthesis. *Focus, 7,* 155–159.
Barden, N. (2004). Implication of the hypothalamic-pituitary-adrenal axis in the physiopathology of depression. *Journal of Psychiatry and Neuroscience, 29,* 185–193.
Campbell, A. J., & Buchner, D. M. (1996). Unstable disability and the fluctuations of frailty. *Age and Ageing, 26,* 315–318.
Cook, J. D., & Bickman, L. (1990). Social support and psychological symptomatology following a natural disaster. *Journal of Traumatic Stress, 3,* 541–556.
Fick, D. M., Cooper, J. W., Wade, W. E., Waller, J. L., Maclean, J. R., & Beers, M. H. (2003). Updating the Beers criteria for potentially inappropriate medication use in

older adults: Results of a U.S. consensus panel of experts. *Archives of Internal Medicine, 163,* 2716–2724.

Fink, S. (2009, August 30). The deadly choices at Memorial. *The New York Times Magazine,* pp. 28–46.

Forbes, A., & Roger, D. (1999). Stress, social support, and fear of disclosure. *British Journal of Health Psychology, 4,* 165–179.

Foster, J. R. (1997) Successful coping, adaptation, and resilience in the elderly: An interpretation of epidemiologic data. *Psychiatric Quarterly, 68,* 189–219.

Katz, S., Downs, T. D., Cash, H. R., & Grotz, R. C. (1970). Progress in the development of the index of ADL. *Gerontologist, 10,* 20–30.

Lawton, M. P., & Brody, E. M. (1969). Assessment of older people: Self-maintaining and instrumental activities of daily living. *Gerontologist, 9,* 179–186.

McEwen, B. S. (1998). Protective and damaging effects of stress mediators. *New England Journal of Medicine, 338,* 171–179.

Tugade, M. M., Fredrickson, B. L., & Barrett, L. F. (2004). Psychological resilience and emotional granularity: Examining the benefits of positive emotions on coping and health. *Journal of Personality, 72,* 1161–1190.

Vandentorren, S., & Empereur-Bissonnet, P. (2006). Health impact of the 2003 heat-wave in France. In W. Kirch, R. Bertollini, & B. Menne (Eds.), *Extreme weather events and public health responses* (pp. 81–87). Berlin: Springer Publishing.

Varghese, F. P., & Brown, E. S. (2001). The hypothalamic-pituitary-adrenal axis in major depressive disorder: A brief primer for primary care physicians. *Primary Care Companion to the Journal of Clinical Psychiatry, 3,* 151–155.

Wirtz, P. H., Redwine, L. S., Baertschi, C., Spillmann, M., Ehlert, U., & von Känel, R. (2008). Coagulation activity before and after acute psychosocial stress increases with age. *Psychosomatic Medicine, 70,* 476–481.

3

The Geriatric Emergency Preparedness and Response (GEPR) Collaborative: A Successful and Productive Network

JUDITH L. HOWE

The Geriatric Emergency Preparedness and Response (GEPR) Collaborative is an exemplary example of successful national networking for sharing and disseminating information, leveraging resources, and influencing policy. Networking is particularly important in the fields of gerontology and geriatrics where there is often competition for resources due to its interdisciplinary nature, a fragmented delivery system, and funding deficits (Johnson, 2006). The GEPR Collaborative has achieved the goals laid out in its 2002 mission statement and strategy plan—to develop and disseminate curricular material and influence policy—as described in this chapter.

GERIATRIC EDUCATION CENTERS (GECs)

The Geriatric Education Centers (GECs) are the only federally funded programs specifically geared to the education and training of health care professionals in the diagnosis, treatment, and prevention of disease and other health concerns of older adults. Initiated in 1985, there are currently 48 GECs that provide training through continuing education; curriculum development and dissemination; training and retraining of faculty; and clinical training in geriatrics in nursing homes, chronic and acute disease hospitals, ambulatory care centers, and senior centers. Over the last two decades, achievements of the GEC programs include the following:

- Training more than 425,000 health care professionals from 27 health-related disciplines to better serve the growing older adult population
- Developing over 1,000 curricular materials on aging-related topics, including interdisciplinary team care, geriatric syndromes, ethnogeriatrics, cultural competency, health literacy, quality of care, rural health access issues, and bioterrorism and emergency preparedness
- Delivering 282 distance learning programs to 37,000 health care professionals in rural and underserved areas (Advisory Committee on Interdisciplinary and Community-Based Linkages, 2006)

THE DEVELOPMENT OF THE GEC GERIATRIC EMERGENCY PREPAREDNESS AND RESPONSE COLLABORATIVE

The terrorist attacks on the World Trade Center on September 11, 2001, heightened awareness of the vulnerability of older persons in times of bioterrorism and emergencies. As is now well-known, older and disabled persons were trapped for days before help arrived after the Twin Towers collapsed. This led to a citywide effort in the following months to develop a system for ensuring agencies had emergency preparedness plans that included rapid and comprehensive assistance for vulnerable populations, such as older adults (O'Brien, 2003).

Process of Developing the Collaborative

At the national meeting of the Gerontological Society of America (GSA) in November 2003, GEC representatives became aware of potential funding streams in emergency and bioterrorism preparedness that excluded older adults. That knowledge led to a quickly assembled meeting at the GSA conference of the GEC network with the aim of ensuring older persons were included in initiatives in this area (Johnson, 2006). It was a seminal meeting, as it essentially launched the movement of GECs working together to ensure health care providers received the necessary training and education to assist older persons in times of bioterrorism and emergencies.

This heightened awareness led the GECs' national organization, the National Association of Geriatric Education Centers (NAGEC), to form the GEPR Collaborative in response to the identified need for increased attention to older people in times of emergencies or disasters. The goal of the founders of the GEPR Collaborative was to jointly develop, disseminate, and evaluate GEPR curricula and training tools for health providers caring for older adults at risk in the event of a disaster or emergency.

The founding members of the GEPR Collaborative agreed to develop a mission statement, carry out a needs assessment, develop an evidence base, and work together in securing funding and developing and dissemi-

Table 3.1

POSITION STATEMENT

Position Statement of the Bioterrorism Preparedness Committee of the National Association of Geriatric Education Centers (NAGEC) – 2003

Inasmuch as neither the nation's health work force nor older people and their caregivers are adequately prepared to respond quickly and effectively in the event of an attack by bioterrorists, the faculty in all 41 GECs have recognized the major threat that the specter of such a disaster poses to a particularly vulnerable segment of our country's population, the 35,000,000 and rapidly growing number of people over the age of 65, especially those frail elders living alone. Many others live in intergenerational households particularly among ethnic minority communities whose access to urgent information may be delayed because of language, cultural factors, and family caregivers who also work outside their homes. Several GECs have already created and disseminated a number of training curricula, all of which are designed to improve the health care provided to the elderly population in response to an attack by bioterrorists. A Bioterrorism Preparedness Committee of the GECs has met and determined the need to develop more specific and standardized training programs and to ensure that all of these programs are conducted throughout the national GEC network. In addition, there is a need to expand the programs beyond the GECs to their community partners to ensure that culturally appropriate training on the special needs of the elderly and their families is offered to agencies that provide services to the elderly in both emergency situations and over the long-term. Working in concert with HRSA, the GECs' Bioterrorism Preparedness Plan . . . can be implemented in 2004.

From "Geriatric Education Centers Prepare to Combat Bioterrorism," by N. Tumosa, 2003, *Aging Successfully, 13*(1), 20–21.

Table 3.2

GEPR STRATEGIC GUIDELINES

TYPE OF RESPONSE	PURPOSE OF RESPONSE	OUTCOMES
Curriculum Development	To include curricular content on bioterrorism preparedness for older adults in allied health and continuing education training programs. Suggested content includes clinical services and outreach, education, and policy.	Health care workers will know more about the elderly, including their special needs and how those needs should be met. Treatment for exposure to certain toxins will be addressed.
Curriculum Dissemination	Curricular materials will be disseminated through all GEC and community partners (e.g., schools, health facilities) using multiple media (e.g., printed materials, conferences, Website).	GECs will identify local partners (e.g., health departments, AAAs) to assist in the implementation of training. The training programs will be evaluated on an ongoing basis.
Policy Development	GEC networks will work to ensure that policy makers at all levels of government are aware of the special needs of older adults.	Enhanced knowledge should ensure that the needs of older adults are included in programs and policies.

From "Geriatric Education Centers Prepare to Combat Bioterrorism," by N. Tumosa, 2003, *Aging Successfully, 13*(1), 20–21.

nating a national curriculum on bioterrorism and emergency preparedness for older people.

A needs assessment was conducted to determine the extent of programs being offered and future plans of the 51 GECs funded at that time. The assessment found that 21 of the GECs had already developed curricula on the topic, with existing circulation through trainings, curricula, Web sites, and various written materials. The committee formulated a Mission Statement (Table 3.1) and developed a three-pronged Strategy Plan (Table 3.2) to guide the national network of GECs in a coordinated response to the threats facing older adults. Specifically, the GEPR Collaborative suggested that the GEC network engage in curriculum development, curriculum dissemination, and policy development in order to strengthen its capacity to meet the needs of older adults.

In January 2003, GEPR representatives held a meeting with the Senate majority leader's staff and the chairman of the House of Representatives Oversight Committee of the Department of Homeland Security. Other Congressional visits followed, laying the groundwork for responding to a Health Services Resources Administration (HRSA) request for proposals in the summer of 2003 on emergency preparedness and other topics important for training the health care workforce to better serve older adults (Roush & Tumosa, 2004).

HRSA Supplemental Funding for GEPR Projects

The Geriatric Education Centers Supplemental Grant Program *Request for Proposals* (CFDA number 93.969), issued in June 2003, was specifically for the following areas: oral health, mental health/behavioral health, bioterrorism, and/or severe acute respiratory syndrome (SARS). One purpose of the supplemental funding was to develop additional training materials that could be adapted by other GECs; HRSA-funded programs, such as Area Health Education Centers; governmental agencies serving older persons, such as Area Agencies on Aging, housing authorities, and public health agencies; health professions schools; and other organizations serving older adults.

Because the foundation had been laid by the GEPR Collaborative, the GECs that applied for the competitive funding were able to include common objectives and language in their grant proposals, which enabled them to work together to develop a national bioterrorism and emergency preparedness for aging curriculum and to participate in joint dissemination of grant products. Six 1-year curriculum development grants in bioterrorism and emergency preparedness for older adults were awarded in the amount of $2.4 million later in 2003. These grants were awarded to the Consortium of New York GECs (CNYGEC), Case Western Reserve GEC, Ohio Valley/Appalachia GEC, the Gateway GEC of Missouri and Illinois, the Texas Consortium GEC, and the Stanford GEC.

The project goals of the six GECs receiving funding were as follows:

- CNYGEC: Offer geriatric mental health and disaster preparedness for interdisciplinary health care providers serving older adults
- Case Western Reserve GEC: Teach the principles of emergency preparedness to groups who serve older people and provide resources to students and the community

- Ohio Valley/Appalachia GEC: Develop Internet GEPR database, create curriculum training modules, conduct community focus groups, and provide interdisciplinary distance and traditional learning opportunities (Johnson et al., 2006)
- Gateway GEC of Missouri and Illinois: Provide interdisciplinary modules to train health care providers to care for frail older people in emergencies
- Texas Consortium of GECs: Develop consensus on what needs to be taught to front-line health care workers regarding bioterrorism and aging and conduct continuing education programs
- Stanford GEC: Provide ethnogeriatric training on mental health aspects and special needs of older ethnic minorities with diabetes and sensory impairment

Developing Consensus

In January 2004, a few months after the HRSA funding was granted, a Consensus Conference was convened by the Miami Area GEC. The 2-day conference, attended by representatives from the six funded GECs, resulted in an outline of a *White Paper on Bioterrorism and Emergency Preparedness* and the focus of the national GEPR curriculum. The Consensus Conference participants identified the necessary information that interdisciplinary health care providers needed to know about bioterrorism and emergency preparedness, which included the following: (1) knowledge of potential threats for older persons and how they may respond differently in a disaster; (2) basic geriatric considerations, such as the unique needs of older persons and common mental health problems; (3) identifying and mobilizing resources, such as coordination between community and health care organizations, including family and friends; (4) communications, such as communicating with non-English-speaking older persons and those with sensory impairments; (5) mental health issues, such as identifying risk factors, knowledge of referral systems, screening and treatment methods, and self-care; (6) ethics, such as the role of ageism and other discriminatory practices, triage, abuse, and neglect; and (7) ethnicity, including special considerations related to ethnicity, race, and class. The group also discussed the most effective means of developing training materials and disseminating those materials for maximum impact. It was decided that the GEPR Collaborative should present at national and regional meetings, publish in various venues, conduct continuing education sessions, partner with groups such as the AARP, and integrate material

Table 3.3

GEC GEPR COLLABORATIVE PRODUCTS

YEAR	PRESENTATIONS AT NATIONAL MEETINGS	CURRICULAR MATERIALS	PUBLISHED ARTICLES	OTHER MATERIALS
2003	(1) Symposium, Gerontological Society of America annual meeting, November, Bioterrorism Policy and Education Issues for Elders and Their Caregivers.	OVAR/GEC Bioterrorism and Emergency Preparedness for Aging Database (http://aging.ukcph.org/gec/bioterrorismandemergency.htm)	Tumosa, N. (Ed.). Geriatric educat on centers prepare to combat bioterrorism. *Aging Successfully, 13*(1), 20–21.	NAGEC GEPR Mission Statement
2004	(1) Poster, Gerontological Society of America annual meeting, November, Emergency Preparedness for Caregivers of Older People (2) Poster, Gerontological Society of America annual meeting, November, Emergency Preparedness: Geriatric Menta Health (3) Pre-conference workshop, Association for Gerontology in Higher Education annual meeting, HRSA-funded GECs: Infusing and Teaching Curriculum Content on Bioterrorism and Emergency Preparedness for the Aging	(1) OVAR/GEC Distance Learning Modules: OVAR/GEC Helping Elders Prepare for Bioterrorism and Emergencies (TRAIN ID: 100647) (2) OVAR/GEC Disaster Preparedness: Developing an Agency Emergency Plan (TRAIN ID: 1007090), OVAR/GEC The Aging Network (TRAIN ID: 1006470) (3) OVAR/GEC Emergency Plans for Individuals and Agencies (http://aging.ukcph.org/gec/bioterrorismandemergency. htm#Emergency_Plans_) (4) WRGEC: Four web-based modules about elders and emergencies:	(1) Tumosa, N. (Ed.). Emergency preparedness. *Aging Successfully, 14*(3), 1–22. (2) Roush, R. E., Fasser, C. E., Schneider, A. W., & Taffet, G. E. (2004). Emergency preparedness for caregivers of older people: Early diagnosis and age-appropriate treatment of Class A biological agents. *The Gerontologist, 44*(1), 502.	

(continued)

Table 3.3

GEC GEPR COLLABORATIVE PRODUCTS (Continued)

YEAR	PRESENTATIONS AT NATIONAL MEETINGS	CURRICULAR MATERIALS	PUBLISHED ARTICLES	OTHER MATERIALS
2004	(4) Pre-conference workshop, American Society on Aging annual meeting, March, Geriatric Education and Neighborhood Planning for Bioterrorism and Emergency Preparedness	biologic agents, frailty, psychological responses, civil rights (http:darla.neoucom.edu/ElderPrepare) (5) Texas: Distance learning modules (http://www.hcoa.org/newsite/tcgec/Distance_Learning_Resources)		
2005	(1) Workshop, Association for Gerontology in Higher Education annual meeting, February, HRSA GECs: Infusing and Teaching Curriculum Content on Bioterrorism and Emergency Preparedness for the Aged (2) Pre-conference workshop, American Society on Aging annual meeting, March, the Neighborhood Plan for GEPR (3) Symposium, Gerontological Society of America annual meeting, November, HRSA GECs: Interdisciplinary	(1) California: Sensory Loss and Emergency Preparedness Strategies with Elders with Diabetes from Diverse Ethnic Backgrounds with a section on emergency preparedness for sensory impaired elders		(1) Gateway GEC: games, including the ETHNIC ELDERS MNEMONIC mnemonic and emergency preparedness kits (2) CA: Interactive and role-play modules, CDs

Year				
2005	Collaborations in Bioterrorism and Emergency Preparedness Reaching Beyond Individual GECs			
2006	(1) Poster, Gerontological Society annual meeting, November, Innovative and Imaginative Methods of Teaching Geriatric Emergency Preparedness (2) Symposium, Association for Gerontology in Higher Education annual meeting, February, Lessons Learned from Katrina, Rita, and Wilma in Emergency Preparedness: Interdisciplinary and Multi-Modal Teaching Methods	(1) CNYGEC: Geriatric Mental Health and Emergency Preparedness curriculum, basis for 40-hour certificate program (2) OVAR/GEC distance learning modules: OVAR/GEC Community Emergency Response Teams–CERT (TRAIN ID: 1005655), OVAR/GEC Pandemic Flu and Aging (Loading; Future TRAIN ID: 1009188)	Johnson, A., Howe, J. L., McBride, M., Palmisano, B., Perweiler, El, Roush, R., et al. Bioterrorism and Emergency Preparedness in Aging (BPEPA): HRSA-funced GEC collaboration for curricula and training. *Gerontology and Geriatrics Education, 26*(4), 63–86.	(1) OVAR/GEC: Mutiple online training resources at http://louisville.edu/sphis/chhp/education--training/distnace-learning.html (2) CNYGEC 40-hour certificate program conducted (Spring) (3) Draft of "A White Paper on Bioterrorism and Aging: Recommendations for the Nation's Health Work Force," a HRSA contract with the Texas Consortium of GECs
2007	(1) Symposium, American Society on Aging annual meeting, Chicago, March, Helping Rural Elders to Pre-pare for Emergencies	OVAR/GEC E-Newsletter for Emergency Preparedness for Aging (http://cwte.louisville.edu/ovar/emergency/fall2007.htm), Preparedness for Long-Term Care (http://cwte.louisville.edu/ovar/emergency/winter2008.htm)	(1) Taylor, S. Disaster plan-ning: Can you ever really be ready? *Aging Successfully, 17*(1), 3, 4, 15.	(1) CNYGEC curriculum posted on POGOe (2) CNYGEC 40-hour certificate program conducted (Spring)

(continued)

Table 3.3

GEC GEPR COLLABORATIVE PRODUCTS (*Continued*)

YEAR	PRESENTATIONS AT NATIONAL MEETINGS	CURRICULAR MATERIALS	PUBLISHED ARTICLES	OTHER MATERIALS
2007	(2) Peer group, American Society on Aging annual meeting, Chicago, March, Emergency Preparedness and Older Adults: Emerging Issues	Health Literacy for Emergency Preparedness and Aging (http://cwte.louisville.edu/ovar/emergency/spring2008.htm), Pandemic Flu and Aging (http://cwte.louisville.edu/ovar/emergency/summer2008.htm)	(2) Tumosa, N. (2007). Disaster: Nursing homes need to be prepared. *Journal of the American Medical Directors Association, 8*(3), 135–137. (3) Roush, R. E. (2007, Winter). Responding to elders during disasters: What healthcare professionals need to know. *Healthcare & Aging* (4), 1–2. http://www.asaging.org/asav2/han/enews/07winter/top.cfm	
2008	(1) Paper, American Society on Aging annual meeting, March, What Health Professionals Need to Know About Emergencies and Vulnerable Groups: Success with ASA, GSA, CDC, DAS, & AGS (2) Special interest group presentation, American		(1) Lamb, K. V., O'Brien, C., & Fenza, P. J. (2008). Elders at risk during disasters. *Home Healthcare Nurse, 26,* 30–37.	(1) CNYGEC 40-hour certificate program conducted (Spring)

Year			
2008	Geriatrics Society annual meeting, May, What Geriatricians Need to Know about Emergencies and Vulnerable Groups: Implications for Curricula and Education (3) Poster, Gerontological Society of America annual meeting, November, Six Model Curricula on Disaster Preparedness: Enhancing Knowledge and Strengthening Elder Resiliency	(2) Roush, R. E. (2008, Summer). Serving ethnic elders during disasters: What healthcare professionals need to know. Diversity Currents, a publication of the American Society on Aging, http://www.asaging.org/asav2/noma/enews/08summer/in_practice.cfm	
2009	(1) Poster, Association for Gerontology in Higher Education annual meeting, February, Safeguarding Better Futures for Older Adults: More Health Providers with Geriatric Training in Disaster Preparedness (2) Peer group, American Society on Aging, Las Vegas, March, Emergency Preparedness for Aging Networks and Collaborations	(1) Bales, C., & Tumosa, N. (2009). Minimizing the impact of complex emergencies on nutrition and geriatric health: Planning for prevention is key. In C.W. Bales & C.S. Richie (Eds.), *Handbook of clinical nutrition and aging* (2nd ed., pp. 635–664). New York: Humana Press. (2) O'Brien, C., Selod, S., & Lamb, K. (in press). A national initiative to train long-term care staff for disaster response and recovery. *Journal of Public Health Management & Practice*.	CNYGEC 24-hour certificate program conducted (Spring)

into existing curricular materials. There was also discussion about measuring outcomes using the following suggested measures: development of emergency plans for older adults, adding questions to certification exams for health care professionals, and including aging issues in emergency preparedness protocols (Bioterrorism and Emergency Preparedness in Aging Collaborative, 2004).

A second meeting of the GEPR Collaborative was held among grantees and HRSA staff in Bethesda, Maryland, on August 25–26, 2004. At this meeting, the six grantees presented progress reports on their HRSA-funded projects as highlighted in Table 3.3, and a nominal group technique was undertaken to develop consensus on recommendations for a new *White Paper* chapter on bioterrorism and aging.[1]

GEPR FOCUS ON THE MENTAL HEALTH EFFECTS OF EMERGENCIES ON OLDER PERSONS

Consortium of New York Geriatric Education Centers

The focus of the CNYGEC GEPR Collaborative project is geriatric mental health and disaster preparedness. The Stanford GEC Bioterrorism and Emergency Preparedness in Aging Collaborative (BTEPA) project also focuses on mental health with an emphasis on ethnogeriatrics. The CNYGEC partners, Mount Sinai School of Medicine Brookdale Department of Geriatrics and Adult Development; Columbia University Stroud Center for Studies of Quality of Life; New York University College of Nursing; and Hunter College, Brookdale Center for Healthy Aging and Longevity, brought together a 13-member panel of experts in April 2004. Representing nursing, social work, medicine, psychology and psychiatry, and public health, the panel was charged with developing a curriculum outline for a training program on the mental health effects of disasters on older persons. The result of the deliberations of this expert group was a curriculum outline with the following content areas:

- Types of man-made and natural disasters
- The story of September 11, 2001
- Definitions and examples of terms such as crisis, emergency, disaster, preparedness, and readiness
- Special considerations of older persons with regard to housing, transportation, psychology, and health
- Overview of aging and mental health, common mental health problems, diagnosis and assessment, and psychosocial factors

■ Geriatric mental health during an event, including individual responses, normal versus abnormal responses, elder abuse in times of crisis, and differential diagnosis of mental disorders
■ Geriatric mental health post-event, including coping strategies, assessment, interventions, pharmacological therapies, and the use of complementary medicine
■ Clinical perspectives and processes in the care of elders during disasters, case finding, and triage/assessment
■ Complementary and alternative modalities of care, spiritual considerations, and rituals
■ Self-care for the health care provider with respect to trauma and burnout

After the consensus meeting, work groups developed curriculum modules that were reviewed by the core project group, composed of Judy Howe, John Toner, and Andrea Sherman, with revisions made as necessary. For instance, the curriculum was updated to reflect the experiences of hurricanes Katrina and Rita. Published in May 2006, the curriculum consists of the following modules:

1. Teaching Guidelines
2. Overview of Disaster Preparedness and Response
3. Clinical Perspectives and Processes in the Care of Older Adults During Disasters
4. Overview of Aging and Mental Health
5. Geriatric Mental Health and Disasters: Individual and Community Mental Health Outcomes
6. Terrorism Elder Mistreatment
7. Geriatric Mental Health and Disasters: Clinical Response (pharmacological and nonpharmacological interventions)
8. Self-Care for the Health Care Provider
9. Disaster Recovery for Older Adults: Holistic Integrative Therapies

To date, this curriculum has resulted in a broad range of geriatric disaster preparedness training sessions. In 2003, the CNYGEC partnered with the Geriatric Research, Education, and Clinical Center (GRECC) of the Department of Veterans Affairs (VA) and the New York City Department for the Aging (DFTA) to host a multi-site videoconference broadcast to 10 VA facilities throughout the nation. The conference, Emerging Issues in Social Work and Aging: Helping Elders Live in Stressful and Uncertain Times, attended by 131 VA and community health care workers, covered the following topics: Recognizing Stress in the Age of Terrorism: Effects on Older Adults, the Personal and Professional Impact of Trauma on Caregivers, the Effect of Aging on Posttraumatic Stress Disorder, Training Volunteers to Help Elderly Deal with Stress, and Spirituality and the Elderly in Stressful Times.

In 2004, the CNYGEC, VA GRECC, and DFTA once again sponsored a multi-site videoconference on the topic of disaster preparedness, Geriatric Mental Health and Disaster Preparedness: Mental Health Interventions and Treatment Plans. Larger in reach than the previous year's conference with 186 attendees, it was broadcast to 20 VA facilities and co-sponsored by the Western Reserve Geriatric Education Center, a BTEPA Collaborative partner at the time. This videoconference was keynoted by Daniel A. Nigro, retired chief of the New York City Fire Department, who survived the collapses of the Twin Towers and became incident commander upon the death of Chief of Department Peter J. Ganci, Jr. He spoke on Disaster Preparedness—Prepare for the Worst by Being at Your Best, followed by presentations on developing emergency plans for older and frail people, structuring a system of mental health response, spiritual assessment in times of crisis, evaluating a bioterrorism preparedness campaign for veterans, and crisis as a revelatory experience.

Beginning in 2006, the CNYGEC curriculum, Geriatric Mental Health and Emergency Preparedness, was piloted in a 40-hour certificate program attended by 21 health care professionals. Based on feedback from these participants, the training program was refined and offered again in 2007 to 20 attendees and in 2008 to 24 attendees. This comprehensive geriatric mental health disaster preparedness curriculum includes learning objectives; an instructor's outline; a teaching guide; resources such as cases, videotapes, ritual, and role-plays; and PowerPoint presentations on CD-ROM. Supplemental curricular materials include a video highlighting the stories of survivors of the September 11, 2001, terrorist attacks and CNYGEC elective workshops entitled the Mental Health and Quality of Life Improvement in Turbulent Times and Spirituality During Times of Stress.

Stanford Geriatric Education Center

The Stanford GEC (SGEC) also targeted its HRSA funding on the mental health effects of disasters and emergencies on older people. Specifically, the SGEC project concentrated on older ethnic minorities, with the following goals: (1) develop, implement, evaluate, and disseminate an ethnogeriatric curriculum module on the mental health needs of ethnic elders known to be at risk for certain conditions such as diabetes and sensory loss and vulnerable in a disaster or emergency situation; and (2) provide training for faculty, primary care providers, interdisciplinary health professionals, and students using classroom and distance methods of learning. In addition to developing a module on emergency preparedness for sensory-impaired ethnic elders with diabetes, SGEC developed a mnemonic, ETHNIC ELDERS (Table 3.4), to guide the development of curriculum content on emergency preparedness for ethnic elders and their families.

SUMMARY

The GEPR Collaborative, through the development of a common goal, protocols, materials, shared information and resources, and a unified dis-

Table 3.4

ETHNIC ELDERS MNEMONIC	
ETHNIC ELDERS Mnemonic	
E	evaluate risk to ethnic elders
T	translate technical information to simple, indigenous terms
H	help the elder communicate special needs
N	negotiate/navigate pathways to trust relationship
I	intervene with culturally appropriate plans
C	collaborate with family, community, and ethnic media
E	explain how to access local/neighborhood resources
L	label survival kits (English and other languages)
D	differentiate stress-induced anxiety and language differences
E	educate elder, family, and community leaders
R	respect traditional healing practices and rituals
S	support with nonverbal behaviors

From "Geriatric Education Centers Prepare to Combat Bioterrorism," by N. Tumosa, 2003, *Aging Successfully, 13*(1), 20–21.

semination strategy, has created a successful and sustainable national education and training program. While $2.4 million in HRSA funding added momentum to the Collaborative's work, there was clearly a will among the GEC network to address the pressing need for older adults to be included in emergency and disaster preparedness plans and to receive appropriate and sensitive care after events such as natural or man-made emergencies. The GEC network demonstrated its connectivity and resourcefulness by mobilizing quickly to effectively train the nation's health care workforce in this critical area.

ACKNOWLEDGMENTS

The author would like to acknowledge the contributions of the Geriatric Education Center Bioterrorism and Emergency Preparedness (BTEPA) Collaborative in not only the success of this joint endeavor but in providing information for the preparation of this chapter: Dr. Arleen Johnson directs the Ohio Valley Appalachia Regional GEC at the University of Kentucky; Dr. Melen McBride is the associate director emerita at the Stanford University GEC; Dr. Robert Roush directs the Texas Consortium GEC at Baylor College of Medicine's Huffington Center on Aging in Houston, Texas; Dr. Nina Tumosa is the co-director of the Gateway GEC at Saint Louis University; and Dr. Karen V. Lamb teaches at Rush University and is also associated with Mather LifeWays in Evanston, Illinois. Mather LifeWays joined the BTEPA Collaborative in 2006 as a non-GEC partner; an original BTEPA partner, the Western Reserve GEC, represented by Barbara Palmisano, MA, RN, and Margaret Sander, MA, LSW, withdrew from the Collaborative at the conclusion of HRSA supplemental funding in 2005.

The author would like to gratefully acknowledge the research and editorial assistance of Annette M. Atanous, MSSW, Bronx VA GRECC education specialist.

NOTE

1. The contract was between HRSA and Robert Roush, PhD, who led a technical advisory group to write this White Paper Chapter. Other members of the group included George Taffet, MD, Robin McFee, MD, Nina Tumosa, PhD, Elyse Perweiler, RN, and Nora O'Brien, MA. Unfortunately, HRSA did not release this chapter upon completion.

REFERENCES

Advisory Committee on Interdisciplinary and Community-Based Linkages. (2006). *Minutes.* Retrieved January 22, 2009, from http://bhpr.hrsa.gov/interdisciplinary/acicbl/072406minutes.htm

Bioterrorism and Emergency Preparedness in Aging Collaborative (2004, January). *Consensus summary GEPR Collaborative meeting.* Annual Meeting of the Association of Gerontology in Higher Education (AGHE), Miami, FL.

Johnson, A. (2006, April). *Networking for success: Expectations, investments, and net results* (Tech. Rep. No. UGAIG-06-004). University of Georgia Institute of Gerontology. Presented at the 17th Annual Southeastern Region Student Mentoring Conference in Gerontology and Geriatrics, University of Kentucky, Lexington, Kentucky. Retrieved January 21, 2009, from http://www.geron.uga.edu

Johnson, A., Roush, R., Howe, J. L., Sanders, M., McBride, M. R., Sherman, A., et al. (2006). Bioterrorism and emergency preparedness in aging (GEPR). *Gerontology & Geriatrics Education, 26*(4), 63–86.

O'Brien, N. (2003, January–February). *Emergency preparedness for older people* (Issue Brief). New York: International Longevity Center-USA.

Roush, R., & Tumosa, N. (2004, March/April). Bioterrorism task force. *GEC Pipeline, 16*(2), 1.

Tumosa, N. (Ed.). (2003). Geriatric Education Centers prepare to combat bioterrorism. *Aging Successfully, 13*(1), 20–21.

Community Response to the Needs of Older Persons in Disasters

4 Coordinating Services: State and Local Networks and Resources

WILLIAM GRANT AND DOUGLAS M. SANDERS

The immediate difficulty in providing services to older persons in both the immediate and recovery phases of disasters is the need to address a wide range of physical abilities, mental acuities, and chronic illnesses that are more highly variable than in other age groups, such as individuals age 18 to 25 years (Aldrich & Benson, 2008). Certainly there is variability in the latter groups, but the number of outlier individuals within any random sampling of these two groups is likely to be significantly different. It is not unexpected that the physical ability of older individuals may range from completely self-sufficient and mobile to highly dependent. As the state of their physical condition approaches high dependence, they often present a complex constellation of physical and psychosocial manifestations requiring multidisciplinary support. As the body ages, individuals have increased vulnerability to the effects of environmental exposures. Their mental status, often compounded by chronic medical conditions, influences their information-processing capabilities. Older individuals, even the relatively independent, are more susceptible to anxiety engendered by changes in daily routine. And they are all at increased risk for the exacerbation of chronic medical conditions as a result of the disruption of medication or other treatment availability (Ford, Mokdad, & Unk, 2006).

The changing mobility of Americans has caused many families to be scattered across a wide range of geographic areas. Since a significant number of older persons living in the community are geographically isolated from family and friends due to migration patterns, disasters pose a particular challenge. Access to disaster areas is often controlled for safety issues; thus, family members seeking to enter an area to provide assistance may not be able to do so. And, as various staging and shelter areas reach capacity, the movement of survivors to outlying areas, sometimes several states away, complicates this access.

Because of the lack of immediate family support systems, older persons become highly dependent upon rescue and recovery personnel for activities ranging from relocation to support for ADLs. Those with higher levels of physical, medical, and/or mental impairment, who may have been able to function reasonably well in their relatively controlled home environment, are at significant risk of becoming highly vulnerable to isolation and underserved in recovery shelters. The shelter environment is often understaffed and relies heavily upon the self-sufficiency of shelter occupants. Vulnerable older individuals often require assistance for even basic survival services such as eating, toileting, and hygiene, and such assistance may not be available on demand (Fernandez, Byard, Un, Benson, & Barbera, 2002; Hurricane Katrina Community Advisory Group & Kessler, 2007; Laditka, Laditka, Cornman, & Chandlee, 2008; Laditka, Laditka, Xirasagar, et al., 2008; Mori et al., 2007; Rami, Singleton, Spurlock, & Eaglin, 2008).

EVOLUTION OF STATE PLANS

During the 2005 rescue and recovery operations for hurricanes Katrina and Rita, the largest displacement of persons in the history of the United States was undertaken. Many older persons from both inner city and rural locations were relocated, often at significant distance from their homes and isolated from other family members (Lamb, O'Brien, & Fenza, 2008). This experience should have been a clear call for the development of appropriate plans for helping all individuals, especially the most vulnerable, in even the most localized disaster. Unfortunately, at the time of this writing in early 2009, only 28 states had official plans specifically addressing preparedness for older persons (U.S. Department of Health and Human Services, 2007).

The county of Santa Clara, California, Department of Emergency Services's *Tips for Preparedness for the Senior Population* (2009), developed at the county level, is reflective of state plans that do exist and offers an excellent summary of the available research regarding older individuals and their preparation for and response to disasters. The following are among the findings highlighted:

■ Older individuals do not use technology to the same degree as younger individuals; older persons are less likely to register in advance of disasters, less likely to register immediately after, and often do not follow-up. The lack of follow-up is largely because many agencies have moved to Web-based information systems, which are not accessed to a high degree by older persons. The Kaiser Family Foundation (2005) found that less than a third (31%) of senior citizens aged 65 and older have ever gone online but that more than two-thirds (70%) of the next generation of seniors, 50–64 years old, have done so.

■ Older persons are not as likely to use formal aid and assistance resources because of an historical pattern of a higher sense of pride in self-reliance.

■ Their social isolation as a result of a lack of family and other social support during recovery may make older persons more vulnerable to mental and physical abuse.

■ Older persons have neither employment options nor other alternatives for obtaining additional funds to deal with the economic impact of a disaster. Further, both their person and their property are typically underinsured.

THE FEDERAL APPROACH

The federal approach centered on amending the Older Americans Act so older persons would receive limited financial assistance. However, this approach has resulted in an often-fragmented response involving multiple agencies, each with their own missions and related administrative costs to cover. Subsequent to the events of September 11, 2001, and hurricanes Katrina and Rita, the method for distribution of federal financial assistance has been to provide funding at the state level rather than the local level, with the provision that each state establish state-level priorities. The process for providing limited financial support included the provision of funds through individual state agencies on aging. Thus, the implementation and distribution of resources is at the sole discretion of individual states and their agencies. This often means funds are initially expended at the state level for administrative and oversight expenses but are not spent for direct service. During disaster recovery, the U.S. Administration on Aging is charged with coordinating with FEMA and individual state emergency management agencies to work with recovery response agencies such as the American Red Cross.

In the event of a mass displacement of individuals during a public emergency, even with prior planning efforts, experience has shown that many older individuals evacuate without appropriate medications, medication records, and/or health records. Because agencies knew that lack of health information would be a problem during the 2005 hurricane recovery efforts, the federal government suspended certain provisions of the federal privacy rule, the Health Insurance Portability and Accountability Act (HIPAA). Among other benefits, this suspension permitted the exchange of information between shelters and health care providers, which would not have been possible in other circumstances. This was particularly critical during the recovery from Katrina and Rita as entire medical offices and their medical records simply no longer existed. The American Medical Association (AMA) estimated that 5,500 physicians were displaced along with all of their patient records. Many of these physicians did not return to the area. Even physicians with electronic medical records had backed up their systems within the damaged region and therefore lost their backups as well as original records (Hurricane Katrina Community Advisory Group & Kessler, 2007).

Funding at the state level does succeed in providing funds closer to the disaster impact area because states are theoretically in a better position to understand their own local and often unique needs. A seemingly coherent federal response can quickly become fragmented in its implementation. At the state level, there are wide variations in individual laws that govern response to emergency situations. Some states utilize broad definitions of what constitutes an emergency; 41 states specifically describe what constitutes a disaster, and 38 states identify what constitutes an emergency (Hodge & Anderson, 2008). Further complicating the situation is that 27 states and the District of Columbia have definitions for what are called disasters/emergencies, as well as for public health emergencies (Hodge & Anderson).

There has been an effort among states to reformulate and redefine their definition of emergency and related emergency powers to match the language provided in the Model State Emergency Health Powers Act (MSEHPA) developed in 2001 by the Centers for Law and the Public's Health (Ridenour, Cummings, Sinclair, & Bixler, 2007; Rosenkoetter, Covan, Bunting, Cobb, & Fugate-Whitlock, 2007; Rosenkoetter, Covan, Bunting, Cobb, & Weinrlch, 2007; Rosenthal, Klein, Cowling, Grzybowski, & Dunne, 2005). The value of the MSEHPA is that agencies seeking to develop specific response strategies for older persons are afforded extraordinary latitude in providing required services. The MSEHPA allows state governors to suspend regulations and laws that may interfere with the provision of needed emergency services, including the following:

- Updating language to allow for expedited access to medications and vaccines
- Enabling responders to provide medical services even with out-of-state licenses
- Providing liability coverage to volunteers and others who provide medical services

The development of appropriate plans for dealing with disasters depends on understanding the nature of a disaster or emergency as well as identifying appropriate responses, including having the right resources in the right place at the right time (Cherniack, Sandals, Brook, & Mintze, 2008; Dorn, Savoia, Testa, Stoto, & Marcus, 2007). Although language differences may differentiate service delivery models and responsibilities, disasters and emergencies have common characteristics. Disaster events are regional, temporal, and in need of external assistance beyond local response resources. By implication, an event is a disaster when local resources are overwhelmed and external resources, including personnel, are required to assist in rescue and recover areas. Under this description, a local apartment fire is not considered a disaster except for the individuals involved since, although it is regional and temporal, it does not usually require assistance beyond the local community for resolution.

In spite of the combined relatively widespread impact of hurricanes Katrina and Rita—which devastated a land area as large as Great Britain—the damage was limited geographically and the impact on resources for dealing with most evacuees was limited almost entirely to the southern United States. While evacuees were dispersed to many cities, there was not a major impact on the daily lives of the vast majority of Americans or American cities.

Disasters are temporal. They have a beginning and an end. Most natural disasters are typically measured in days commencing with the start of the event and concluding with the completion of recovery. Hurricanes, for example, have predictable paths and are more easily forecast—their damage, timing of travel, and estimated duration are well documented. Human-initiated terrorist attacks, in contrast, have a very short *lifetime* and are quantified in terms of the precipitating event.

THE DEVELOPMENT OF RESPONSE PLANS

A common sequence of events surrounding a disaster can be seen in recent large-scale disasters ranging from the September 11, 2001, terrorist attacks; Hurricane Katrina; the 2004 tsunami in Phuket, Thailand; and the 2007 shootings at Virginia Polytechnic Institute and State University. Three distinct phases have been identified. Disaster response planners utilize these phases, which are the basis for any successful disaster preparedness plan, to determine the timing and nature of response actions. Phase I is the preparedness/readiness phase. Activities in this phase involve the identification of resources, the identification of training requirements, and the practicing and evaluation of plan effectiveness. Phase II is the actual response to a disaster. This is when the plans are put into effect. Phase III is the process of recovery and implementation evaluation. Recovery includes not only physical activities, such as rebuilding homes, but also emotional and physical recovery for all who have been affected. Phase III is often longer than initially anticipated.

When a disaster strikes, by definition it is likely to compromise a regional area (Gaynard, 2009). Because a disaster will indiscriminately affect all individuals and services within the region, it is likely to take time for agencies and rescue workers to organize, mobilize, and arrive in the region to begin their work. Depending on the nature and scope of the event, rescuers and emergency management systems may be initially overwhelmed. Disaster communication may be compromised, and road, rail, and air transportation may be limited or curtailed. Thus, immediately following the event, victims within the affected areas typically are on their own. This period of required self-sufficiency can be an hour or two or may be measured in terms of days. Ice storms during the winter of 2008–2009 left many in the mid-South without power for several weeks, and downed trees and power lines made immediate access to many areas impossible for rescue and recovery services.

It can be frustrating for victims, but rescuers and responders are limited in the services they can provide. Power companies moving in after an ice storm will work first to restore power to public health and safety entities: emergency management offices, hospitals, nursing homes, and so forth. Individual homes will be addressed later. Police officers will not be able to stay and guard individual properties. Fire personnel may need to let a building burn if water is not available or if other property is more critical. No one likes to make such decisions. In a disaster, there will not be enough resources initially to go around. The media may be the most reliable source of information while federal, state, and local officials are busy getting organized. Individuals should have a reliable source of medical access that is independent of direct power access.

The development of age-specific disaster response plans must recognize not only the large numbers of older persons but also their complex needs. By 2030, approximately 20% of the American population will be aged 65 or older. This almost doubling of the over-65 population represents the fastest growth for any segment of the population. Furthermore, this population is highly susceptible to chronic disease. Almost 50% of older adults have at least one chronic medical or physical condition (Federal Interagency Forum on Aging-Related Statistics, 2008). These conditions often affect their ability, even in the best of circumstances, to perform routine daily activities. Due to limited physical capacity; mental limitations; and reductions in vision, hearing, and balance in older adults, compounded by limited social support systems and income, many will not be able to prepare adequately for emergencies even when they have received assistance through gathering needed supplies.

Research related to natural disasters, most recently post-Hurricane Katrina research, suggests that older persons with chronic illness have a higher probability of hospitalization immediately following disasters—29.2% for those with chronic disease and related conditions compared to 10.9% for those without (Sharma, et al., 2008). The good news is that the recovery process for this population tends to follow a course consistent with the general population. For example, chronic disease at 18 months post incident was not a statistical risk factor for either impaired health-related quality of life or mental health problems (den Ouden, et al., 2007). Of more importance in predicting mental health sequelae was the development of PTSD due to life disruptions including relocation, as well as the complexity of predisaster chronic health issues (Mori, et al., 2007).

The development of state or local plans for providing rescue and recovery services for older persons should include appropriate triaging systems. Dyer, Regev, Burnett, Festa, and Cloyd (2008) developed and validated the SWiFT (Seniors Without Families Triage) program while caring for displaced older persons from Hurricane Katrina entering shelters. This one-page system quickly triages individuals into one of three groups:

- SWiFT 1 are those who are unable to perform daily activities and need immediate placement where direct care can be provided—nursing homes, care homes, or assisted living locations.
- SWiFT 2 are those individuals who need assistance in accessing benefits or in fund management and who can be linked to appropriate services.
- SWiFT 3 are individuals who simply need to be connected to families or who have issues easily addressed by volunteer agencies.

The SWiFT form quickly assembles information on physical and mental health issues and status and information on case management needs.

Working with the AMA, the SWiFT team also evaluated the effectiveness of the response in relation to the services provided to older persons. Their recommendations for best practices in the management of older disaster victims were derived from their experiences in dealing with over 10,000 cases and include designating separate shelter areas for older persons, using a triage system like the SWiFT, and protecting older persons from abuse and fraud (Baylor College of Medicine and the American Medical Association, n.d.).

Research related to large-scale man-made disasters in the United States is limited to events surrounding the September 11, 2001, combined terrorist attacks on the Twin Towers. These events did not result in large-scale population evacuation or large disruption in living spaces. However, they did result in changes in employment and movement within the affected areas. But these impacts were largely limited to the New York City area. Similarly, the airplane collision into the Pentagon did not affect residential areas, and the impact in Pennsylvania occurred in a largely rural area. This research suggests that for this type of event, adults of all ages are largely resilient, with low evidence of PTSD or low evidence of increase in substance abuse. Resilience was found to be related to complex interactions of sex, age, race, level of education, degree of exposure to the trauma, income and subsequent change in income, social support, chronic disease presence, and recent and past life stressors (Bonanno, Galea, Bucciarelli, & Vlahov, 2007). This complexity of mitigating variables makes it very difficult to develop targeted preparedness plans.

Even in high-risk natural disaster areas, there remains insufficient planning for dealing with older persons (Dosa, Grossman, Wetle, & Mor, 2007; Lach, Langan, & James, 2005). There is a lack of preparedness in identifying vulnerable individuals, noting specific anticipated needs and mobility issues, providing for the protection of important medical and personal property records, providing for tracking individuals who may be required to move to alternative locations, and coordinating disaster planning and response across community and regional agencies (Mangum, Kosberg, & McDonald, 1989; Reed, 1998). A study of the evacuation plans of 213 nursing homes, for example, found that only 31% had specified evacuation routes (Castle, 2008).

Adequate planning for evacuation also requires consideration for provision, transportation, reinstallation, and use of any specialized equipment. A post-Katrina study conducted in the New Orleans region identified 24,938 community-dwelling older persons who would require assistance to evacuate as well as shelter in sites that could accommodate special equipment such as wheelchairs, oxygen units, and other specialized health equipment (McGuire, Ford, & Okoro, 2007).

The U.S. Centers for Disease Control and Prevention's (CDC) January 2008 bulletin reported their review of the best recommendations for communities to consider in preparing for disasters. The report placed specific emphasis on addressing the needs of vulnerable older Americans and those with chronic disease (Aldrich & Benson, 2008). The first and most obvious CDC recommendation was to develop strong formal relationships between various agencies, including public health, aging, and first responders. A strategy for fulfilling this recommendation remains elusive.

Two other important recommendations made by the CDC were to develop backup communication systems and to provide storage for redundant medical and personal information. This includes the storage of medical and personal information at locations other than in the immediate region.

To enhance response rates, the use of geographic information systems (GIS) and other mapping systems can provide first responders with invaluable information on the location of individuals likely to need assistance and less likely to be self-sufficient. Comprehensive GIS systems can link responders to data banks that contain relevant patient medical information such as the need for oxygen concentrators, wheelchairs, and other devices, which will allow them to arrive with appropriate equipment.

The development of alternative shelter locations should include design alternatives including accessible locations for older persons and those with special needs. To get older persons to the shelters, there must be planning for the transportation of critical medical equipment and locating and securing medications and medical supplies. It is critically important that pharmacological services are included in plan development as it is likely evacuees will not have direct access to full medical and prescription drug histories without a GIS system.

Many older individuals have either working or nominal companion animals that require simultaneous transportation and subsequent sheltering. Shelters typically do not provide for the inclusion of household pets, which are housed at separate nearby facilities. Federal guidelines require that owners provide cages, food, and water for their pets. This may present an obstacle for older persons since not all older individuals have separate animal cages for their pets. The evacuation of animals is an issue that can be distressing for older persons and has caused some to refuse evacuation (ESAR-VHP, 2007).

Older persons often have sensory deficits, such as impaired eyesight or hearing, and require that all information on emergency preparedness be presented in a variety of appropriate formats. As previously noted, many older individuals do not have direct access to or facility with the Internet, so information must be provided in written and other forms that can be readily accessed and used. The statement "Go to our Web site" will not suffice for many older individuals.

During the immediate response to a regional disaster, law enforcement will establish control perimeters to assure that recovery can occur and that individuals other than first responders are not put at unnecessary risk. Many professional health care and senior service workers do not necessarily have universally recognized identification cards. It is important to establish a secure system of photo identification and permits to ensure access to homebound clients by health care and senior service workers when an emergency occurs.

Related to this is the often-contentious issue of requiring personal identification cards for individuals. The rapid identification of individuals with specific health care requirements ensures these individuals are quickly and appropriately provided care and services. *Smart cards*—electronic medical records stored on cards similar to credit cards—can also be used to provide a repository of critical medical information that may not be otherwise available.

Caregivers who must go into disaster areas or shelters to provide care must be provided relief as well as reliable communication systems to allow them to be in contact with physicians, pharmacists, and other health specialists. There are formal volunteer groups that can be accessed through the U.S. Freedom Corps, including the health-specific Medical Reserve Corps. It is also important to tap local volunteers who may be willing to assist health care providers in an emergency.

There are no consistent national or state emergency preparedness plans that detail how to provide services to older persons. Most plans provide general advice and direction. This is likely due to the understanding that in a large-scale emergency response, much of the recovery will rely on the self-sufficiency of individuals. It is incumbent on each individual and family to be proactive in the planning stage (Scherr, 1996; Torgusen & Kosberg, 2006). Specific recommendations for assisting older persons who are not living in the immediate vicinity of family have been prepared by the AARP (2006).

It is this level of familial, proactive planning that best individualizes preparedness. While more global, community-based responses with organized structure are essential, a family and/or individual can inform a more personally nuanced plan of action in event of a disaster. It is this relational context that often provides the impetus for individuals to engage and cooperate with a disaster mental health response protocol. At the core of effective and organized service delivery is personalized coordination that incorporates an individual's mental health and his or her ability to trust and follow the guidance of disaster responders.

SERVICE COORDINATION, MENTAL HEALTH, AND THERAPEUTIC RAPPORT

Prior mental health history is another significant risk factor that must be addressed by the disaster mental health service provider. A significant predisaster mental health history may not only be a poor prognostic indicator relative to a person's clinical response to disaster, but it may also interact with conditions and circumstances that may impede effective planning. For example, a SWiFT 1–assessed individual with a prior trauma history and a diagnosis of paranoid schizophrenia would present a very unique challenge to a relocation demand induced by an event. The latter would likely require a very nuanced intervention. Historically depressed individuals whose symptoms are exacerbated by disaster may be resistant to engage in anything that promotes recovery or even safety due to maladaptive thoughts that nothing will help. Underscoring each of these examples is a basic premise that standard recovery efforts may need to be individualized for the mental health population. In addition, developing a trusting rapport with a recovery worker also can be a significant facilitative factor in improving the chances the recovery services offered are received and utilized by this population.

Even without prior history or diagnosis, many psychological variables play an influential role in whether or not a system's response to a person's needs is helpful. For example, a perception of racism or unjust delivery of services during a disaster can decrease the likelihood of a person's engagement of those services provided. If the government or disaster response agency is perceived as not doing the right thing or not having an individual's best interest in mind, people are unlikely to follow its suggestions. This frame of thinking, unfortunately, was prominent within the African American population when Hurricane Katrina struck New Orleans. Weems, et al. (2007), while not finding any significant relationship between degree of perceived racism and expressed symptoms as measured by the Brief Symptom Inventory, report finding a negative relationship between perceived level of social support and symptomatology. Perceived racism would likely disrupt a person's sense of social connectedness and likely have deleterious effects on his or her recovery over a longer period of time.

A strategy that mitigates the risk posed by past or current psychological issues, and that likely facilitates recovery across a broad range of other services, is the establishment of working relationships with survivors. In fact, one might say it is paramount to synergize most, if not all, recovery efforts. Whether buffering the effects of perceived racism, providing hope and interpersonal connection, or taking the edge off a person with a paranoid disposition, engagement in recovery-oriented behavior is embedded in an interpersonal context. While treatment options for the mentally ill are discussed in chapter 10, they are mentioned here due to their potential effect on basic operational engagement to promote basic safety. The dissemination of accurate information, for example, is a critical component of disaster management under any circumstance; it is rendered ineffective by an individual who rejects it. The acceptance of information implies trust, and strong interpersonal connections at many levels are instrumental in this process.

Given this context, the preparation of disaster responders in the areas of mental health, and in particular geriatric mental health, is critical. This training should not only emphasize specific techniques of psychological first aid and supportive communication at the level of individual intervention, but it should also reflect the larger context within which disaster mental health unfolds. A representative example of such a training model was initiated and carried out in New York State via a joint effort of the respective departments of mental health (NYSOMH) and health (NYSDOH) in conjunction with the University of Rochester's Disaster Mental Health Program. The *Disaster Mental Health: A Critical Response* (University of Rochester, 2005) curriculum is a train-the-trainer initiative that incorporated the big picture scope of disaster along with more nuanced training in specific, individualized intervention strategies to promote recovery from disaster. This model first covered the macroscopic aspects of disaster—including the definition of disaster, classification of subtypes of disaster, and planning and response phases of disaster planning—before focusing on typical and atypical human responses to disaster and disaster management. While comprehensive, the curriculum was not overly technical, allowing the information to be disseminated by instructors who received 3 days of intensive training in the material and manual. These trained instructors were expected to reach across the state and re-perform 2 days of training for those deemed disaster mental health responders in the event of significant disaster and deployment. This model has the distinct advantage of including a detailed registry, periodically updated to ensure adequate responder resources.

As this training model highlights, there is a need for disaster mental health responders who are aware of and know how to utilize and participate in large-scale, systemic responses to disaster. While this macroscopic viewpoint is critical, it is also essential to acknowledge that individual nuance, family and cultural background, previous mental health history, and prior disaster exposure or experience will all color an individual's response to disaster, as well as their response to intervention efforts. This highlights the critical and instrumental nature of the helping relationship/process, the bedrock of all successful disaster mental health response.

REFERENCES

AARP. (2006). *Emergency preparedness, develop a disaster plan for older, distant relatives.* Retrieved July 7, 2009, from http://www.aarp.org/family/housing/articles/preparing_for_emergencies.html

Aldrich, N., & Benson, W. F. (2008). Disaster preparedness and the chronic disease needs of vulnerable older adults. *Preventing Chronic Disease, 5, A27.*

Baylor College of Medicine and the American Medical Association. (n.d.). *Recommendations for best practices in the management of elderly disaster victims.* Retrieved September 2, 2009, from http://www.bcm.edu/pdf/bestpractices.pdf

Bonanno, G. A., Galea, S., Bucciarelli, A., & Vlahov, D. (2007). What predicts psychological resilience after disaster? The role of demographics, resources, and life stress. *Journal of Consulting and Clinical Psychology, 75*(5), 671–682.

Castle, N. G. (2008). Nursing home evacuation plans. *American Journal of Public Health, 98,* 1235–1240.

Cherniack, E. P., Sandals, L., Brook, L., & Mintzc, M. J. (2008) Trial of a survey instrument to establish the hurricane preparedness of and medical impact on a vulnerable, older population. *Prehospital Disaster Medicine, 23,* 242–249.

County of Santa Clara (CA) Office of Emergency Services. (2009). *Tips for preparedness for the senior population.* Retrieved July 9, 2009, from http://www.sccgov.org/portal/site/oes/agencyarticle?path=%2Fv7%2FEmergency%20Services%2C%20Office%20of%20(DEP)%2FPeople%20with%20Special%20Needs&contentId=accc38c39eb74010VgnVCMP230004adc4a92

den Ouden, D. J., van der Velden, P. G., Grievink, L., Morren, M., Dirkzwager, A. J., & Yzerrnans, O. (2007). Use of mental health services among disaster survivors: Predisposing factors. *BMC Public Health, 7,* 173.

Dorn, B. C., Savoia, E., Testa, M. A., Stoto, M. A., & Marcus, U. (2007). Development of a survey instrument to measure connectivity to evaluate national public health preparedness and response performance. *Public Health Reports, 122,* 329–338.

Dosa, D. M., Grossman, N., Wetle, T., & Mor, V. (2007). To evacuate or not to evacuate: Lessons learned from Louisiana nursing home administrators following hurricanes Katrina and Rita. *Journal of the American Medical Directors Association, 8,* 142–149.

Dyer, D. B., Regev, M., Burnett, J., Festa, N., & Cloyd, B. (2008). SWiFT: A rapid triage tool for vulnerable older adults in disaster situations. *Disaster Medicine and Public Health Preparedness, 2,* 545–550.

Federal Interagency Forum on Aging-Related Statistics. (2008). *Older Americans 2008: Key indicators of well being.* Washington, DC: U.S. Government Printing Office.

Fernandez, L.S., Byard, D., Un, C. C., Benson, S., & Barbera, J. A. (2002). Frail elderly as disaster victims: Emergency management strategies. *Prehospital Disaster Medicine, 17,* 67–74.

Ford, E. S., Mokdad, A. H., & Unk, M. W. (2006). Chronic disease in health emergencies: In the eye of the hurricane. *Preventing Chronic Disease, 3,* A46.

Gaynard, S. T. (2009, May 18). All disasters are local. *New York Times,* p. A23.

Hodge, J. G., & Anderson, E. D. (2008). Principles and practice of legal triage during public health emergencies. *NYU Annual Survey of Law, 64,* 249–292.

Hurricane Katrina Community Advisory Group, & Kessler, R. C. (2007). Hurricane Katrina's impact on the care of survivors with chronic medical conditions. *Journal of General Internal Medicine, 22,* 1225–1230.

Kaiser Family Foundation. (2005, January). *Health and the elderly: How seniors use the Internet for health information.* Menlo Park, CA: Author.

Lach, H. W., Langan, J. C., & James, D. C. (2005) Disaster planning: Are gerontological nurses prepared? *Journal of Gerontological Nursing, 31,* 21–27.

Laditka, S. B., Laditka, I. N., Cornman, C. B., Davis, C. B., & Chandlee, M. J. (2008). Disaster preparedness for vulnerable persons receiving in-home, long-term care in South Carolina. *Prehospital Disaster Medicine, 23,* 133–142.

Laditka, S. B., Laditka, I. N., Xirasagar, S., Cornman, C. B., Davis, C. B., & Richter, J.V. (2008). Providing shelter to nursing home evacuees in disasters: Lessons from Hurricane Katrina. *American Journal of Public Health, 98,* 288–293.

Lamb, K. V., O'Brien, C., & Fenza, P. J. (2008). Elders at risk during disasters. *Home Health Nurse, 26,* 30–38.

Mangum, W. P., Kosberg, J. I., & McDonald, P. (1989). Hurricane Elena and Pinellas county, Florida: Some lessons learned from the largest evacuation of nursing home patients in history. *Gerontologist, 29,* 388–392.

McGuire, L. C., Ford, E. S., & Okoro, C. A. (2007). Natural disasters and older U.S. adults with disabilities: Implications for evacuation. *Disasters, 31*(1), 49–56.

Mori K., Ugai, K., Nonami, Y., Kirimura, T., Kondo, C., Nakamura, T., et al. (2007). Health needs of patients with chronic diseases who lived through the great Hanshin earthquake. *Disaster Management and Response, 5,* 8–13.

Rami, J., Singleton, E. K., Spurlock, W., & Eaglin, A. R. (2008). A school of nursing's experience with providing health care for hurricane Katrina evacuees. *Association of Black Nursing Faculty in Higher Education Journal, 19,* 102–106.

Reed, M. K. (1998). Disaster preparedness pays off. *Journal of Nursing Administration, 28,* 25–31.

Ridenour, M., Cummings, K. J., Sinclair, J. R., & Bixler, D. (2007). Displacement of the underserved: Medical needs of Hurricane Katrina evacuees in West Virginia. *Journal of Health Care for the Poor and Underserved, 18,* 369–381.

Rosenkoetter, M. M., Covan, E. K., Bunting, E., Cobb, B. K., & Fugate-Whitlock, E. (2007a). Disaster evacuation: An exploratory study of older men and women in Georgia and North Carolina. *Journal of Gerontological Nursing, 33,* 46–54.

Rosenkoetter, M. M., Covan, E. K., Cobb, B. K., Bunting, S., & Weinrlch, M. (2007b). Perceptions of older adults regarding evacuation in the event of a natural disaster. *Public Health Nursing, 24,* 160–168.

Rosenthal, M. S., Klein, K., Cowling, K., Grzybowski, M., & Dunne, R. (2005). Disaster modeling: Medication resources required for disaster team response. *Prehospital Disaster Medicine, 20,* 309–315.

Scherr, S. (1996). Residential living: Preparing your assisted living facility for a disaster. *Provider, 21*(4), 35–36.

Sharma, A. J., Weiss, E. C., Young, S. L., Stephens, K., Ratard, R., Straif-Bourgeois, S., et al. (2008). Chronic disease and related conditions at emergency treatment facilities in the New Orleans area after Hurricane Katrina [Electronic version]. *Disaster Medicine and Public Health Preparedness, 2*(1), 27–32.

Torgusen, B. L., & Kosberg, J. I. (2006). Assisting older victims of disasters: Roles and responsibilities for social workers. *Journal of Gerontological Social Work, 47,* 27–44.

University of Rochester. (2005). *Disaster mental health: A critical response.* Rochester, NY: University of Rochester. Retrieved August 30, 2009, from http://www.omh.state.ny.us/omhweb/countyguide/

U.S. Department of Health and Human Services. (2007). *Emergency Systems for Advance Registration of Volunteer Health Professionals (ESAR-VHP) Program.* Washington, DC: U.S. Department of Health and Human Services.

Weems, C., Watts, S. E., Marsee, M. A., Taylor, L. K., Costa, N. M., & Cannon, M. F. (2007). The psychosocial impact of Hurricane Katrina: Contextual differences in psychological symptoms, social support and discrimination. *Behavior Research and Therapy, 45,* 2295–2306.

5

National and Cross-National Models of Geriatric Disaster Preparedness: The Canadian Context

TRISH DRYDEN AND LYNDA ATACK

Concerns have emerged worldwide about the heightened vulnerability of older persons in natural and man-made disasters (HelpAge International, 2006). The Canadian Disaster Database (Public Safety Canada, 2007), maintained online by Public Safety Canada, lists detailed information on over 700 natural, technological, and conflict events that have directly affected Canadians over the past century. Relatively recent disasters such as a Quebec ice storm, which caused power outages for more than 30 days in some areas; floods in Manitoba and Quebec; and a firestorm in British Columbia highlight the risks older persons encounter in emergency situations (Plouffe, 2008).

In this chapter, we draw on Statistics Canada data to provide a snapshot of the current older adult population in Canada, review the impact of three disasters on older Canadians, and describe governmental, community-based, and academic initiatives under way in Canada. This broad perspective reflects a combination of literature review and the results of key informant interviews conducted with emergency preparedness coordinators, academics, consultants, and policy analysts in aging and disaster management as we prepared the chapter (see Chapter Acknowledgments for the names of these informants). These experts provided important observations on planning and disaster management, education, research, and knowledge exchange that have informed our analysis and discussion of the issues.

A SNAPSHOT OF OLDER CANADIANS

Statistics Canada recently published *A Portrait of Seniors in Canada* (Turcotte & Schellenberg, 2007). This report characterizes the current generation of older Canadian citizens and provides relevant demographic data about the vulnerability and resilience of older persons in emergency situations.

There are differences among the 10 provinces and 3 territories within Canada with respect to the proportion of the population comprised of older persons (aged 65 and older). For example, the population of older persons is 14.8% in Saskatchewan, 12.8% in Ontario, and 2.6% in Nunavut. Similar to the geographic distribution of all age groups, the older adult population in Canada is increasingly urban. In 2001, 7 out of every 10 older people lived in urban centers with at least 50,000 residents. Almost one-third of Canadians over age 65 live in the largest Canadian cities: Toronto, Vancouver, or Montreal.

The majority of older persons (93%) live in their own homes. Older women are much more likely to live alone than older men, reflecting differences in life expectancy. Among Canadians aged 85 and older, 34% live alone. Only 7% live in collective dwellings, primarily nursing homes and hospitals. The likelihood of institutional residency increases with age, from 2% among those 65 to 74 years of age to 32% among those 85 years of age or older.

The majority of older people are able to carry out daily activities on their own until at least age 75. In 2003, 1 in 10 persons aged 75 or older and living in a private household needed some level of assistance with personal care and one-quarter needed assistance with housework. For those with long-term health problems, a combination of informal and formal support is common. In 2005, 85% of people under age 75 and 60% of those 75 and older reported they had a valid driver's license. Eighty-nine percent of those under age 75 and 73% of those aged 75 and older reported they or someone in their household leased or owned a vehicle. In 2003, more than 80% of older persons were considered to have prose literacy skills below the desired threshold for coping well in a complex knowledge society.

In general, older Canadians have vibrant social networks. They are more likely than younger individuals to report not having close friends or other friends but slightly more likely to report knowing their neighbors and having many immediate family members to whom they feel close. Older people under age 75 are more likely to report having provided help in the past month than having received help from others. Self-reported psychological distress declines as people age while self-reported well-being increases for older persons up to age 75. Declines in self-reported psychological distress and self-reported well-being continue in those aged 75 and older. A sense of mastery—the level of control a person feels they have over their life—declines with age.

Falls are a leading cause of injury for older persons. In 2000–2001, 53% of injurious falls in older people were the result of slipping, tripping, or stumbling on a non-icy surface. Age-related physiological changes do not necessarily result in disease, but many older people have at least one chronic condition. The prevalence of chronic conditions increases with age for older persons. Overall, arthritis or rheumatism is the most frequently reported chronic condition in those aged 65 and older (47%), followed by high blood pressure (42.8 %). Cataracts are also common (20.7%). Compared to younger adults, older persons have a lower prevalence of mood disorders (4.2 %) and anxiety disorders (2.9%) but a higher prevalence of dementia (2%). Cancer and heart disease are the main causes of death for older persons. In 2003, the life expectancy for a Canadian at birth was about 80 years. Mortality rates are declining for all but the oldest age group (90 years and older). For example, in 2002, for every 1,000 people aged 80–84, 64.8 persons died.

This demographic snapshot helps explain why older persons may be vulnerable in emergency situations. The developmental changes that accompany aging and the associated health problems may result in a reduced ability to prepare for, manage, and recover from disasters.

CANADIAN DISASTER RESEARCH

While Canadian disasters cannot compare with recent global disasters in terms of lives lost or economic impact, losses in just over the past 10 years have been significant. Three major disasters took place in Canada in the space of 3 years (1996 to 1998): the Red River Manitoba floods, the Quebec ice storm, and the Saguenay-Lac St. Jean floods. Key observations regarding older persons, including observations that pertain to mental health issues, have been extrapolated from research studies on these events, as well as from a major study on emergency response capacity conducted by the Canadian Red Cross. We have chosen to highlight these studies given their explicit inclusion of older persons as a population of interest rather than conduct a comprehensive review of all disaster-related literature on Canadian situations. That said, it should be noted that the Canadian disaster literature regarding older persons is relatively sparse overall.

Red River Manitoba Floods

In 1997, the Red River in Manitoba, a province in Canada, flooded, resulting in the evacuation of 28,000 people and $500 million in damage to property and infrastructure (Etkin, Haque, & Brooks, 2003). Buckland and Rahman (1999) conducted a study to examine the relationship between community preparedness for the disaster and the level and pattern of community development in three rural communities. Research was conducted through key informant interviews that included elderly residents, focus groups with emergency personnel, and a household survey. The communities differed significantly in their ethnicity and level of community development, and results indicate the level of community development did indeed have an impact on the communities' response to disaster. One community of First Nations' peoples was particularly affected. First Nations' communities are under federal jurisdiction in Canada, whereas the central disaster planning agency is a provincial responsibility, which complicates disaster preparation and management. Researchers suggested this community's long-standing social isolation and the weak relationship between the community and different government levels meant there were fewer resources for managing disaster response and a less robust population, from a public health perspective, to manage disaster recovery. The two communities described as having stronger social capital had the resources to better manage the disaster.

Study participants agreed that the mandatory government evacuation order, which applied to the young, elderly, and disabled, was necessary; however, they raised concerns about the process by which the order was communicated and implemented. Buckland and Rahman (1999) concluded their study by emphasizing the critical need for close connections and more respectful and open communication between communities and government.

Communication problems were also identified in Lindsay and Hall's (2007) report on older persons and the Red River flood. These authors noted that 75 news releases and 41 public service announcements were distributed in relation to the disaster; however, none of these messages were directed to older persons or other high-risk populations. The province developed a lengthy list of recommendations for change in the wake of the floods; however, notably absent were any recommendations that the public, including high-risk groups such as older persons, be included in disaster planning. Lindsay and Hall (2007) also reported results from the *Aging in Manitoba (AIM) Study,* a longitudinal study of Manitoba older persons. By chance, older persons had been surveyed 10 months before the flood; they were contacted again after the disaster to collect post-event comparison data regarding their physical, cognitive, and mental health. The majority of the older flood victims reported the same level of physical functioning pre- and post-flood.

The findings on mental health are informative—the flood had a notable impact. Stress levels for evacuated individuals were higher 10 months after the disaster than for those who did not experience the flood. Results were not all negative; some older persons who had been evacuated showed gains in terms of cognitive status and self-rated health. The authors suggest that successfully coping with a disaster later in life may provide some protection, perhaps temporary, against cognitive decline and contribute to a perception of better overall health in older persons.

Quebec Ice Storm

In 1998, a major ice storm struck central Canada (Quebec and Ontario) and the Maritime provinces, causing massive power blackouts lasting from a few days to nearly a month. Because it was winter, the loss of power had a major impact and affected 67% of Quebecers (Maltais, 2006). Thirty deaths were attributed to the disaster, and persons 65 and older made up half of those who died. Deaths in the early days of the storm—from burns, carbon monoxide poisoning, and hypothermia—were largely preventable. Death from respiratory disease also rose in the older population from the improper use of generators, stoves, and faulty heating devices.

Local community organizations had not been included in provincial emergency response plans and had to cope as best they could. As a result, organization at some relief centers was poor, particularly for older persons, as the centers struggled to cope in the early days of the disaster. A lack of communication and planning between the municipalities and local health agencies resulted in overcrowded shelters with inadequate sanitation. Some older persons reported having to sleep on the floor and experiencing disturbed sleep by noise from those around them.

Maltais, Robichaud, and Simard (2001) conducted a study with older persons, the majority (61%) of whom remained in their homes during the ice storm. These older persons advocated that more practical support and safety information should be made available by radio for those who choose to stay at home. More outreach to older persons was also recommended. Neighborhood patrols by police and door-to-door checks by relief personnel made older persons feel safer and provided hands-on assistance with heavy jobs. Some older persons noted that they continued to receive their regular home health care; however, many older persons who lived alone or had health problems but who were not known to relief organizations were overlooked.

Improved coordination between municipalities, community groups, public health departments, and social service organizations; reliable, up-to-date record keeping on high-risk individuals; and better communication with victims were among the authors' recommendations (Maltais, et al., 2001).

The focus on mental health issues in this study was directed to resilience more than vulnerability. Older persons identified a number of supports that helped them during the disaster. Older persons who worked as volunteers reported it was a beneficial experience for themselves as well as others. They believed they had been useful and that the work had kept them busy throughout the stressful time. Psychological support, a patient attitude, and compassion from health and allied workers were also viewed as having made an important difference.

Flooding in Quebec Saguenay Region

In July 1996, major flooding took place in Saguenay-Lac St. Jean, a part of Quebec. No lives were lost; however, 2,000 elderly were evacuated from their homes, 426 homes were destroyed, and more than 2,000 homes were damaged (Maltais & Lachance, 2007).

Mental health issues related to this disaster have been explicitly studied by Maltais and colleagues. Lalande, Maltais, and Robichaud (2000) conducted research using a case study approach to describe the experiences of the disaster on flood victims' psychological health. Participants included 15 men and 15 women between 33 and 74 years of age. Of the 30 participants, 19 lost their homes completely or suffered major damage to their home. All those interviewed reported that the floods had disrupted their lives greatly and that they had experienced emotional difficulties. They described periods of overwhelming fatigue and a sense of isolation as they embarked on major cleanup and renovations. The majority reported new health problems or the exacerbation of existing problems. The authors recommended that the consequences of disasters be studied in a holistic, comprehensive manner, bringing together researchers and health, mental health, social service, and community organizations.

Maltais and Lachance (2007) reported the results of several longitudinal studies conducted in the years following the Saguenay-Lac St. Jean floods. Data were collected using questionnaires and interviews with flood victims and nonvictims. Two years after the floods, there were significant differences in the physical and psychological health of victims when compared with nonvictims. Eight years after the disaster, psychological differences persisted; however, the overall physical health of victims had improved. Interestingly, older persons reported some positive outcomes of the disaster. Some reported changes in their values and perspectives—for example, becoming less materialistic and recognizing the importance of life, family, and friends. Perceptions of support received during the disaster were also reported. However, some older persons thought the amount of help received was inadequate, particularly from family members. This contributed to their anxiety; they feared help would not be sufficient in the event of another disaster. The authors note that in the future, relief agencies would do well to clarify the degree and type of support that could realistically be provided from various sources.

CANADIAN RED CROSS STUDY

The Canadian Emergency Management and High-Risk Populations Study was conducted in 2007 by the Canadian Red Cross (Enarson & Walsh, 2007) to examine existing relationships and activities between voluntary and emergency management organizations with respect to the needs and capacities of high-risk populations. Online surveys were conducted with 48 federal, provincial, and territorial organizations and 89 volunteer organizations that service high-risk populations, including older persons, to promote disaster planning. Respondents were asked to comment on the current and intended service provided to these populations. The results were encouraging in part: approximately two-thirds of respondents indicated they address older persons' concerns in their activities. Sixty-seven percent of the emergency response organizations indicated they routinely conduct outreach activities with older persons. However, more grassroots organizations were less likely to have the resources to maximize emergency management planning and service to older persons and other high-risk groups. Forty-three percent of respondents from local organizations stated half of their job relates directly to emergency management. That finding contrasted considerably with the 73% of provincial level respondents who reported that 90% or more of their job relates directly to emergency management activities. Ninety percent of federal respondents indicated greater than 90% of their duties relate directly to emergency management. While many best practices are under way, major gaps are present in meeting the needs of high-risk populations. While local emergency and voluntary organizations aim to meet the needs of these groups, they often do not have the necessary connections to other groups or resources. The report also emphasized the importance of relationship building between emergency management and voluntary organizations, connecting with local organizations that know their high-risk groups best. The authors proposed that while work is needed at all levels, the federal or highest level of government should "provide a cross-cutting and integrated framework at the national level and ensure that emergency management systems are accountable to those least able to help themselves" (Enarson & Walsh, p. 43).

The results of research on these three relatively recent Canadian disasters as well as the Canadian Red Cross study on vulnerable populations concur in the identification of several major themes. The coordination of planning and relief and improved communication consistently present as key issues. Resource gaps are a crosscutting issue. The mental health implications of disasters are significant for older persons and may manifest in a variety of ways over time. Older persons demonstrate both vulnerability and resilience in response to disasters, and it is clear that the gaps in coordination and resources extend to the mental health arena.

GOVERNMENT INITIATIVES

Consistent with the aforementioned findings, authors of a recent governmental review identified an urgent need for increased focus on emergency management and disaster preparedness in Canada (Standing Committee on National Security and Defense, 2008). Despite the very real need for more attention to the issues of emergency and disaster preparedness at municipal, provincial, and federal levels in Canada, it is important to recognize the groundwork that has already been laid with respect to older persons. There is a growing legacy of leadership on this issue by the Public Health Agency of Canada (Public Health Agency of Canada [PHAC], February 2008, March 2008), which began at the Presidential Symposium on the 2004 Tsunami and Older People convened by Simon Fraser University professor Gloria Gutman, outgoing president of the International Association of Gerontology and Geriatrics at the June 2005 International Association of Gerontology and Geriatrics (IAGG) World Congress. The symposium confirmed that few programs developed by humanitarian agencies are designed to specifically target older persons. Subsequent to the IAGG congress, PHAC hosted two international meetings, including one for participants attending the White House Conference on Aging in December 2005, which resulted in a commitment to collaborate internationally. A working meeting of disaster and emergency experts held in Toronto in February 2006 identified the need for an international workshop.

In 2007, the government of Canada and the government of Manitoba, in collaboration with the World Health Organization (WHO), hosted the International Workshop on Seniors and Emergency Preparedness in Winnipeg, Manitoba, Canada. A synthesis of research on recent Canadian disasters was among the resources commissioned for this event (Gutman, 2007). This workshop brought together over 100 experts from around the world to identify priorities to better address older persons' needs and utilize older persons' capacities as a component of emergency management. The report on this event, *Building a Global Framework to Address the Needs and Contributions of Older People in Emergencies,* was presented to the United Nations Commission for Social Development in February 2008 (PHAC, February 2008). Following the workshop, national and international steering committees and working groups were created to address key issues. The Second International Workshop on Seniors and Emergency Preparedness was held in Halifax, Nova Scotia, Canada, a year later in March 2008 (PHAC, March 2008) with the goals of sharing tools, information, and resources; identifying gaps; discussing effective communication strategies; strengthening networks/partnerships; and setting in motion activities for ongoing collaborative work.

The Division of Aging and Seniors (DAS) at PHAC serves as a central coordinating body for the three working groups that continue to collaborate on the development and dissemination of resources, promising practices, and guidelines as well as knowledge exchange, policy, and program development (P. Gorr, PHAC, personal communication, December

2008). PHAC has also brought key stakeholders together to raise awareness of the functional needs framework (D. Hutton, PHAC, personal communication, December 2008).

Collaboration among PHAC, Help the Aged (UK), and WHO has resulted in the development of a report based on case studies that examine the impact of 16 emergencies in developed and developing countries around the world, including 4 Canadian events (Plouffe, 2008). This report is a response to the call in the 2002 United Nations Madrid International Plan of Action on Ageing (MIPAA) for signatories (including Canada) to pay attention to the particular vulnerabilities and capacities of older persons in emergency situations (United Nations, 2002). This report positions the analysis and discussion of older persons and emergency management within the WHO Active Ageing policy framework (World Health Organization, 2002). PHAC was also instrumental in the development of a recent WHO report on policy issues relevant to older people in emergencies, *Older People in Emergencies: Considerations for Action and Policy Development* (Hutton, 2008).

Mental health issues for older persons have been acknowledged as an important aspect of disaster management initiatives in Canada. For example, the priorities for action that emerged from the first international conference on seniors and emergency preparedness in Winnipeg included "support qualitative and quantitative research on older persons' mental health needs in emergency situations that will lead to practical applications and guide interventions for health service and care providers and practitioners" (PHAC, February 2008, p. 20). The second international conference in Halifax included a concurrent session on gaps in emergency preparedness training for health professionals related to older persons and the frail elderly (PHAC, March 2008). One ongoing focus of the three PHAC-sponsored working groups has been advocacy for increased awareness of mental health issues through participation in national and international health care, aging, and disaster management conferences.

ACADEMIC INITIATIVES

There is increasing recognition in Canada, as elsewhere, that disaster management [DM] education plays a vital role in helping communities plan and recover from disaster. As Canada's baby boomers age and DM field professionals retire, there will be a pressing need for DM-trained professionals over the next decade. Unfortunately, students are not always welcome at clinical sites during a disaster as agencies struggle to respond. During the SARS outbreak in Ontario, health science students were removed from clinical placements. This sharply limits resource availability and students' ability to prepare for emergency situations, a key competency for future practice.

Falkiner (2003) surveyed 38 of Canada's largest universities and schools to determine if the necessary programs were in place to meet the anticipated DM education gap. Results indicated the distribution of courses was poor. Geography departments offered the majority of DM courses; however, most focused on the physical aspect of hazards. There were almost no courses that examined disaster planning, management, or mitigation. Falkiner concluded that DM representation in disciplines such as political science, psychology, and economics was very limited, a surprising finding given the broad social impact of disasters on individuals and communities. Falkiner recommended that these disciplines increase course offerings on DM by developing DM education modules that could be integrated into existing curricula. He also called for more research on courses in the natural science fields and graduate programs as a baseline for planning and curriculum development.

Cummings, Corte, and Cummings (2005) surveyed Canadian medical schools to determine the number of programs offering disaster medicine education before and after the events of September 11. The results were surprising: 22 programs were offered at nine sites before September 11 compared with 14 programs after, representing a 37% decrease. Eighty percent of survey respondents felt DM should be taught to undergraduates, and all respondents agreed DM should be core content in fellowship programs.

In Canada, DM education has traditionally been included in the Emergency Medicine and Public Health curriculae; the Royal College of Physicians and Surgeons of Canada does not require competency in DM. After September 11, the number of DM programs dropped from nine to three. One major online program in Alberta closed, and DM medical education shifted away from emergency medicine to infectious disease management with the outbreak of SARS. Cummings and colleagues (2005) concluded that Canada has a social obligation to prepare physicians for disaster management and that at least a basic program should be mandatory for undergraduates and fellows at all Canadian medical schools.

Bruce, Donovan, Hornof, and Barthos (2004) conducted a study to examine emergency/disaster management postsecondary courses and programs in Canada and generated recommendations for education and research. The situation had improved since the Falkiner (2003) study with the advent of several new programs including Brandon University's two 4-year baccalaureate applied disaster and emergency studies programs, which offer a disaster science concentration and a planning and management concentration. The results of the study by Bruce and colleagues (2004) indicated, however, that Canada still has an insufficient number of DM education programs to meet the country's needs. Two contributing factors are the lack of an established body of literature in emergency response management in Canada and the difficulty in finding educators with both the necessary field and academic preparation. The authors recommended Canada immediately take action to ensure sufficient resources will be in place to meet the education gap. They called for the establishment of a working group to determine Canada's particular needs and to develop education standards for emergency managers. They also recommended that the national research institutes recognize DM as a research program and designate funds for this emerging field. Educational programs and support are essential for the emerging discipline of DM.

Since the Bruce and colleagues (2004) report, there have been further encouraging developments in DM education. A continuum of programs is gradually being developed across the country to meet the needs of busy working professionals as well as students new to the field. Part-time certificate programs such as Centennial College's emergency management program, which is delivered executive-style over nine weekends, or Cape Breton University's postgraduate emergency management program, which is offered through distance education for those with an existing diploma or degree, make educational upgrading more accessible. Full-time baccalaureate and master's programs have recently been developed. Royal Roads University in western Canada now offers a 2-year interdisciplinary master of arts in disaster and emergency management and York University in central Canada offers a master of arts in disaster and emergency management.

The Red Cross report referenced earlier (Enarson & Walsh, 2007) highlights the training gap regarding the DM needs and capabilities of high-risk groups in Canada and the lack of emergency preparedness training in organizations that work with these groups. The authors recommended that a major review of training and postsecondary teaching materials be conducted to assess their sensitivity to high-risk population groups in Canada. They also argued for strengthening the social vulnerability perspective on disasters and emergency management policy and practice in educational programs across all disciplines.

In response to the DM education gap, which became apparent when health science students were excluded from clinical settings during the SARS outbreak in Canada, the Interprofessional Disaster/Emergency Preparedness Action Studies (IDEAS) Project Group was formed in 2006. The group consists of nine member hospitals of the Toronto Academic Health Science Network; five educational institutions; and municipal, provincial, and federal government policy representatives. Their objective was to develop, deliver, and evaluate an 8-week online program in disaster management and emergency preparedness combined with a live mass-casualty exercise that would promote interprofessional collaboration and team building among undergraduate students. The course can be integrated as an elective in numerous undergraduate programs. Students from medicine; nursing; medical, respirator, and radiation technology; paramedicine; pharmacy; law enforcement; and media are eligible to enroll. Embedded in the course are four multilayer games based on four disasters that affect progressively larger communities: Moscow Theatre hostage taking, Katrina, tsunami, and pandemic. The online modules include topics such as preparing for disasters, sharing information, directing information, sharing resources, skills inventory and simulation preparation, team cohesion, accountability, and systems analysis. The needs of the frail and elderly are addressed in the Hurricane Katrina module. Students also participate in a 1-day community mock-disaster simulation involving professionals from emergency response and health organizations. Students work with elderly community volunteers who act as family health unit patients on site during the simulation. The students also deliver telehealth visits to older persons in their homes as part of the mock disaster.

A study was conducted to examine changes in disaster management competency and interprofessional attitudes after students completed the course. Results indicated the students made significant gains in DM competencies and improved their attitudes toward interprofessional education and practice. The students also reported gaining insight and empathy into the experiences of patients and families who had participated in the mock disaster. The IDEAS network team has already made changes to the curriculum regarding high-risk groups for the next iteration of the course, which commenced in January 2009 with 400 students. Building on experiences with IDEAS, a workplace-based interprofessional DM course will be created in a compressed flexible format that could be delivered as in-service professional development or long-distance continuing education to providers currently in practice. The new program will include a geriatric curriculum thread to address the needs of the elderly in acute, chronic, and community health care.

COMMUNITY INITIATIVES: LESSONS LEARNED

Community resilience is the bedrock for emergency resilience (Hutton, 2001). Resiliency is defined in the *Emergency Management Framework for Canada* (Ministers Responsible for Emergency Management, 2007, p. 12) as "the capacity of a system, community or society potentially exposed to hazards to adapt, by resisting or changing in order to reach and maintain an acceptable level of functioning and structure." Disasters affect whole families and communities, with severe repercussions for the disaster victims' ability to care not only for themselves but also for each other (Norris, 2002). Lindsey (2003) reports that health researchers have studied a number of social, economic, and physical factors that could be utilized for identifying those who might be vulnerable in disasters.

In this section we highlight several community-based initiatives that exemplify this spirit of building disaster resiliency at the grassroots level. Much of the excellent work of local municipalities and communities does not appear in the professional or academic research literature, and so we drew on contacts within the Canadian emergency preparedness community, especially PHAC, to identify a sample of community initiatives for illustrative purposes.

John Webb, director of emergency social services, Nova Scotia (interviewed December 2, 2008)

On Monday, September 29, 2003, Hurricane Juan made landfall in Nova Scotia and left a trail of extensive damage across the central part of the province. Isolated older persons and persons with disabilities were found to be particularly vulnerable as emergency responders were unable to get to these populations as quickly as needed. As a consequence, older persons' groups approached the government to inquire how they could become better prepared for future disasters. Several innovative programs were developed and piloted with funding from the province and nonprofit organizations. One of the first initiatives created a network of individuals who produced a preparedness guide for persons with disabilities and frail older persons. This was followed by a train-the-trainer program whereby older persons and persons with disabilities were trained to conduct a 2-hour emergency preparedness presentation for various community and at-risk groups based on the guide. The third program to emerge, the Joint Emergency Management System (JEMS), is currently delivered in 10 communities in Nova Scotia. JEMS networks community stakeholders with emergency personnel to learn more about emergency preparedness. This program is also designed to facilitate the creation of comfort centers (in churches or fire halls) so older persons and persons with disabilities can more easily access equipment like generators. John Webb emphasized that each of the programs focuses on increasing community resiliency.

> Randy Hull, City of Winnipeg emergency preparedness coordinator, and Joe Egan (retired), City of Winnipeg emergency social services coordinator, Manitoba (interviewed November 6, 2008, and November 13, 2008)

An enhanced local network of older persons' groups emerged from the 2007 Winnipeg International Workshop on Seniors and Emergency Preparedness. The enhanced network created an easy to read paper presentation for older persons on how to become better prepared. A core group of older persons was trained to give presentations on managing in emergencies and the essential components of an emergency kit. In 2008, 15 presentations were given to over 400 participants. Older persons are also involved as actor evacuees in local disaster simulation exercises. Older persons' participation in these events increased their awareness of what could happen during a disaster and educated them on preparedness topics such as what to include in an emergency kit. Other programs initiated by the City of Winnipeg focus on building personal service plans. For example, in planning for relatively small-scale disasters involving 100–200 people, 30 to 35 social service workers were trained to specifically attend to individual older persons' needs, including locating and transferring them to temporary housing and implementing a frequent check-in program for displaced individuals. For larger scale disasters, the city is working with emergency responders (fire services) to ensure lists of most-at-risk individuals in buildings are maintained in the building's firebox to assist in rapid identification in the event of a disaster or emergency.

> Wayne Dauphinee, consultant with the Health, Emergency Management Unit, BC Ministry of Health Services, and Dave Hutton, FPT coordination and emergency social services, Public Health Agency of Canada (interviewed December 2 and 3, 2008)

In preparation for the Second International Workshop on Seniors and Emergency Preparedness held in Halifax, Nova Scotia, in March 2008 (PHAC, March 2008), older persons in British Columbia were randomly surveyed on what their concerns would be if confronted by a disaster. The survey gave clear indications of issues that need to be addressed. Older persons were most concerned by potential disruptions in routine, the loss of family and friends, and the loss of other support networks. Older persons also wanted to be recognized for their capacity to be active as volunteers in emergency preparedness and planning and to have their experience and skills utilized. The concept of resilient older persons shifted the focus of emergency preparedness planning from a vulnerable population perspective to a functional needs framework. The functional needs framework looks at mobility, communication, and supervision needs, among other key dimensions of functionality. This framework allows planners to look at all at-risk groups in a coherent, integrated manner without isolating one specific population. Work surrounding the framework to develop best practice guidelines is being led by Karen Martin, emergency preparedness coordinator, BC Coalition of People with Disabilities.

THE FUTURE OF DISASTER MANAGEMENT AND PREPAREDNESS AND THE OLDER ADULT POPULATION IN CANADA

Disasters do not occur in isolation; they have major social consequences. Increased attention to the issues of emergency and disaster preparedness for older persons in Canada has also focused attention on several conceptual and pragmatic issues warranting continuing study and discussion. We suggest that the various activities on older adult disaster management under way in Canada—government initiatives, academic developments, community projects, and the many and varied activities of numerous experts—reflect some common directions for the future of disaster management in general as well as specific to geriatric mental health. These include the following factors.

Shared Accountability

Canadians are relatively well prepared to respond to disaster situations. Federal, provincial, and territorial agencies have historically addressed disaster management as an individual departmental responsibility. While progress has been made, recent Canadian studies support the critical need for strong partnerships between government, community, and volunteer organizations in disaster management (Health Canada, 2003). Networking and support in particular should take place with local organizations.

There is an emerging consensus that to be effective, emergency management must reflect an understanding of the determinants of health and vulnerability within community infrastructures. The Canadian research emphasizes learning what individuals and community groups need and can offer and encouraging their participation in disaster planning. Lindsay (2007, p. 8) notes, "emergency managers must accept that decreasing community vulnerability will require more than just better response plans. Dealing with vulnerability requires emergency management to become integrated in community decision-making." It is recommended that researchers examine initiatives at different levels of government, provide support for local initiatives, and evaluate best practice strategies over time (Public Health Agency of Canada, March 2008).

The coordination of planning and relief, improved communication, and attention to resource gaps are important issues requiring a community-level response. Mental health issues, including factors that increase vulnerability and factors that promote resilience, must be mainstreamed within this response, with due consideration for determinants of health including age and stage of life.

Vulnerable Populations

A consensus emerging from recent Canadian conferences on older persons and emergencies, held in 2007 in Winnipeg and 2008 in Halifax, is that research related to high-risk groups needs to be extended and supported. Recommendations from the Red Cross report highlight the need for research regarding the experiences of high-risk populations as well as assessing the impact disasters have on society, which in turn affects the capabilities and needs of high-risk groups.

There is currently no consensus on how to mainstream the needs of vulnerable populations within emergency management operations. In Canada, one can find online emergency preparedness resources developed by federal provincial and municipal authorities targeted specifically to older persons (e.g., British Columbia Ministry of Health, *Community Evacuation Information for Seniors,* 2007), as well as resources that include older persons within a broader target audience focused on specific functional disabilities (e.g., Emergency Management Ontario, *Emergency*

Preparedness Guide for People with Disabilities/Special Needs, 2007). Some advocates argue for the identification of older persons as a distinct vulnerable group, while others, pointing to the heterogeneity with the older age category, argue it is functional limitations that create vulnerability, not age. Neither the community of older persons nor those with disabilities are necessarily happy to be co-identified. One approach to addressing this issue is the aforementioned functional needs framework for emergency preparedness.

The Mental Health Commission of Canada recently proposed a framework for developing a comprehensive mental health strategy for Canada (Mental Health Commission of Canada, 2009). The framework identifies and challenges the negative impact of stigma and discrimination on people who live with mental health problems and illnesses. The principle that discrimination should not be tolerated in policies, practices, and laws also has important implications for the development of emergency services and the mainstreaming of older persons with mental health needs within emergency management operations.

Building Capacity

A third issue pertains to the need to build capacity both to respond to older persons' heightened vulnerability in emergencies and to more effectively utilize the contributions older persons can make to emergency management. Capitalizing on older persons' potential contributions requires a sociopolitical culture receptive to the skills, knowledge, and wisdom of older persons (HelpAge International, 2006; the Sphere Project, 2004; United Nations, 2002). The integration of older persons within emergency management initiatives is identified as a key target for future research and development, along with developing community organizations, strengthening public education, and encouraging individual responsibility in disaster preparation (Sérandour & Beauregard, 2007).

Communication is central to integration and capacity building. The research on Canadian disasters presented here highlights the critical importance of communication. Historically, older Canadians had less access to education and have corresponding lower literacy skills (Turcotte & Schellenberger, 2007). It is essential that emergency management information is developed and disseminated in ways that will reach the older adult population (Gibson, 2007). A failure to be responsive to the varying communication needs of population subgroups can exacerbate emergency management challenges unnecessarily. This issue is addressed in the various community-based initiatives described earlier, in which enhancing communication is a central feature. In addition, a research project recently funded by the Social Sciences and Humanities Research Council of Canada (SSHRC), titled *Seniors and Emergency Preparedness: Applying a Senior-Friendly Lens to Emergency Planning in Canada*, addresses this issue (principal investigator M. Kloseck, personal communication, November 2008).

As a complement to building capacity at the community level, it is critical that Canada continue to make steady progress in DM education. A higher-education strategy that supports program development, while avoiding duplication, is needed. The continuum of course and program offerings under development is an excellent approach and will permit increased access and flexibility for beginning students and practitioners interested in upgrading or formalizing their credentials. Enhancing portability and laddering between the various programs will be the next important step for educators who wish to support students and the development of this rapidly evolving profession. An admirable job has been done surveying disaster management curriculae across the country. Identifying the precise content and curriculum gaps related to the geriatric population is another necessary step to improve DM programs in Canada.

CONCLUSION

Canadians are working to strengthen their capacity to respond to disaster situations. Current research, education, and policy initiatives are helping build disaster management capacity for older persons. While trends are moving in the right direction, recent Canadian studies and results from key informant interviews support the critical need for strong partnerships between government, community, and volunteer organizations. Further, the consequences of disasters—including mental health consequences—need to be studied in a holistic, comprehensive manner, bringing together researchers; health, mental health, social service, and community organizations; and older persons themselves.

ACKNOWLEDGMENTS

We extend our thanks to those experts who participated in interviews for this chapter, including the following:

Wayne Dauphinee—consultant, Health Emergency Management Unit, BC Ministry of Health Services

Joe Egan—[retired] emergency social services coordinator, City of Winnipeg

Patti Gorr—policy analyst, PHAC, Division of Ageing and Seniors

Gloria Gutman—fellow of the Gerontological Society of America, founding president of the Gerontology Association of BC, past president of the Canadian Association on Gerontology and the International Association of Gerontology, member of the board of directors of the International Institute on Ageing–UN Malta, and WHO's Expert Advisory Panel on Ageing and Health

Randy Hull—emergency preparedness coordinator, City of Winnipeg

Dave Hutton—FPT coordination and emergency social services, PHAC

Marita Kloseck—director, Aging and Community Health Research Lab; scientist, Lawson Health Research Institute; faculty of health sciences, University of Western Ontario

John Lindsay—chair of the department of applied disaster and emergency studies, Brandon University

Danielle Maltais—professor, Université du Québec à Chicoutimi, département des sciences humaines

Laurie Mazurik—strategic lead, disaster and emergency preparedness, Sunnybrook Health Science Centre; faculty of medicine, University of Toronto; innovation lead IDEAS Project, Centennial College, Toronto

John Webb—director of emergency social services, Nova Scotia

REFERENCES

British Columbia Ministry of Health. (2007). *Community evacuation information for seniors.* Retrieved January 30, 2009, from http://www.healthlinkbc.ca/healthfiles/pdf/hfile103a.pdf

Bruce, J. A., Donovan, K. F., Hornof, M. J., & Barthos, S. (2004). *Emergency management education in Canada.* Prepared for Public Safety and Emergency Preparedness Canada. Ottawa, Ontario: Queen's Printer.

Buckland, J., & Rahman, M. (1999). Community-based disaster management during the 1997 Red River flood in Canada. *Disasters, 23,* 174–191.

Cummings, G. E., Corte, F. D., & Cummings, G. G. (2005). Disaster medicine education in Canadian medical schools before and after September 11, 2001. *Canadian Journal of Emergency Medicine, 7,* 399–405.

Emergency Management Ontario. (2007). *Emergency preparedness guide for people with disabilities/special needs.* Retrieved January 30, 2009, from http://www.scics.gc.ca/cinfo07/830903005_e.pdf

Enarson, E., & Walsh, S. (2007). *Canadian Red Cross: Integrating emergency management and high-risk populations: Survey report and action recommendations.* Prepared for Public Safety Canada. Retrieved January 2, 2009, from http://www.redcross.ca/cmslib/general/dm_high_risk_populations.pdf

Etkin, D., Haque, C. E., & Brooks, G. R. (Eds.). (2003). *An assessment of natural hazards and disasters in Canada.* The Netherlands: Kluwer Academic Publishers.

Falkiner, L. (2003). *Inventory of disaster management education in major Canadian universities.* University of Western Ontario Institute for Catastrophic Loss Reduction. London, Ontario: Queen's Publisher.

Gibson, M. (2007). *Psychosocial issues pertaining to seniors in emergencies.* Ottawa, Ontario: Centre for Emergency Preparedness and Response, Public Health Agency of Canada.

Gutman, G. (2007). *Seniors and disasters: A synthesis of four Canadian case studies.* Paper presented at the Winnipeg International Workshop on Seniors and Emergency Preparedness, February 2007, Winnipeg, Manitoba.

Health Canada. (2003). *Centre for Emergency Preparedness and Response: Report of Activities 2001–2002.* Ottawa, Ontario: Minister of Health.

HelpAge International. (2006). Neglect in emergencies. *Ageing and Development, 19*(1), 1. Retrieved November 2009 from http://www.helpage.org/Resources/Regularpublications/AgeingandDevelopment/main_content/tnRY/ad19eng.pdf

Hutton, D. (2008). *Older people in emergencies: Considerations for action and policy development.* Geneva, Switzerland: World Health Organization.

Hutton, D. (2001). *Psychosocial aspects of disaster recovery: Integrating communities into disaster planning and policy making* (Paper #2). University of Western Ontario Institute for Catastrophic Loss Reduction, London, Ontario. Retrieved November 2008 from http://www.iclr.org/pdf/research%20paper%2016%20-%20paper%202%20david%20hutton.doc.pdf

Lalande, G., Maltais, D., & Robichaud, S. (2000). Les sinistrés des inondations de 1996 au Saguenay: Problémes vécus et séequelles. *Santé mentale au Québec, 25*(1), 95–115.

Lindsay, J. (2003). The determinants of disaster vulnerability: Achieving sustainable mitigation through population health. *Natural Hazards, 28*(2–3), 291–304.

Lindsay, J. (2007). *Vulnerability—Identifying a collective responsibility for individual safety: An overview of the functional and demographic determinants of disaster vulnerability* (Report for the Centre for Emergency Preparedness and Response). Ottawa, Ontario: Public Health Agency of Canada.

Lindsay, J., & Hall, M. (2007). *Older persons in emergency and disaster: A case study of the 1997 Manitoba flood.* Unpublished manuscript prepared for the World Health Organization.

Maltais, D. (2006). *The ice storm and its impact on seniors.* Paper presented at the Winnipeg International Workshop on Seniors and Emergency Preparedness, February 2007, Winnipeg, Manitoba.

Maltais, D., & Lachance, L. (2007). The medium- and long-term consequences of the July 1996 floods on the bio-psycho-social health of the elderly. *Vie et Vieillissement, 6*(2), 30–36.

Maltais, D., Robichaud, S., & Simard, A. (2001). *Les conséquences de la tempête de verglas sur la santé biopsychosociale des familles, des personnes âgées et des agriculteurs de la Montérégie.* Chicoutimi, Québec: Université du Québec á Chicoutimi.

Mental Health Commission of Canada. (2009). *Toward recovery and well-being: A framework for a mental health strategy for Canada.* Draft document for public discussion. Retrieved April 2009 from http://www.mentalhealthcommission.ca/SiteCollectionDoc uments/Key_Documents/en/2009/Mental_Health_ENG.pdf

Ministers Responsible for Emergency Management. (2007). *An emergency management framework for Canada.* Public Safety and Emergency Preparedness Canada. Retrieved November 2008 from http://www.scics.gc.ca/cinfo07/830903005_e.pdf

Norris, F. H. (2002). Psychosocial consequences of disasters. *PTSD Research Quarterly, 13*(2), 1–8.

Plouffe, L. (2008). *Older persons in emergencies: An active ageing perspective.* Geneva, Switzerland: World Health Organization.

Public Health Agency of Canada. (2008, February). *Building a global framework to address the needs and contributions of older people in emergencies* (Report based on the 2007 Winnipeg International Workshop on Seniors and Emergency Preparedness, February 2007, Winnipeg, Manitoba). Ottawa, Ontario: Minister of Public Works and Government Services Canada.

Public Health Agency of Canada. (2008, March). *Second international workshop on seniors and emergency preparedness* (Report based on the Halifax, Nova Scotia, Workshop, March 16–19, 2008). Ottawa, Ontario: Public Health Agency of Canada Division of Ageing and Seniors.

Public Safety Canada. (2007). *Canadian disaster database.* Retrieved January 30, 2009, from http://ww5.ps-sp.gc.ca/res/em/cdd/search-en.asp

Sérandour, B., & Beauregard, F. (2007). Canada's commitment to emergency preparedness for seniors. *Vie et Vieillissement, 6*(2), 49–55.

The Sphere Project. (2004). *The sphere project: Humanitarian charter and minimum standards in disaster response.* Retrieved October 2008 from http://www.sphere-project.org/component/option,com_docman/task,doc_download/gid,12/Itemid,26/lang,english/

Standing Committee on National Security and Defense. (2008). *Emergency preparedness in Canada.* Retrieved November 2008 from http://www.parl.gc.ca/39/2/parlbus/commbus/senate/com-e/defe-e/press-e/02sep08a-e.htm

Turcotte, M., & Schellenberg, G. (2007). *A portrait of seniors in Canada 2006.* Statistics Canada (Catalogue No. 89-519-XIE). Ottawa, Ontario: Minister of Industry.

United Nations. (2002). *Madrid international plan of action on ageing.* Report of the Second World Assembly on Ageing, April 8–12, 2002, Madrid, Spain.

World Health Organization. (2002). *Active ageing: A policy framework* (Report No. WHO/NMH/NPH/02.8). Geneva, Switzerland: World Health Organization.

6

Supervision and Facilitated Reflective Practice as Central to Disaster Preparedness Services to the Older Adult: A National and Cross-National Model

PHILIPPA SULLY, MALCOLM WANDRAG, AND JENNY RIDDELL

This chapter addresses the use of facilitated reflective practice as central to the preparation for and delivery of interprofessional, client-centered services to older persons and the communities in which they live during major disasters. It explores the value of dual supervision for the team facilitators' own reflective practice upon conscious and unconscious processes evoked within interprofessional groups when working with practitioner anxiety. The central tenet of this chapter is the crucial role of reflection in the planning, delivering, and evaluating of professional, interprofessional, interagency, and possibly international responses to older persons in civil emergencies and disasters. A key assumption in this chapter is that the ownership and valuing of lived experience is an essential component of reflection and, hence, practice, service development, and delivery. What practitioners bring to their experiences of working with individuals and communities—including their perceptions of older adults facing civil emergencies and disasters—will consciously and unconsciously influence how they regard themselves and their roles. Their responses and the manner in which they interact with colleagues in their own and other disciplines, as well as how they interact with the individuals and communities they serve, will also be influenced.

THE INFLUENCE OF PRACTITIONER
TRAUMA ON SERVICE DELIVERY

Rothschild (2006) provides examples of practitioners who have been affected by vicarious trauma through the interaction of client experiences on their own histories. The emotional foundations of these experiences are frequently related to profound human suffering, loss, and distress. These personal, family, and/or community histories have shaped practitioners and their practice. It is the authors' view that these experiences will overtly, as well as unconsciously, influence the work of practitioners in the development and delivery of services in emergencies and disasters.

The violence inherent in disasters violates boundaries. When practitioners work alongside or with communities involved in civil emergencies, merely listening to the survivors' stories may reawaken their own early trauma or their community's history of trauma. The transference of practitioners will have an impact on attitudes and values across teams and disciplines, both nationally and internationally, and on the processes of service development and delivery. In the same way, this transference will influence individual and community responses to those who aim to offer help and support.

Warren, Lee, and Saunders (2003) and Herman (1992), among others, identify the effects on practitioners who work with people and communities involved in traumatic events. There is also an extensive literature on the development of unconscious organizational defenses that enable practitioners to deal with the painful nature of much that human service provision entails (Huffington, Armstrong, Halton, Hoyle, & Pooley, 2004; Hughes & Pengelly, 1997; Obholzer & Roberts, 1994). Since violence and loss are associated with civil emergencies and disasters, it is likely that practitioners, their teams, and organizations will have developed effective defenses to the anxiety evoked by their teamwork. If these defenses impede effective service delivery, however, it can be detrimental to the well-being of individuals and the community (Hughes & Pengelly; Obholzer & Roberts). Herman (p. 141) states in relation to therapists who work with traumatized people:

> The therapist's adverse reactions, unless understood and contained, also predictably lead to disruptions in the therapeutic alliance with patients and to conflict with professional colleagues. Therapists who work with traumatised people require an ongoing support system to deal with these intense

reactions. Just as no survivor can recover alone, no therapist can work with trauma alone.

The authors argue this is also the case with practitioners whose work involves assisting individuals and communities to cope with disasters and the resulting trauma. They, too, need support. Close supervision or well-contained reflective practice and supervision sessions must be offered as an integral component of the development, delivery, and evaluation of emergency preparedness.

TOOLS FOR TEAMS: NARRATIVES AND FACILITATED REFLECTION

Narratives

Narratives enable individuals and groups to make sense of their experiences and, if necessary, reframe them to accommodate new experiences of and perspectives on the events in which they have been involved. Stories can be a useful means of learning to understand one's own experiences, as well as the experiences of others.

Indeed, some cultures use this form of information sharing more than others, as has been highlighted in research undertaken by Voulgaridou, Papadopoulos, and Tomaras (2006). Voulgaridou and colleagues discussed the value of cultural therapeutic mediators, who worked with them to understand the needs of refugee communities in Greece and the cultural influences and implications in service delivery and client adjustments to new environments. The authors suggest older persons would benefit from opportunities to discuss their own stories of survival within an atmosphere of mutual cooperation and respect as a form of inoculation. It is possible, therefore, to transfer this model of reflection and supervision to older persons who are part of at-risk communities rather than solely to the workers in order to help the elders learn from previous experiences, bring them into the present, and make plans for the future (Wilson, 2008).

The authors' experiences of using narrative and relating it to here-and-now group processes are supported by the literature (Clarke & Rowan, 2009). Narrative—the recounting of experience—can bring an event to life in the here-and-now (Wood, 2007). It can therefore be argued that narrative can be used to enable teams to learn from their processes of working together (Reeves & Sully, 2007), both nationally and internationally, across disciplines. Thus, narratives can enable teams to distinguish the processes that will support and/or hinder the development and delivering of client- and community-centered services, which are their primary task, as well as identify those areas where they might be going off task.

Many teams can be perceived as powerful and intimidating because of their extensive experience facing life-and-death situations and their success in making a difference in people's lives. This perception, in the authors' experiences, can be effectively contained and may be used as an excellent resource to inform practice when narratives are part of reflective practice. The model outlined in the next section shows the parallel processes demonstrated in team behavior and reflection when the practitioners are away from the immediacy of responding to emergencies. In this way, it is possible to allow team members to anticipate events and the manner in which they might respond to them, as well as to enable them to learn from previous experiences.

Reflective Practice

Reflective practice is defined as the capacity to review practice by reflection-in-action-and-on-action (Schön, 1987) in order to gain new perspectives and insights. Reflective practice as a means of examining past actions in a structured manner is well documented. What is not so well documented is the use of facilitated reflection to monitor and develop delivery of services by organizations as well as individuals. However, reflective practice as a means of establishing therapeutic direction is receiving more attention now than it did when Max van Manen named it "anticipatory reflection" in 1991 (as cited in Wilson, 2008, p. 180).

Facilitated reflective practice, the model the authors propose, has been shown to have a beneficial effect upon practice. The model uses co-facilitated reflective practice sessions as an integral part of the planning process to specifically address the needs of client groups and workers. In this mutual supervision model, reflection is used to convert previous experiences into knowledge and insight. Practitioners are then assisted to transform this new learning into sound practice. Their organizations, in turn, change individual practice and insight into true interprofessional responses focusing on survivors' needs rather than delivering a service solely prescribed and led by procedures. Through these processes, open systems that make clear the parameters for service provision and provide clear guidelines for practice within and across organizational boundaries can be developed (Roberts, 1994).

Different professions that form an interprofessional team can have different or even conflicting views of the primary task of the group. In order to overcome this phenomenon, it is essential each professional understand the perspectives of the other professionals in the team. Reframing perspectives by focusing on the task can help practitioners to explore new viewpoints and agree on practice interventions. Schön (1987, p. 128) describes this process as the "capacity for framed reflection."

As groups and teams meet to develop professional, interprofessional, and collaborative services that will be sensitive to the particular needs of older adults caught up in civil emergencies and disasters, reflection on the group processes of working together in the here and now can be a rich source for understanding diverse strengths in the team, as well as possible pitfalls and barriers to effective service provision. In the processes of service delivery, the *what-goes-on-in-here* mirrors or is a parallel course to the *what-goes-on-out-there*. For example, a team experiencing anxiety about a forecast of severe weather is reflecting and acting out the anxiety also present in the community they serve.

Planning for and responding to disasters demands flexible responses to those in need. Procedure- and/or protocol-led responses that do little to deliver a service to individuals can stifle creative approaches to practice that consider the needs of individuals or groups with common or shared experience. The authors suggest that such inelastic systems are more likely to produce off-task behaviors such as basic assumption mentalities (Bion, 1961), the unconscious tendency to avoid work on a primary task, particularly when providing care to vulnerable groups where the emotional impact might be more intense.

The use of the reflective practice technique ensures that practitioners from a variety of backgrounds and nationalities respond sensitively to the needs of individuals and communities, rather than creating procedures that result in a one-size-fits-all response. Therefore, the particular needs of older adults are more likely to be acknowledged and addressed. By adopting this model, unconscious processes, beliefs, attitudes, stereotypes, and values and their influence on practice in disasters can be uncovered and explored. It also provides an excellent opportunity to highlight incompatible interprofessional and international structures, priorities, and procedures that could potentially result in conflicting actions when responding to disasters.

This technique has been used by the authors to assist their students in developing insight and considering how their individual practice fits with the primary task of their home organization and with the delivery of true, interprofessional services to clients caught up in violent episodes. As a result of their own work with students in master's programs delivering services to victims of intentional, interpersonal acts of violence such

as bombings or gang violence and unintentional violence such as tsu-
namis, gas explosions, or rail crashes, the authors suggest that reflective
practice can aid the delivery of services centered upon the needs of the
client group, be it an individual, a community, or a nation.

Reflective practice is, then, a vital component at all stages of the disaster continuum from the early stages of contingency planning through
postrecovery. It is not enough to see reflection as a luxury or something to
be indulged in once in a while, when time allows, or when funds are available. The process is cyclical, and the cycle can be entered at any point. The
advantage of these sessions is that they benefit practitioners as well as individuals and communities who might be involved in a passive role and
perceive the disaster as happening to them.

All reflective practice sessions must be structured carefully with clear
working agreements, boundaries, focus, and supports (Proctor, 2000) in
order to examine task-focused processes and basic assumption mentalities
(Bion, 1961) and how they are manifest. The sessions can then be used to
construct responses from interprofessional and international service providers because they provide a mirror of the realities of practice (Hawkins &
Shohet, 2006) in the field of disaster management. This process also enables professional; cultural, including the cultures of individual professions/
services; and national perspectives, which might not be readily acknowledged in the immediate responses to disasters, to be identified earlier in
the process. Earlier identification leads to earlier accommodation; the impact of these perspectives during disaster responses can be foreseen, understood, and addressed wherever possible.

Reflective practice initiated from the first stage of any planning effort
assists not only in the formation of the planning group as a team but also
in ensuring all necessary interests are represented. The reflective practice
sessions use the existing knowledge, skills, and experiences of the group
members and guarantee that the primary task is addressed and that any
off-task behaviors will be identified for the team to consider. Reflective
practice sessions continue to be held throughout the preparedness process—through completion of the plans in the first stage, through later test-
ing/exercising, and then in subsequent reviews, either as a result of testing
or periodic reviews.

The supervisory element is a key component of facilitated reflective
practice. Proctor (1986) identifies three processes of professional supervision, one of which is restorative (Howard, 2008). This process is integral
to sound facilitated reflection; its relevance in emergency responses is
therefore a valid reason for the inclusion of facilitated reflective practice

in service development and delivery, as has been suggested by Hawkins and Shohet (2006). The other two processes are the normative, which deals with the maintenance of appropriate standards of practice, and the formative, which educates the practitioner.

The authors are of the view that embedding cofacilitated group and/or team supervision throughout the processes of planning, disseminating, responding, recovering, and returning to the nonemergency state offers the opportunity to review practice in the here and now as well as reviewing experience by "returning to the experience" (Boud, Keogh, & Walker, 1985, p. 12). There also is an opportunity for addressing practice, including practitioners' own feelings and attitudes, thus leading to the possibility of transforming practice through a "commitment to action" (Boud, et al., p. 12).

Supervision can not only identify what is available for the future through looking at the past, but it can also be used to conduct a review of each stage of the process in the left-hand column of Figure 6.1 in order to achieve best practice and learn from each experience. The supervisory process also provides an effective form of containment for the facilitators, which they in turn pass on so that the practitioner group is also contained. The parallel, or mirroring, in the supervision processes (Clarke & Rowan, 2009; Hawkins & Shohet, 2006; Hughes & Pengelly, 1997)—in which the processes of service provision are enacted in the here-and-now processes of supervision as well as in individual or group behavior—is a valuable resource on which to explore and elucidate service provision. An example is the exploration of the functioning of an interprofessional team and, thus, the development of these services.

The power of disasters and emergencies can be overwhelming, a reaction that can be manifest in team or group behavior. To avoid this, facilitators also are supported by their own practice supervision, which provides them with a containing environment (Agass, 2000). In supervision, they too can explore their practice and transfer their learning into their facilitative roles, rather than becoming overwhelmed and responding inappropriately. Facilitated reflective practice sessions allow for the normative, formative, and restorative processes (Proctor, 1986, 2000) that structured facilitated reflection offers. It allows for "mutual supervision-in-action" (Sully, Wandrag, & Riddell, 2008, p. 135).

Within this context, the supervision of reflective practice facilitators acts not only to monitor and develop their practice but also to provide a means of processing their perceptions and understanding of the group process. It also allows for safety in practice by addressing the possibility of

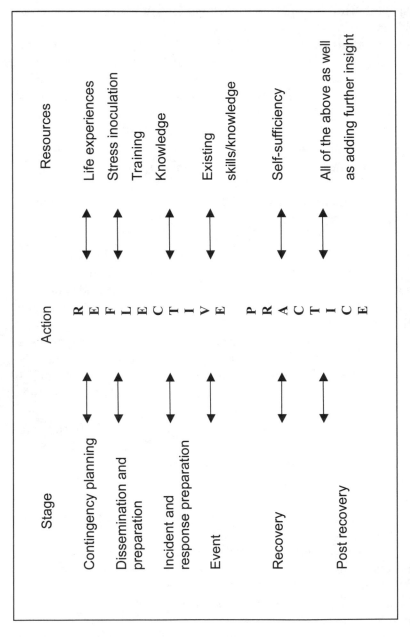

Stage	Action		Resources
Contingency planning	R	↕ ↔	Life experiences
Dissemination and preparation	E F L	↕ ↔	Stress inoculation
	E	↕ ↔	Training
Incident and response preparation	C T	↕ ↔	Knowledge
Event	I V E	↕ ↔	Existing skills/knowledge
Recovery	P R A	↕ ↔	Self-sufficiency
Post recovery	C T I C E	↕ ↔	All of the above as well as adding further insight

Figure 6.1 Reflective practice as a link in disaster preparedness.

unconscious collusion with the team and the possibility of missing vital aspects of interprofessional working that could be inadvertently detrimental to the overall team task. In this way, the supervision of the facilitators supports their maintenance of professional boundaries such that they mirror safe practice and containment to the team while they enable practitioners to explore their work together.

The safety provided by supervision enables the growth and sensitivity of the internal supervisor (Casement, 1985) within the facilitators and practitioners, with resulting transformation of practice (Reeves & Sully, 2007). The *internal supervisor* is the capacity of the practitioner to reflect during the practice process on how clients might experience their situation and their relationship with the practitioner and, thus, how they might receive, perceive, and construe the practice interventions offered. This ability to try to see the world from the client's point of view can enable the practitioner to gain insight into how the client might be feeling and what help might be worthwhile. The authors suggest that the internal supervisor involves more than reflection-in-action (Schön, 1987) as it involves the *whole person* of the practitioner—thoughts, feelings, interactions, physical sensations, posture, and gesture.

Once the supportive supervisory relationship, which is central to sound supervision (Hawkins & Shohet, 2006; Hazler, 2001; Hughes & Pengelly, 1997; Sawdon & Sawdon, 1995; Wood, 2007) has been established, the two facilitators are then available to conduct reflective practice sessions should an incident occur. The benefit of reflective practice sessions during all phases of an incident is that practitioners will have an arena in which to consider professional, interprofessional, national, and international processes as well as actions.

Reflective Practice Benefits the Community

It is not only practitioners who can benefit from the use of reflective practice but also individuals and communities who might be involved in a passive role. True preparation requires sufficient knowledge of a variety of factors including but not limited to type of emergency, likelihood, imminence, level of response, and expected assistance. Preparation for disasters in communities at high risk is a "form of psychological immunization" (Hoff, Hallisey, & Hoff, 2009, p. 468) for practitioners and communities who face the likelihood of disastrous events. At the stage of information provision, practitioners, both individual and organizational, can identify and draw upon the resources available to them and to the community that might be of benefit in the event of an incident. Figure 6.1 shows the two-way process the authors suggest can lead to a parallel process as discussed in the following. The benefits of such a parallel process are described in Hawkins and Shohet (2006) and Hughes and Pengelly (1997). The authors suggest that the community's identified resources in disaster management not only involve consultation with the communities served but also include an identification of their abilities to help themselves and the support for self-help.

In adopting the model as suggested here, practitioners can use a structured process that will benefit both sides. This model provides a link between what is going on in the here and now and what might happen out there in the future. At each point along the way, the supervisor will encourage the use of reflective practice both to identify previous experiences and existing coping mechanisms and to link them to future, possible actions (Wilson, 2008). This use of *anticipatory reflection* to identify future courses of action (Sully, et al., 2008) can be used to promote self-help within communities and individuals. While this model is unlikely to be used widely, it would be possible to use it in *closed* communities such as residential homes, retirement complexes, and so forth.

Figure 6.2 shows how the mirroring processes can inform the development and delivery of services during an emergency or disaster. The process is contained by a semipermeable boundary that allows such things as national and international law to have an impact upon the reflective process and on the experiences of practitioners, who in turn influence national and international agreements, protocols, and codes of practice. For this reason, it is important that the containing boundary is not rigid and inflexible. It is imperative throughout the process that the core conditions of facilitative relationships (Hazler, 2001; Rogers, 1961; Wood, 2007) are strictly observed.

CONCLUSION

Reflective practice is a means of enabling practitioners to hone their skills in understanding group process and their interprofessional and interagency responses and address shared spoken and unspoken group choices, especially the displacement of anxiety (Obholzer, 1994), when preparing for and responding to major disasters.

The supervisory process is a key element of this model. Supervision can identify what is available for the future through looking at the past,

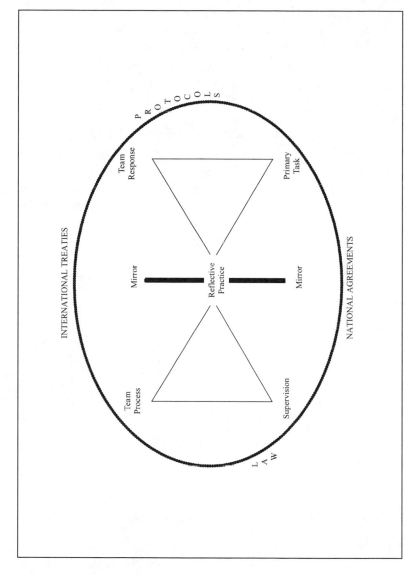

Figure 6.2 The mirror as the catalyst for anticipatory reflection and reflection-in-action-and-on-action. From *The Mirror as the Catalyst for Anticipatory Reflection and Reflection-in-and-on Action*, by P. Sully, M. Wandrag, and J. Riddell, 2009, London: Personal Professional Records. © Copyright 2009 Sully, P., Wandrag, M., & Riddell, J. Reprinted with permission.

and it can also be used to conduct a review of each stage of the service process in the left-hand column of Figure 6.1 in order to achieve best practice and to learn from each experience.

The authors' way of facilitating this focuses on the people involved—client groups and practitioners—rather than procedures, thus ensuring the services delivered are sensitive to the needs of survivors and their communities. The use of anticipatory reflection (Sully, et al., 2008; Sully & Dallas, 2005) enables practitioners to use their past experiences and knowledge together with their present experiences in writing contingency plans to prepare themselves for future action, as described in more detail by Wilson (2008).

The inclusion, as part of the protocols of structured cofacilitated reflective practice sessions during all phases of the service provision cycle—from contingency planning to service evaluation—along with the evidence base for practice, is arguably one of the foundations on which person- and community-centered emergency responses can be developed and sustained. It also provides a container in which practitioners can explore their anxieties about teamwork and service delivery within and across disciplines, communities, and nations.

REFERENCES

Agass, D. (2000). Containment, supervision, and abuse. In U. McCluskey & C. A. Hooper (Eds.), *Psychodynamic perspectives on abuse: The cost of fear* (pp. 209–222). London: Jessica Kingsley Publishers.

Bion, W. R. (1961). *Experiences in groups: And other papers.* New York: Basic Books.

Boud, D., Keogh, R., & Walker, D. (Eds.). (1985). *Reflection: Turning experience into learning.* London: Kogan Page.

Casement, P. (1985). *On learning from the patient.* London: Tavistock.

Clarke, G., & Rowan, A. (2009). Looking again at the team dimension in systemic psychotherapy: Is attending to group process a critical context for practice? *Journal of Family Therapy, 31*(1), 85–107.

Hawkins, P., & Shohet, R. (2006). *Supervision in the helping professions* (3rd ed.). Basingstoke, UK: Oxford University Press.

Hazler, R. (2001). Somehow therapy works: Core conditions of the facilitative therapeutic environment. In R. Hazler & N. Barwick (Eds.), *The therapeutic environment* (pp. 4–12). Buckingham, UK: Oxford University Press.

Herman, J. L. (1992). *Trauma and recovery.* London: Pandora.

Hoff, L. A., Hallisey, B. J., & Hoff, M. (2009). *People in crisis: Clinical and diversity perspectives* (6th ed.). New York: Routledge.

Howard F. (2008). Managing stress or enhancing well-being? Positive psychology's contributions to clinical supervision. *Australian Psychologist, 43*(2), 105–113.

Huffington, C., Armstrong, D., Halton, W., Hoyle, L., & Pooley, J. (Eds.). (2004). *Working below the surface*. London: Karnac.

Hughes, L., & Pengelly, P. (1997). *Staff supervision in a turbulent environment*. London: Jessica Kingsley Publishers.

Obholzer, A. (1994). Managing social anxieties in public sector organizations. In A. Obholzer & V. Z. Roberts (Eds.), *The unconscious at work: Stress in the human services* (pp. 169–178). London: Routledge.

Obholzer, A., & Roberts, V. Z. (Eds.). (1994). *The unconscious at work: Stress in the human services*. London: Routledge.

Proctor, B. (2000). *Group supervision: A guide to creative practice*. London: Sage.

Proctor, B. (1986). Supervision: A co-operative exercise in accountability. In M. Marken & M. Payne (Eds.), *Enabling and ensuring supervision in practice* (pp. 23–34). Leicester, UK: National Youth Bureau and Council for the Education and Training in Youth and Community Work.

Reeves, S., & Sully, P. (2007). Interprofessional education for practitioners working with the survivors of violence: Exploring early and longer-term outcomes on practice. *Journal of Interprofessional Care, 21*(4), 1–12.

Roberts, V. Z. (1994). The organization of work: Contributions from open systems theory. In A. Obholzer & V. Z. Roberts (Eds.), *The unconscious at work: Stress in the human services* (pp. 28–38). London: Routledge.

Rogers, C. (1961). Significant learning: In therapy and education. In C. Rogers, *On becoming a person* (pp. 279–296). London: Constable.

Rothschild, B. (2006). *Help for the helper*. New York: Norton.

Sawdon, C., & Sawdon, D. (1995). The supervision partnership: A whole greater than the sum of its parts. In J. Pritchard, *Good practice in supervision* (pp. 3–19). London: Jessica Kingsley Publishers.

Schön, D. (1987). *Educating the reflective practitioner: Toward a new design for teaching and learning in the professions*. San Francisco, CA: Jossey-Bass.

Sully, P., & Dallas, J. (2005). *Essential communication skills for nurses*. Edinburgh: Mosby.

Sully, P., Wandrag, M., & Riddell, J. (2009a). *Reflective practice as a link in disaster preparedness*. London: Personal Professional Records.

Sully, P., Wandrag, M., & Riddell, J. (2009b). *The mirror as the catalyst for anticipatory reflection and reflection-in-and-on action*. London: Personal Professional Records.

Sully, P., Wandrag, M., & Riddell, J. (2008). The use of reflective practice on masters programmes in interprofessional practice with survivors of intentional and unintentional violence. *Reflective Practice, 9*(2), 135–144.

Voulgaridou, M. G., Papadopoulos, R. K., & Tomaras, V. (2006). Working with refugee families in Greece: Systemic considerations. *Journal of Family Therapy, 2,* 200–220.

Warren, T., Lee, S, & Saunders, S. (2003). Factors influencing experienced distress and attitude toward trauma by emergency medicine practitioners. *Journal of Clinical Psychology in Medical Settings, 10*(4), 293–296.

Wilson, J. P. (2008). Reflecting-on-the-future: A chronological consideration of reflective practice. *Reflective Practice, 9*(2), 177–184.

Wood, J. (2007). *Models of reflective practice*. Unpublished doctoral dissertation, City University London, England.

7

Making the Community Plan: A Public Health Perspective

ANDREA VILLANTI

DISASTERS: A COMMUNITY-LEVEL EVENT

Disasters are events that "seriously [disrupt] the functioning of a community or society and [cause] human, material, and economic or environmental losses that exceed the community's or society's ability to cope using its own resources" (International Federation of Red Cross and Red Crescent Societies, 2008a). While disaster research has focused on the impact of personal loss, property damage, and individual trauma, community destruction may also result in a collective trauma with broad public health implications (Norris, 2002). Research on disasters has shown the community-level impact of these destructive events on mental health across the life span (Galea, et al., 2002; Galea, Tracy, Norris, & Coffey, 2008; Norris, Friedman, & Watson, 2002; Norris, Friedman, Watson, et al., 2002; Thompson, Norris, & Hanacek, 1993) as well as the ways individuals turn to their communities to cope (Schuster, et al., 2001).

In 2004, the International Federation of Red Cross and Red Crescent Societies focused their annual *World Disasters Report* on community resilience, asserting that disaster preparedness and response should adopt the sustainable livelihoods framework central to international development work (International Federation of Red Cross and Red Crescent Societies, 2004). The report argued that shifting the risk approach by

119

focusing on community assets, competence, and capacities rather than needs, hazards, and vulnerabilities strengthens local resilience and the capacity of communities to adapt better and cope with disasters. The sustainable livelihoods framework approaches development by assessing natural capital, financial assets, human capital, social capital, and physical capital in a community, building awareness of these resources and catalyzing consensus for community action (International Federation of Red Cross and Red Crescent Societies).

Surveys conducted within 8 weeks of the September 11, 2001, attacks showed that residents of Manhattan reported elevated levels of symptoms consistent with PTSD and depression (Galea, et al., 2002). While rates of postdisaster psychiatric symptoms were higher among persons directly affected by the disaster, persons indirectly affected also experienced a higher prevalence of PTSD and depression than national benchmark estimates, and elevated levels of psychological distress were also seen in respondents with low social support (Galea, et al.). National surveys of stress reactions reported that 44% of U.S. adults experienced substantial stress following the September 11, 2001, attacks (Schuster, et al., 2001), Together, these studies confirm that the psychological sequelae of disasters reach far beyond those who are directly affected. By framing disasters as community-level events with psychological implications for all involved, regardless of direct personal loss (Norris, 2002), we can tailor disaster preparedness to meet the needs of specific communities, prevent the erosion of community cohesion, and provide the means for communities to take control of disaster and emergency planning and response.

This chapter critiques existing preparedness activities, describes the importance of community preparedness for older adults, and presents a conceptual model of the relationship between community preparedness, psychological well-being, and positive adaptive functioning to promote quality of life.

GAPS IN TRADITIONAL EMERGENCY PREPAREDNESS

Preparedness activities focus on reducing or mitigating the impact of a disaster on a population and developing an effective response to its consequences (International Federation of Red Cross and Red Crescent Societies, 2008b). Traditional emergency preparedness has focused on training for police, fire, and public works departments; emergency medical services; and emergency management personnel (Office of Domestic Preparedness, 2002) and risk communication for citizens involving individual preparedness kits and plans (Department of Homeland Security, 2008c). As a result, emergency preparedness activities have largely existed at the civic and individual levels, apart from the community context in which they are both embedded. The lack of an organizing notion of community as the level of disaster preparedness and recovery has produced gaps in existing preparedness efforts.

Lack of Training for Nongovernmental Entities

Public safety organizations, such as police and fire departments, have, for decades, incorporated disaster preparedness into their operational activities, and federal and state governments have developed extensive competencies in emergency preparedness and response. Emergency responder guidelines published in 2002 by the Office of Justice Programs Office of Domestic Preparedness identified five main groups responsible for emergency response, often referred to as *first responders:* law enforcement, fire services, emergency medical services, emergency management, and public works (Office of Domestic Preparedness, 2002).

Following the terrorist attacks of September 11, 2001, and Hurricane Katrina in 2005, the U.S. Department of Homeland Security acknowledged the role of nongovernmental organizations in emergency preparedness and response in its National Response Framework (Federal Emergency Management Agency [FEMA], 2008a). FEMA has compiled a catalog of training programs on domestic preparedness for "state and local first responders to prevent, protect, respond to, and recover from manmade and natural catastrophic events" (FEMA, 2008c). Though the FEMA catalog describes extending training offerings to the private sector and U.S. citizens, these groups are not identified as a target audience of any training in the catalog, and few of the trainings mention the private sector or U.S. citizens in their descriptions (FEMA, 2008d).

FEMA's community and citizen-related preparedness efforts focus on two partnered programs: Citizen Corps (Department of Homeland Security, 2008a) and Community Emergency Response Teams (Department of Homeland Security, 2008b). These programs focus on local capacity to provide coordination and training on emergency preparedness; using a train-the-trainer model, FEMA offers the curriculum for Community Emergency Response Team (CERT) training and relies on local communities for implementation via traditional first responders. Despite a national effort to provide community preparedness coverage through these programs, coordinated communication about program training and effectiveness was only initiated in September 2008 (Community Emergency Response Team, 2008). While FEMA has acknowledged the need for including nongovernmental entities, citizens, and communities in emergency preparedness (i.e., in its National Response Framework, training course catalog, Citizen Corps, and CERT program), the lack of focused, coordinated, or integrated training for these groups reflects a gap in existing preparedness efforts.

Focus on Citizen Preparedness Kits Rather Than Skills

Emergency preparedness messages for individual citizens in the United States have focused on concrete actions and checklists. The Department of Homeland Security's *Ready America* Web site lists three steps to preparedness: 1) get a kit, 2) make a plan, and 3) be informed (Department of Homeland Security, 2008c). Rather than viewing preparedness as an evolving process (Perry & Lindell, 2003), these messages limit preparedness activities to household-level kits, emergency plans, and a readiness quotient quiz. While there is a need for individual-level preparedness, these activities cannot end with a document or a bag of supplies; training, drills, and critique must provide the opportunity to develop skills vital to emergency planning and response (Perry & Lindell). Additionally, the isolation of individuals from the community in disaster planning ignores the experience of disaster as a community-level phenomenon (Norris, 2002) and the importance of social and family networks in emergency response, especially for vulnerable populations. Without developing skills to accompany a preparedness kit or emergency plan, and without making links to broader networks, individual preparedness activities based on existing federal messages fail to ensure adequate preparedness for safety and response.

Lack of Community-Level Drills

Despite the demonstrated importance of community in disaster response, emergency response simulation exercises have been targeted to first responders and emergency management officials in local, state, and federal jurisdictions (FEMA, 2008d). While multiagency drills are vital to developing an emergency response infrastructure, the inclusion of communities in these programs could greatly improve morale, cohesion, and trust in government preparedness efforts. Although a few studies on community-based preparedness drills indicate a profound and encouraging effect on community residents, existing research on preparedness activities largely focuses on the role of drills for emergency managers. This work shows that community-based preparedness organizations can have a very positive effect on individual and neighborhood preparedness activity, that programs on preparedness can increase feelings of social support, and that these groups can serve as new models for collaborative public- and private-sector preparedness (Simpson, 2002).

Lack of a Designated Community Role in Emergency Planning and Response

Studies following disasters indicate that disaster victims are more likely to seek assistance or support services from informal or community resources than from relief workers (North & Hong, 2000; Perry & Lindell, 2003). A Rand survey published in November 2001 showed that Americans, who self-identified as experiencing stress after the September 11 attacks, turned to their communities to cope: 98% said they talked to others, 90% turned to religion, 60% joined in group activities, and 36% made donations or did volunteer work (Schuster, et al., 2001). By providing immediate and long-term assistance with disaster response and recovery, community groups are often informal partners in disaster response efforts, leveraging existing ties to community members to address gaps in services for those affected by the disaster.

A White House report on lessons learned from the federal response to Hurricane Katrina described nongovernmental and faith-based community groups as "the foot soldiers and armies of compassion that victims of Katrina so desperately needed" (White House, 2006, p. 49). Despite the essential support provided by these groups, they were unable to coordinate their response efforts with those at the local, state, and federal levels because they had limited access to local emergency operations centers and limited information about the response efforts (White House). This lack of a designated role for nongovernmental groups in the National Response Plan hindered the coordination and integration of Katrina response efforts

(White House); to improve the efficiency and effectiveness of emergency response, these groups must be systematically included in emergency planning.

Special Concerns for Emergency Preparedness in the Geriatric Population

Older adults face unique challenges in disasters. In addition to the physiological, sensory, and cognitive changes that occur during aging, older adults have an increased burden of chronic disease, making them more physically and emotionally vulnerable than healthy adults (Aldrich & Benson, 2008). The experiences of the 1995 Chicago heat wave; the terrorist attacks of September 11, 2001; the 2003 European heat wave; and Hurricane Katrina in 2005 also highlight social isolation as an important risk factor for mortality as many older disaster victims were forgotten by their families and neighbors (Aldrich & Benson; Gibson, 2006; International Federation of Red Cross and Red Crescent Societies, 2004). Similar to recommendations for individual preparedness, materials on emergency preparedness for older adults and the disabled published by AARP, FEMA, and the American Red Cross focus on the development of a preparedness kit and a disaster plan and discussion of the plan with family, friends, and caregivers (AARP, 2006; FEMA & American Red Cross, August 2004). One component of these plans is identifying a personal support network—several individuals who will help prepare the older adult for a disaster and check in with the older adult in the event of a disaster (FEMA & American Red Cross). Preparedness materials also encourage older adults with disabilities to register with a local police or fire department and with the utility company if they need electricity for medical reasons. While preparedness recommendations for older adults and the disabled do encourage planning and thinking through disaster situations, they place most of the responsibility for these actions on the individual, again ignoring the surrounding community and alternate caregivers.

Relying on frail older adults to be able to activate a personal support network, be evacuated, and receive appropriate care is shortsighted given the numerous challenges experienced in a disaster setting. Disability, disease, and social isolation signal the need for better location and evacuation strategies for frail older adults in disasters; emergency planning must include a detailed plan for locating older adults who are confined to their homes or nursing homes and ensuring shelter, an appropriate diet, adequate water, and routine medical care (including prescription medication) throughout the duration of disaster recovery.

WHAT IS COMMUNITY PREPAREDNESS?

The community is an essential organizing unit in disasters and the level at which both immediate disaster response and long-term recovery occur. Past experience has shown that the best and most efficient means of implementing public health initiatives and changes brings together those from whom the collective response will be required. At the community level, this includes traditional first responders as well as local government representatives, health care providers, schools, religious organizations, community organizations, and community members. Norris, Stevens, Pfefferbaum, Wyche, and Pfefferbaum (2008, p. 131) described community resilience as "a process linking a set of networked adaptive capacities to a positive trajectory of functioning and adaptation in constituent populations after a disturbance." With this definition, community resilience and community preparedness may be interchangeable; community resilience could also be interpreted as an intended outcome of preparedness efforts. Drawing upon the sustainable livelihoods framework and Norris and colleagues' work, community preparedness is a process focused on harnessing and coordinating the assets, capabilities, and competence of existing communities to adapt and respond to a disturbance (Norris, et al.; and also, International Federation of Red Cross and Red Crescent Societies, 2004). Through community preparedness planning, community members discuss how to address the physical and mental health sequelae of disasters and the social functioning of the collective, define goals and decision-making processes by consensus, and collaborate on plans of action (Norris, 2002; Norris, et al.). In the wake of a disaster, community preparedness can set resilient communities on a positive trajectory of functioning through improved and appropriate response and recovery efforts. Community preparedness is not a documented plan (Perry & Lindell, 2003) shared among first responders and community members but rather the process of thinking through how to utilize existing community resources to meet needs and address vulnerabilities in a disaster.

Community Preparedness, Social Support, and Social Capital

In the wake of a disaster, as fatigue and financial difficulties set in, the immediate effect of community cohesion and mutual helping may yield to interpersonal conflict, disharmony, and a deterioration of support; the experience of communal pain, therefore, may provide communities initially with cohesion and, later, with conflict (Vlahov, 2002). While the degree of integration in a social network is postulated to have a direct effect on overall well-being, regardless of stress (Kawachi & Berkman, 2001), positive social support is vital to psychological wellness following a disaster (Norris & Kaniasty, 1996).

Studies of social support typically delineate three phenomena: social integration, social network structure, and the functional quality of social relationships (Gottlieb, 1985; House, Umberson, & Landis, 1988). The operation of social support at the community, social network, and interpersonal levels maps to different effects on mental health via belongingness (community level), bonding (social network level), and binding (interpersonal level; Lin, Ye, & Ensel, 1999). The functions of social support have been described as providing instrumental or tangible aid, emotional support, informational support, and appraisal support (House, 1981). In a study of social support mobilization following Hurricane Hugo in 1989, Kaniasty and Norris (1995) found that disaster victims received and provided more support than nonvictims, that those with greater disaster-related losses received more support, and that instrumental support was the most relevant type of support provided. In a subsequent study of Hurricane Hugo and Hurricane Andrew, Norris and Kaniasty (1996) found that perceived social support mediated the relationship between received social support and psychological distress following exposure to a disaster. Received support exerts a long-term positive effect on psychological distress after a disaster when individuals perceive that social support continues to be available to them; if, in the stress of disaster, individuals perceive their support network has deteriorated, the stress-buffering effects of social support may not operate (Norris & Kaniasty). These studies point to the importance of maintaining community relations during a disaster, mobilizing social support, and maintaining network ties to maximize received and perceived support available to the affected community.

In addition to social support, social capital is thought to buffer the effects of stress by providing access to benefits through social networks, thereby enhancing an individual's coping skills (Hawe & Shiell, 2000). Social capital develops from trust and reciprocity and operates at both the micro and macro levels, allowing the exchange of assets, opportunities, and other benefits to network members (Hawe & Shiell). At the micro level, social capital is a function of integration in a network and linkages outside an immediate network while at the macro level it can be seen as a synergy between the interests of network members and the actions of the larger society and the integrity of institutions to act independently of vested interests (Hawe & Shiell; Woolcock, 1998). In the context of disasters, social capital can reduce psychological distress by bringing about mutually beneficial collective action (Nakagawa & Shaw, 2004); in addition to the ability of social capital to promote a flow of support through and between social networks, the integrity and synergy (Woolcock) of larger social institutions in disaster response can engender distress or recovery.

Norris and colleagues (2008) identified social capital as one of the four networked capacities central to community resilience in times of disaster. In their model, social capital is linked with economic development, information and communication, and community competence. It is made up of social network structure, social support, social embeddedness, organizational linkages and cooperation, citizen participation, attachment to place, and sense of community (Norris, et al.). In the wake of Hurricane Katrina, many people were displaced from their homes and communities for an extended period (Galea, et al., 2008). In addition to experiencing eroding existing social support networks, sense of community, and attachment to place, Katrina victims lost trust in governmental assistance due to confusing or incomplete public announcements regarding federal financial assistance available to disaster victims (White House, 2006). The result of this deterioration of social capital and other stressors was an increased burden of PTSD among those living in disaster-affected areas at the time of Hurricane Katrina (Galea, et al.). Strategies for community preparedness and resilience rely upon the development of multilevel social networks, social capital, and linkages between the local, political, legal, and economic sectors to improve positive functioning after a disaster (Adger, Hughes, Folke, Carpenter, & Rockstrom, 2005; Norris, et al.).

Older Adults and Social Support

Exposure to disasters impacts the health status of older adults and results in greater physical health effects when there are greater personal losses and community destruction (Phifer, Kaniasty, & Norris, 1988). In addition to the vulnerability created by physiological, cognitive, sensory, and medical needs (Aldrich & Benson, 2008), older adults may be more susceptible to the effects of disaster due to their lower economic resources and weaker social support (Thompson, et al., 1993). In one study of Hurricane Hugo, older adults were the least likely to provide and receive support compared to younger and middle-aged adults following a disaster (Thompson, et al.). As such, older adults can either experience a pattern of neglect—where they receive less help than their younger counterparts, as seen with Hurricane

Katrina (Gibson, 2006)—or a pattern of concern, where societal norms of aiding the most needy, reciprocity, and filial ties overcome the pattern of neglect (Kaniasty & Norris, 1995). After Hurricane Hugo, older adults who experienced disaster injury or threat received as much instrumental and informational support as younger adults, following a pattern of concern; this points to the ability of older adults to draw from their lifetime bank of social support and recruit the support they need in times of stress (Kaniasty & Norris). On the other hand, older adults with property and financial loss in a community affected by similar losses following Hurricane Hugo were less likely to be recognized as needing assistance, following a pattern of neglect (Kaniasty & Norris).

Conceptual Model of Community Preparedness

Figure 7.1 introduces the conceptual model of community preparedness and its relationship to psychological well-being and positive adaptive functioning to promote quality of life. Community preparedness reduces the mental health sequelae of disasters by directly providing knowledge and

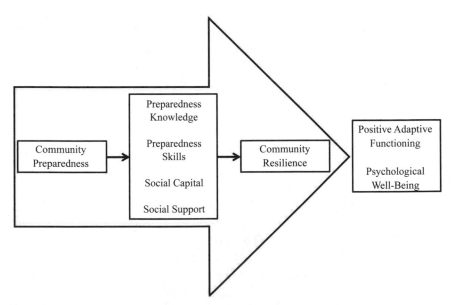

Figure 7.1 Community preparedness conceptual framework.

skills in addition to improving social cohesion, trust, and communication within a community.

In the first stage of the model, community preparedness efforts provide emergency preparedness knowledge to community members and organizations; through discussion and drills in the preparedness planning process, knowledge translates into applicable skills. In addition to tangible skills, the process of planning enhances the community's social capital and social support networks. The coordination of efforts among various stakeholders and engagement with the community creates organizational linkages, extends social support networks, and strengthens existing network ties at many levels in the community. With the explicit participation of the local government, increased synergy between state and society leads to shared goal setting, improved trust, and social cohesion in a community. The community networking prompted by community preparedness planning leads to the actual and perceived availability of support resources in a community, thereby increasing positive psychological functioning. Through the development of knowledge, skills, social capital, and social support, community preparedness efforts lead to community resilience; by planning for an emergency situation, a community develops and harnesses the adaptive networked capacities (Norris, et al., 2008) needed for response. In the last stage of the model, community resilience improves the positive adaptive functioning and psychological well-being of a community at all times, and especially in times of crisis.

MAKING A COMMUNITY PLAN

Federal disaster response plans support short-term recovery following a disaster (FEMA, 2008a), requiring that longer term needs and recovery be assessed and met by the community itself. The development of shared goals, articulated roles, and preparedness resources at the local level is imperative for positive community functioning following a disaster. At their core, community preparedness efforts are a public health intervention; by building and strengthening ties among those from whom disaster response and recovery will be expected, community resilience and capacity will improve, leading to better community health.

The following recommendations outline several ways in which community preparedness can be established through partnership with the many stakeholders in a given community, including older adults, for improved community health.

Define the Role of Community Organizations in Emergency Preparedness and Response

The White House report *Lessons Learned from Hurricane Katrina* recommended the inclusion of nongovernmental organizations (NGOs) in the broader national response effort and called upon state and local governments to "engage NGOs in the planning process, credential their personnel, and provide them the necessary resource support for their involvement in a joint response" (White House, 2006, p. 49). Under the 2008 National Response Framework, nongovernmental organizations and the private sector have designated roles based on the National Incident Management System, a template for emergency response to be used nationwide (FEMA, 2008a). The private sector role is "protecting critical infrastructure systems and implementing plans for the rapid restoration of normal commercial activities and critical infrastructure operations in the event of disruption," and the nongovernmental role is "performing essential service missions in times of need" (FEMA, p. 7). While the National Response Framework emphasizes the need for the systematic integration of the private sector and nongovernmental organizations in its unified, multilayered emergency response, it provides little information on how to integrate these groups in planning or how they will function within the National Incident Management System in an emergency. Ongoing delays in the publication of FEMA's Response Partner Guides, which detail the key roles and actions for these groups, also hinder the ability of communities to implement emergency response plans based on these guidelines or incorporate these groups in existing preparedness efforts (FEMA, 2008a, 2008b).

Provide Preparedness Training
Specific to Community Organizations

To be successful, all partners in the response plan must be trained to meet a baseline level of performance and certification standards (FEMA, 2008a). While many training programs exist for first responders (FEMA, 2008c), new training activities should address the contributions and capacities of nongovernmental and private-sector organizations in emergency preparedness and response and how these organizations will operate within the National Incident Management System.

Recognize the Role of Community and Community Organizations in Preparedness and Recovery

The experience of September 11, 2001, taught us that 90% of those experiencing stress after the World Trade Center attacks sought support from religious and community activities (Schuster, et al., 2001). Community caregivers, including teachers, clergy, and community leaders, are considered *gatekeepers* who serve as a first line of assistance to communities at all times and especially during times of crisis (Neighbors, Musick, & Williams, 1998). For groups who traditionally underutilize mental health services—such as older adults, Black Americans, and those of low socioeconomic status—community outreach is necessary to improve access to care following a disaster (Kaniasty & Norris, 1995; Neighbors, et al.; Van Citters & Bartels, 2004). Recognizing the essential role of community caregiving—such as religious coping and spiritual care—as a first line of mental health response (Roberts, Flannelly, Weaver, & Figley, 2003), and more broadly as a positive element of disaster response (Meisenhelder, 2002), could improve communication between traditional mental health providers and community-recognized mental health providers, thus improving services for entire communities. Additionally, since long-term disaster recovery occurs in the community, recognizing community organizations for their efforts would be a step toward improving group relations with the public health community and the government.

Develop Community Mental Health Programs in Partnership With Community Organizations

Following the 1995 Oklahoma City bombing, an innovative community mental health program was developed to intervene in the short-to-medium term with survivors of this major terrorist event (Call & Pfefferbaum, 1999). Funded by FEMA and the Federal Center for Mental Health Services, which together form the Crisis Counseling Assistance and Training Program (CCP), Project Heartland provided crisis counseling, support groups, outreach, and education for individuals affected by the bombing (Call & Pfefferbaum). While the program was successful, it did encounter some major problems: repeated exposure to trauma and secondary traumatization eroded the staff's morale, the program encountered criticism from professionals because of a "perceived failure to refer individuals in need of more traditional and intensive services," and the program failed to systematically evaluate its effectiveness (Call & Pfefferbaum, p. 955). Nonetheless, when the World Trade Center attacks occurred in 2001, CCP funded a similar short-term program for public education, outreach, and crisis counseling services in New York City named Project Liberty, which, like Project Heartland, did not specialize in long-term mental health treatment (Felton, 2002).

According to program logs, Project Liberty conducted 42,025 service encounters with 91,146 clients between October 2001 and March 2002 (Felton, 2002). The gap in assistance between the number served and the 527,790 New York City area residents projected to experience PTSD as a result of September 11, 2001 (Herman, Felton, & Susser, 2002), signaled the need for community-based and community-centered approaches, in addition to individual-based approaches like Project Liberty, to promote recovery and healing (Vlahov, 2002). While people seemed more willing to seek support services after September 11, 2001, the disconnect between community organizations and the institutions, like Project Liberty, offering such services may explain why only one in three people in the Greater New York area had sought any kind of help or assistance by April 2002 (American Red Cross in Greater New York, 2002).

Develop Procedures for Defusing and Debriefing Community Caregivers

Following a disaster, relief workers may be exposed repeatedly to high levels of trauma and stress and can experience secondary trauma, compassion fatigue, or burnout (Roberts, et al., 2003). Following the World Trade Center attacks on September 11, 2001, the American Red Cross instituted a *shift defusing* system for its spiritual care volunteers that included shift rotations and end-of-shift debriefing for the clergy involved per standard operating procedure (American Red Cross, 1995; Roberts, et al.). A 2002 study of clergy and other disaster relief workers found that participants who volunteered for the American Red Cross in New York City following the World Trade Center attacks had a lower incidence of compassion fatigue compared to those who had volunteered for other relief agencies (Roberts, et al.). The American Red Cross prioritizes the mental health of their volunteers, asserting that the response effort may be compromised if the responders do not function well (Marcus, 2000). Consideration must be given to the extent of the disaster and the length of the recovery processes. Additionally, systems must be developed to protect the mental health of the many individuals involved in the response. Mental health caregivers, traditional first responders, local government, and other community organizations will require caregiver services to prevent fatigue and burnout.

Develop Links and Bridges Between Civic, Business, Academic, Health, and Community Organizations to Build Social Capital

One of the lessons learned after September 11, 2001, was that public health providers must extend beyond health institutions to schools, religious organizations, community groups, the military, and public service organizations to reach the vast majority of the population (Susser, Herman, & Aaron, 2002). Connecting traditional first responders to other service providers in a given community would engage its members and organizations to create a tailored and appropriate plan for public health preparedness and response. It would also empower communities to develop plans based on their assets, competences, and capacities (International Federation of Red Cross and Red Crescent Societies, 2004); improve risk communication, surveillance, and emergency response within communities; build social cohesion; and bolster morale.

Multiagency networking and familiarity must become central features of community preparedness as the collective response to disaster requires coordination by diverse groups at many levels. Fostering a trusting relationship between civic, health, business, academic, and community organizations would improve social capital by creating linkages and extending the reach and capacity of a community's support network. The expectation of exchange and reciprocity between diverse organizations within a community would improve synergy and integrity at the macro level (Woolcock, 1998) and greatly improve the effectiveness of preparedness planning and implementation. By reaching consensus, developing plans of action, practicing skills needed in disaster response, and establishing communication plans, communities will begin to develop the adaptive capacities indicative of community resilience (Norris, et al., 2008). While the process of community preparedness may serve as a catalyst for creating bonds between organizations, these linkages can be harnessed for collective action on other fronts.

Use Community Resources in Innovative Ways to Improve Preparedness

Use Community Organizations as Safe Spaces in Times of Emergency

In times of disaster, workplaces and homes are often not accessible or are uninhabitable, and communications may be disrupted. Religious and service organizations, however, are likely to remain open. After September 11, 2001, many people sought refuge—physical and emotional—in these places. Community organizations may have space to provide, and religious organizations, in particular, have leaders trained in basic counseling. By recognizing these organizations as *safe spaces* during times of emergency, people would be able to visit and receive basic crisis counseling from community members, fostering a sense of cohesion and community with others that could bolster their coping and healing.

House Emergency Supplies in Community Organizations in Exchange for Teaching Community Leaders and Other Caregivers How to Use Them

In the event of a disaster causing mass casualties, the hospital system could be overwhelmed. By housing emergency medical supplies in community organizations, health providers could be dispatched to communities to conduct triage and provide basic health services within the community, thus reducing the stress on the hospital system. Additionally, providing CPR equipment (like automatic defibrillators) and basic first aid training to leaders of community organizations could greatly improve their response efficacy to common health emergencies and empower them to take a more active role in the community's public health efforts.

Include Community Leaders in Emergency Alert Systems to Improve Information Dissemination

Religious and other community leaders have the power to disseminate information to masses of people during services, in bulletins, or through other channels. As a trusted source of information, their messages may be considered more relevant and salient by neglected or hard-to-reach populations such as older persons. Including these caregivers in the distribution list of emergency alert communications would enable them to disseminate applicable information widely and to groups who may not hear it otherwise.

Provide Preparedness Training in Partnership With Community Organizations

The benefit of locating preparedness efforts in the community is the links created among diverse organizations. One way to bring these groups into increasing contact is to identify specific community agencies (e.g., police and fire departments) as preparedness trainers and require local precincts to offer basic preparedness training with community organizations. By moving preparedness training into the community, more individuals will have the opportunity to become engaged in the process and participate actively in community preparedness efforts. By interacting outside of traditional work roles or settings, the agencies designated as preparedness trainers will connect with community stakeholders and gain perspective on community assets, resources, and competencies.

Include Older Adults in Community Preparedness Planning

Older adults bring prior experience, coping strategies, and wisdom to the community preparedness process. In a study of older adults after serious flooding in Kentucky, Norris and Murrell (1988) found that prior experience with a disaster reduced the impact of a subsequent disaster on anxiety. While older adults are not immune to the negative effects of stress, the ability to deal with stressful situations across a lifetime may reflect successful coping strategies. Community efforts would benefit from the wisdom, experience, and perspective of older adults, and older adults would benefit from finding a role in disaster planning and response and in developing their social support networks. While physical disaster recovery work may not be appropriate, older adults are poised to provide other forms of tangible, emotional, informational, and appraisal support to disaster victims (Norris & Murrell; Thompson, et al., 1993). In fact, older persons may be excellent resources for helping to evaluate impairments in disaster victims' quality of life by utilizing methods (Banerjee, Willis, Graham, & Gurland, 2009; Barrett & Gurland, 2001; Gurland & Gurland, 2008a, 2008b) for evaluating restrictions of older victims' choice and choosing processes, thus facilitating the preservation and/or improvement in quality of life during disasters. With an opportunity to provide social support in times of crisis, older adults may be more likely to perceive that assistance will be available to them in crisis and, thus, experience improved psychological health.

The unique perspective of older adults could also inform provisions for special housing, evacuation, and medical needs in preparedness planning. A report on recommendations for best practices in the management of older disaster victims describes the importance of replicating a coordinated community-based caregiving system for older adults during disasters, including preparing portable medical records and developing shelter settings to accommodate their special needs (Baylor College of Medicine & American Medical Association, 2006). A coordinated approach to preparedness for older adults would include the participation of older adults in community-wide disaster planning, the enumeration and location of older adults coordinated by the local emergency operations center prior to a disaster, a unified database of special needs available to all partners in emergency planning and response, and the development of a multilayered support network to ensure the health and safety of older adults in their homes or after evacuation.

SUMMARY

In times of disaster, resources are scarce and groups with the greatest needs, such as older persons and the disabled, are often neglected (Aldrich & Benson, 2008; Gibson, 2006; Kaniasty & Norris, 1995; Thompson, et al., 1993). While a *pattern of concern* may improve the provision of assistance to the most needy in a disaster (Kaniasty & Norris), it does not ensure the mobilization of assistance to older adults as evidenced by the disproportionate burden of mortality among older adults following Hurricane Katrina (Gibson). Embedding older adults within the network of community preparedness will allow for planning to address their unique challenges, incorporate their capacities and competence, and leverage their abilities to call upon long-standing reciprocal relationships for social support.

REFERENCES

AARP. (2006). *Dealing with disaster.* Washington, DC: Author.

Adger, W. N., Hughes, T. P., Folke, C., Carpenter, S. R., & Rockstrom, J. (2005). Social-ecological resilience to coastal disasters. *Science, 309*(573), 1036–1039.

Aldrich, N., & Benson, W. F. (2008). Disaster preparedness and the chronic disease needs of vulnerable older adults. *Preventing Chronic Disease, 5*(1), A27.

American Red Cross. (1995). *Disaster mental health services—Participant workbook.* Washington, DC: Author.

American Red Cross in Greater New York. (2002). *Critical needs in the aftermath of September 11, findings from surveys: Two months and five months later.* New York: Strategic Surveys International.

Banerjee, S., Willis, R., Graham, N., & Gurland, B. J. (2009). The Stroud/ADL Dementia Quality Framework: A cross-national population-level framework for assessing the Quality of life impacts of services and policies for people with dementia and their family carers. *International Journal of Geriatric Psychiatry, 25,* 26–32.

Barrett, V. W., & Gurland, B. J. (2001). A method for advancing quality of life in home care. *Home Health Care Management and Practice, 13*(4), 312–321.

Baylor College of Medicine & American Medical Association. (2006). *Recommendations for best practices in the management of elderly disaster victims.* Washington, DC: Baylor College of Medicine, Harris County Hospital District, American Medical Association, Care for Elders, and AARP.

Call, J. A., & Pfefferbaum, B. (1999). Lessons from the first two years of Project Heartland, Oklahoma's mental health response to the 1995 bombing. *Psychiatric Services, 50*(7), 953–955.

Community Emergency Response Team. (2008). Local certification training. *Community Emergency Response Team (CERT) National Newsletter, 1*(1), 6–8.

Department of Homeland Security. (2008a). *About citizen corps.* Retrieved November 1, 2008, from http://www.citizencorps.gov/about.shtm

Department of Homeland Security. (2008b). *Community Emergency Response Teams (CERT).* Retrieved November 1, 2008, from http://www.citizencorps.gov/cert/index.shtm

Department of Homeland Security. (2008c). *Ready America.* Retrieved October 5, 2008, from http://www.ready.gov/america/index.html

Federal Emergency Management Agency. (2008a). *National response framework* (FEMA Pub. No. P-682). Washington, DC: Author.

Federal Emergency Management Agency. (2008b). *National response framework resource center: Response partner guides.* Retrieved November 23, 2008, from http://www.fema.gov/emergency/nrf/responsepartnerguides.htm

Federal Emergency Management Agency. (2008c). *Training and exercise integration (TEI) course catalog.* Retrieved November 1, 2008, from http://www.fema.gov/pdf/government/training/tei_course_catalog.pdf

Federal Emergency Management Agency. (2008d, June 10, 2008). *Training and exercises.* Retrieved November 1, 2008, from http://www.fema.gov/government/training/index.shtm

Federal Emergency Management Agency, & American Red Cross. (2004, August). *Preparing for disaster for people with disabilities and other special needs* (No. FEMA476 or A4497). Jessup, MD: Federal Emergency Management Agency.

Felton, C. J. (2002). Project Liberty: A public health response to New Yorkers' mental health needs arising from the World Trade Center terrorist attacks. *Journal of Urban Health, 79*(3), 429–433.

Galea, S., Ahern, J., Resnick, H., Kilpatrick, D., Bucuvalas, M., Gold, J., et al. (2002). Psychological sequelae of the September 11 terrorist attacks in New York City. *New England Journal of Medicine, 346*(13), 982–987.

Galea, S., Tracy, M., Norris, F., & Coffey, S. F. (2008). Financial and social circumstances and the incidence and course of PTSD in Mississippi during the first two years after Hurricane Katrina. *Journal of Traumatic Stress, 21*(4), 357–368.

Gibson, M. J. (2006). *We can do better: Lessons learned for protecting older persons in disasters.* Washington, DC: AARP.

Gottlieb, B. H. (1985). Social networks and social support: An overview of research, practice, and policy implications. *Health Education & Behavior, 12*(1), 5.

Gurland, B. J., & Gurland, R.V. (2008a). The choices, choosing model of quality of life: Description and rationale. *International Journal of Geriatric Psychiatry, 24,* 90–95.

Gurland, B. J., & Gurland, R. V. (2008b). The choices, choosing model of quality of life: Linkages to a science base. *International Journal of Geriatric Psychiatry, 24,* 84–89.

Hawe, P., & Shiell, A. (2000). Social capital and health promotion: A review. *Social Science and Medicine, 51*(6), 871–885.

Herman, D., Felton, C., & Susser, E. (2002). Mental health needs in New York State following the September 11th attacks. *Journal of Urban Health, 79*(3), 322–331.

House, J. S. (1981). *Work stress and social support.* Reading, MA: Addison Wesley.

House, J. S., Umberson, D., & Landis, K. R. (1988). Structures and processes of social support. *Annual Reviews in Sociology, 14*(1), 293–318.

International Federation of Red Cross and Red Crescent Societies. (2004). *World disasters report: Focus on community resilience.* Sterling, VA: Kumarian Press.

International Federation of Red Cross and Red Crescent Societies. (2008a). *Disaster management: About disasters.* Retrieved November 1, 2008, from http://www.ifrc.org/what/disasters/about/index.asp

International Federation of Red Cross and Red Crescent Societies. (2008b). *Disaster management: Preparing for disasters.* Retrieved November 1, 2008, from http://www.ifrc.org/what/disasters/preparing/index.asp

Kaniasty, K., & Norris, F. H. (1995). In search of altruistic community: Patterns of social support mobilization following Hurricane Hugo. *American Journal of Community Psychology, 23*(4), 447–477.

Kawachi, I., & Berkman, L. F. (2001). Social ties and mental health. *Journal of Urban Health, 78*(3), 458–467.

Lin, N., Ye, X., & Ensel, W. M. (1999). Social support and depressed mood: A structural analysis. *Journal of Health and Social Behavior, 40*(4), 344–359.

Marcus, E. H. (2000). Disaster mental health services. *The Internet Journal of Rescue and Disaster Medicine, 1*(2).

Meisenhelder, J. B. (2002). Terrorism, posttraumatic stress, and religious coping. *Issues in Mental Health Nursing, 23,* 771–782.

Nakagawa, Y., & Shaw, R. (2004). Social capital: A missing link to disaster recovery. *International Journal of Mass Emergencies and Disasters, 22*(1), 5–34.

Neighbors, H. W., Musick, M. A., & Williams, D. R. (1998). The African American minister as a source of help for serious personal crises: Bridge or barrier to mental health care? *Health Education and Behavior, 25*(6), 759–777.

Norris, F. H. (2002). Disasters in urban context. *Journal of Urban Health, 79*(3), 308–314.

Norris, F. H., Friedman, M. J., & Watson, P. J. (2002). 60,000 disaster victims speak: Part II. Summary and implications of the disaster mental health research. *Psychiatry, 65*(3), 240–260.

Norris, F. H., Friedman, M. J., Watson, P. J., Byrne, C. M., Diaz, E., & Kaniasty, K. (2002). 60,000 disaster victims speak: Part I. An empirical review of the empirical literature, 1981–2001. *Psychiatry, 65*(3), 207–239.

Norris, F. H., & Kaniasty, K. (1996). Received and perceived social support in times of stress: A test of the social support deterioration deterrence model. *Journal of Personality and Social Psychology, 71*(3), 498–511.

Norris, F. H., & Murrell, S. A. (1988). Prior experience as a moderator of disaster impact on anxiety symptoms in older adults. *American Journal of Community Psychology, 16*(5), 665–683.

Norris, F. H., Stevens, S. P., Pfefferbaum, B., Wyche, K. F., & Pfefferbaum, R. L. (2008). Community resilience as a metaphor, theory, set of capacities, and strategy for disaster readiness. *American Journal of Community Psychology, 41*(1–2), 127–150.

North, C. S., & Hong, B. A. (2000). Project CREST: A new model for mental health intervention after a community disaster. *American Journal of Public Health, 90*(7), 1057–1058.

Office of Domestic Preparedness. (2002). *Emergency responder guidelines.* Washington, DC: Office of Justice Programs.

Perry, R. W., & Lindell, M. K. (2003). Preparedness for emergency response: Guidelines for the emergency planning process. *Disasters, 27*(4), 336–350.

Phifer, J. F., Kaniasty, K. Z., & Norris, F. H. (1988). The impact of natural disaster on the health of older adults: A multiwave prospective study. *Journal of Health and Social Behavior, 29*(1), 65–78.

Roberts, R. S. B., Flannelly, K. J., Weaver, A. J., & Figley, C. R. (2003). Compassion fatigue among chaplains, clergy, and other respondents after September 11th. *The Journal of Nervous and Mental Disease, 191*(11), 756.

Schuster, M. A., Stein, B. D., Jaycox, L., Collins, R. L., Marshall, G. N., Elliott, M. N., et al. (2001). A national survey of stress reactions after the September 11, 2001 terrorist attacks. *New England Journal of Medicine, 345*(20), 1507–1512.

Simpson, D. M. (2002). Earthquake drills and simulations in community-based training and preparedness programmes. *Disasters, 26*(1), 55–69.

Susser, E. S., Herman, D. B., & Aaron, B. (2002). Combating the terror of terrorism. *Scientific American, 287*(2), 70–77.

Thompson, M. P., Norris, F. H., & Hanacek, B. (1993). Age differences in the psychological consequences of hurricane Hugo. *Psychology and Aging, 8*(4), 606–616.

Van Citters, A. D., & Bartels, S. J. (2004). A systematic review of the effectiveness of community-based mental health outreach services for older adults. *Psychiatric Services, 55*(11), 1237–1249.

Vlahov, D. (2002). Urban disaster: A population perspective. *Journal of Urban Health, 79*(3), 295.

The White House. (2006, February). *The federal response to Hurricane Katrina: Lessons learned* (Report to the president of the United States). Retrieved October 5, 2008, from http://www.whitehouse.gov/reports/katrina-lessons-learned/

Woolcock, M. (1998). Social capital and economic development: Toward a theoretical synthesis and policy framework. *Theory and Society, 27*(2), 151–208.

8

Self-Help Tools for Older Persons and Their Caregivers

NINA TUMOSA

In 2006, 37 million people aged 65 and over—or just over 12% of the total population—lived in the United States (National Center for Health Statistics, 2008). Their median age was reported as 74.8 years (U.S. Census Bureau, 2009). The size of the oldest-old population—those aged 85 and over—was just over 5.3 million. Once all of the Baby Boomer generation—those born between 1946 and 1964—reach or surpass age 65 in 2030, the proportion of people aged 65 and over will remain relatively stable at around 20% of the population, even though the absolute number of people in that cohort will continue to grow. The oldest-old population is projected to grow rapidly after 2030 as the Baby Boomers move into this age category.

The portion of the U.S. population who are more than 65 years old, a population whose ages span almost 50 years, are not a homogeneous group, but as a group they do differ from the overall U.S. population in many significant ways as presented in Table 8.1.

Compared to the overall population, they are more likely to be female, White, widowed, disabled, living alone, living in the same house as the previous year, owning their home, a veteran, disabled, and foreign born. Older persons are less likely to have a high school diploma and be in the labor force but are also less likely to live in poverty. About 4.3% reside in a nursing

Table 8.1

COMPARISON OF CHARACTERISTICS OF THE TOTAL U.S. POPULATION AND THE POPULATION AGE 65 AND OVER

SUBJECT	TOTAL POPULATION	≥65 POPULATION
Female	50.8%	58.0%
Average age	36.4 years	74.8 years
White race	74.1%	85.2%
Living alone	27.3%	44.9%
Widowed	6.4%	31.6%
Living in same house as last year	83.4%	93.1%
Owning their house	57.5%	88.4%
Veteran status	10.4%	24.5%
Disabled	15.1%	40.9%
Less than high school education	16.0%	27.2%
Foreign born	12.5%	13.0%
Speak English less than "very well"	8.6%	8.1%
In the labor force	64.5%	14.5%
Living in poverty	13.3%	9.9%

From U.S. Census Bureau, 2009. *Population 65 years and over in the United States, 2005–2007 American Community Survey 3-year estimates* (Table S0103).

home at any one time, some only temporarily for rehabilitation from injury or surgery. Eighty-five percent live without any disability, and 80% live at or above 150% of the poverty level. Seventy-five percent are White, and 12% are African American. Only 8.6% do not speak English very well.

No single aforementioned trait marks a person as having a reduced quality of life, but the existence of multiple traits does tend to increase a person's chances of requiring assistance to live safely. Approximately 20% of the community-dwelling older population of the United States is vulnerable older persons aged 65 and older who are considered at increased risk of functional decline or death over 2 years (Saliba, et al, 2001; Wenger, et al, 2003). In addition, the 4.3% of older persons living in nursing homes at any one time are also vulnerable (Pandya, 2001).

Therefore, about one quarter of all persons age 65 or older should be considered to be unable to provide self-help during an emergency or disaster. Many of these vulnerable older persons, especially those over age 85, have informal unpaid caregivers.

Interestingly, many of these caregivers are over age 65 themselves (Spillman & Black, 2005). This underscores the fact that during an emergency or disaster, 75% of all persons aged 65 or older are available not only to provide self-help but also to assist vulnerable elders and otherwise provide assistance and guidance as required.

Most individuals regardless of age or level of disability are resilient; when faced with disaster or adversity they manage to recover functionally and psychologically. Some, however, experience prolonged episodes of hopelessness, helplessness, and PTSD (Blcich, Gclkopf, & Solomon, 2003; Maguen, Papa, & Litz, 2008). They require assistance with developing successful coping strategies. Strategies that increase feelings of self-sufficiency (Bleich, Gelkopf, & Solomon) and normal routine (Maguen, Papa, & Litz) are thought to contribute to recovery.

This chapter presents examples of self-help programs that have been used successfully to promote optimal health, assess the likelihood of recurrence of disease, and manage disease. Ideas will be presented about self-help tools that can be easily adopted to assist vulnerable older persons to prepare for, survive during, and recover from disasters or emergencies. This chapter is dedicated to those vulnerable older persons who do not recover easily from disasters.

DETERIORATION OF HEALTH RESULTING FROM DISASTERS OR EMERGENCIES

Resiliency is defined as a process by which persons cope and acquire skills that allow them to overcome adversity (Gerrard, Kulig, & Nowatzki, 2004) and can be easily measured (Connor, 2006). Even under normal circumstances, older persons are not as resilient as younger persons because of their reduced reserve capacity (Finkelstein, Petkun, Freedman, & Antopol, 1983; Katz, et al., 2004). Older persons are more likely to die of infectious diseases than are younger persons (Morens, Folkers, & Fauci, 2004). A compromised immune system makes older persons more susceptible to stress, regardless of the source (Barakat, et al., 2002; Bradley,

1999; Helget & Smith, 2002; Katz, et al.; Madjid & Casscels, 2004; Salerno & Nagy, 2002; Solana & Mariani, 2000). Even as long as 2 years post trauma, the physical and psychological well-being of victims are affected (Maltais, et al., 2000).

Victims of emergencies or disasters are more likely to rate their overall health as poor or average than are nonvictims and are also more likely to present with more symptoms of posttraumatic stress and higher levels of depression and anxiety. These symptoms are exacerbated by prior trauma and poverty (Chen, et al., 2007), language and cultural differences between victims and rescuers (Shiu-Thornton, Balabis, Senturia, Tamayo, & Oberle, 2007), economic loss (Acierno, Ruggiero, Kilpatrick, Resnick, & Galea, 2006), displacement (Acierno, et al., 2007; Chung, Dennis, Easthope, Farmer, & Werrett, 2005), and preexisting health conditions (Somasundaram & van de Put, 2006). Strong social support prior to the emergency or disaster protects against deteriorating physical and mental health (Acierno, et al., 2007; Lating & Bono, 2008), as does a perceived degree of control over events (Gerrard, Kulig, & Nowatzki, 2004). One approach that has been used successfully is self-help programs, which provide persons with increased control over their medical conditions.

SELF-HELP MODELS IN MEDICINE

Self-help programs have a respectable history in the management of medical conditions. Many of the programs consist of small interactive groups led by trained professionals and are designed to encourage sharing personal experiences and improving health literacy about a disease. Well-known self-help groups of this type include the 12-step model for dealing with overcoming different types of addictions, such as Alcoholics Anonymous, Eating Orders Anonymous, and Nicotine Anonymous. The effectiveness of such 12-step programs at sustaining behavior change has been confirmed (Vederhus & Kristensen, 2006).

Other programs are more educational and concentrate on teaching participants to manage chronic diseases by showing them how to actively participate in their own health care, work more effectively with their health care providers, and handle the day-to-day challenges of their disease. Arthritis is a disease for which an effective self-help program with sustained health benefits and reduced medical costs has been developed (Arthritis Foundation, 2007; Kowarsky & Glazier, 1997; Lorig, Mazonson, & Holman, 1993). Outcomes for the participants of the arthritis self-help groups include increased knowledge about their disease, increased self-confidence, decreased feelings of isolation and depression, decreased pain, and decreased physician visits.

The value of self-help groups for eating disorders is not as clear, and the level of perceived success may depend upon the goal of the group. A self-help program with face-to-face counseling sessions has been shown to be less effective than a structured commercial program for weight loss in overweight and obese people (Heshka, et al., 2003). However, active participation in an online program for the prevention of eating disorders shows promise in predicting reduced levels of eating disorder attitudes and behaviors (Manwaring, et al., 2008). A study of group-based lifestyle programs on obesity management (Pettman, et al., 2008) showed improvements in body composition and cardio-metabolic and physical fitness that were similar to one-on-one interventions, which are more resource-intensive to deliver. The study concluded that programs were more successful if they included social support and self-management techniques.

SELF-CARE PROGRAMS

Many self-care programs do not rely upon group participation but involve a person acting alone or in conjunction with a caregiver. A comprehensive Tool Chest of assistive tools for diabetics with hearing, manual, and visual disabilities (Bartos, et al., 2008) can be accessed privately by diabetic patients to make them self-sufficient in their disease management. The tool chest includes such information as where to locate blood glucose monitors, magnifiers for syringes and pumps, injection devices, and talking label prescriptions, as well as lists of relevant phone numbers and Web sites. Another promising new assessment tool is the Therapy-Related Symptom Checklist, an innovative checklist for cancer patients. A study by Williams and colleagues (2006) suggests this checklist gives patients the opportunity to play an important role in their own comfort care and pain management. Users of the checklist reported it gave them a sense of structure that helped them cope with their illnesses and treatments.

Self-rated instruments for patients suffering from mental trauma have also been shown to be useful in disease management. Several self-report instruments that can be used on patients with depression—for example, the Zung Self-Rating Depression Scale (Zung, Richards, & Short, 1965) or, with suicide ideation, the Hopelessness Scale (Beck, Weissman, Lester, & Trexler, 1974)—are described by Valente and Saunders (2005). Because these tools rely upon self-report, informal caregivers can easily administer them to their charges to determine depression or suicide risk. The information can then be shared with health care providers. These instruments have been shown to improve clinical decision making because of improved patient/provider communication and the ability of the patient to know when to seek professional care because a crisis is looming (Valente & Saunders).

Zimmerman and colleagues (2006) have developed and validated a brief, single-item assessment of three domains important to consider when treating depressed patients: symptom severity, psychosocial functioning, and quality of life. The assessment was determined not to be burdensome for patients to complete, and informal caregivers can administer it. Patient providers reported that the patient-administered assessment was incorporated easily into clinical practice and was used to collect data on treatment effectiveness. Postal questionnaires (delivered by mail) that require patients to self-report depressive symptoms have been shown to be as effective as questionnaires administered by physicians (Mallen & Peat, 2008). Self-rated instruments are now available for individuals who are at risk for the development of PTSD (Connor, Foa, & Davidson, 2006).

Web-based self-help therapy is also popular with people with anxiety disorders (Farvolden, Denisoff, Selby, Bagby, & Rudy, 2005). Participants self-report on screening questionnaires and then complete dynamic sessions weekly. Upon completion, they are asked to self-report on a second screening assessment and are encouraged to continue to use an online diary and support group along with individualized email support. This program has been shown to reduce panic attack frequency and severity. Depression self-help and information programs can be delivered effectively online (Griffiths & Christensen, 2007).

FOSTERING RESILIENCY

Morbidity and mortality can be minimized by enhancing and promoting resilience (Lating & Bono, 2008; Nucifora, Langlieb, Siegal, Everly, & Kaminsky, 2007). Fostering resiliency in older persons concerning disasters can occur along a disaster timeline by developing confidence inspired by careful precrisis preparation (Boscarino, Figley, & Adams, 2003), developing interventions early in a crisis (Lating & Bono), carefully monitoring persons and their health post crisis (Bryant, 2006; Chung, Werrett, Easthope, & Farmer, 2004; Connor, 2006), and encouraging victims to confront their trauma (Foa, 2006). Confidence heightens resiliency, and there is a need for confidence building in emergency preparedness. Currently, there is little confidence that health care systems in the community (Alexander, Larkin, & Wynia, 2006), in hospitals (O'Sullivan, et al., 2008), or in nursing homes (Castro, Persson, Bergstrom, & Cron, 2008) are well prepared for natural or man-made disasters. Therefore, there is an overwhelming need to develop individualized tools as part of the older person's overall emergency plans. These tools can help individuals better control fear levels (Boscarino, Figley, & Adams, 2003; Salcioğlu & Başoğlu, 2008), minimize disruption in their quality of life (Ross & Bing, 2007), enhance personal safety (Johnson, et al., 2006), provide peace of mind (Blessman, et al., 2007), provide culturally and ethnically appropriate information (Bryant & Njenga, 2006; Carter-Pokras, Zambrana, Mora, & Aaby, 2007; Constantine, Alleyne, Caldwell, McRae, & Suzuki, 2005; Eisenman, et al., 2006), and improve coping with posttraumatic stress (Chung, Werrett, Easthope, & Farmer), including reducing the stigma of mental health problems (Carlos-Otero & Njenga, 2006). Each of these components plays an important role in decreasing morbidity and mortality in the older population both during and after a crisis.

In order to ensure these individualized self-help tools will be used, they should be developed with input from older persons (Arsand & Demiris, 2008). Several such programs have been developed already, although few have been studied for long-term effectiveness. For example, four community-based emergency preparedness programs have been developed in Canada, and two have been successfully tested during a crisis (PHAC, 2008). These programs all use older persons as community resources by including them in the planning, development, promotion, and execution of community-wide disaster preparedness plans that both engage and empower older persons.

Red River, Manitoba, a rural farming community, developed a District Guardian Program in 2004. This program maintains a database that identifies residents, their special needs, and available resources. Community members were included in the planning stages so everyone participated in providing information for the database. This system was tested during a flood that threatened the town's water supply in 2007 and worked well to maintain order and a sense of control (PHAC, 2008).

The Groupe d'Action Communautaire de Sante Benevole (GACSB) in Ferland-et-Boillear, Quebec, works to improve the quality of life for the town's citizens. The GACSB played a pivotal role in a flood in 1996 by serving as a liaison between older persons and authorities. Older persons play a critical role in running the GACSB (PHAC, 2008).

St. Christopher House, a community-based program, has been in Toronto, Ontario, since 1912. Because of the multicultural and multilingual nature of its clients, St. Christopher House must communicate with its clients through a multitude of formats. The three most successful formats by which programming in emergency preparedness is delivered by and to older persons include a Health Action Theatre (HATS), which puts on a nonverbal play about emergency preparedness; a program called In the Picture, which provides translation services about disasters for older persons; and a program called Group Effective Leadership, which shows older persons how to provide responsible leadership during emergencies (PHAC, 2008).

For Seniors, By Seniors, a project in Winnipeg, Manitoba, was created to foster resiliency and community networks for older persons. The program focuses on developing support networks with senior groups. Its goal is to reduce the burden on the 911 system during a crisis. Elements of the project include a 30-minute presentation on disaster intended to inform rather than alarm older persons. Another component involves seniors assembling older person–specific home survival kits (PHAC, 2008).

All these programs are examples of how older persons are taught to be providers and first responders during emergencies. These are also examples of training that targets older persons and is provided by older persons themselves. The social networks supporting these training programs ensure compliance with the training.

Certain tools have been developed to enhance independence in frail older persons. The successful adoption of these tools relies upon a somewhat different social dynamic, usually that of family pressure. These tools include the Vial of LIFE (Lifesaving Information for Emergencies; Vial of LIFE Project, 2006), a container that often resembles a prescription bottle but may also look like a bifold wallet. This container contains preprinted forms for recording medical information such as the individual's medical condition, prescriptions, and allergies. This allows critical emergency medical information to be found in a single place. The container can be stored in the refrigerator, in a purse or wallet, or in the glove compartment of an automobile. Indeed, copies of the vial and its contents can be kept in all of these places, thereby enabling health professionals to access the information regardless of where the emergency takes place. The Vial of LIFE Project has a mission of donating the vials to all seniors. The forms can be downloaded from the Internet for no cost. The perceived value of this program can be appreciated by an Internet search on "Vial of Life." Thousands of examples of Vial of LIFE programs that have been adopted by Boy Scout troops, hospitals, Area Agencies of Aging, and fire departments are available for review.

Medical alert services, of which Lifeline® is the best recognized, are telephone-based systems designed to summon help for homebound people who are injured and unable to help themselves. In the event of a fall or other emergency, the wearer pushes a button to activate a telephone call to an agency, which summons local assistance previously identified by the person in distress. This system is designed to extend the social network of isolated older persons through technology. Even though there are no research papers studying its effectiveness, many copycat programs have been developed, suggesting a demand for such programs. What amount of the demand is from concerned family members rather than the users themselves is undocumented.

Another person-centered tool, endorsed by the Red Cross Web site (http://www.redcross.org/general/0,1082,0_91_4440,00.html), is the emergency preparedness kit. The Web site provides instructions on creating kits for several different populations. None are specifically for older persons, but there is an ability to mix and match components. Emergency kits for older persons should be compact, light, and user specific (Tumosa, 2004). They must contain at least one week's worth of medications, information about health care and social contacts, and safety products like flashlights, name badges, and reflectors. The Red Cross in St. Louis, Missouri, has developed a peer group train-the-trainer program where older persons educate other groups of older persons on how to assemble such kits. A quality improvement study that looked at the effectiveness of a Gateway Geriatric Education Center train-the-trainer model for encouraging the production of these kits uncovered an unexpected patient outcome (Bales & Tumosa, 2009). Those who received the training were given two kits: one to use when training others and the other to give to an older person of their choice. Nine months later, the trainers reported that the recipients of their kits used them when they went to emergency shelters during three extended power outages. In addition, the trainers themselves reported using their training kits in order to feel more secure when traveling back and forth to work on icy roads during those times of crisis. This suggests that the presence of the kits increased confidence in personal safety.

One resource that can be used to encourage older persons to use self-help tools is the public service announcement (PSA). A very effective use of PSAs has been developed by the U.S. Department of Veterans Affairs (VA) (2009). The VA is distributing to its veterans, of which over

50% are age 65 or older, a 2009 Salute to Our Veterans calendar. The 2009 calendar has 12 PSAs that address issues such as accessing the VA Web site for health information, using an emergency kit, and accessing supportive information about dealing with combat stress and suicidal thoughts. The overall message of the calendar is that veterans are part of a valued community and that the VA is there to help them in a crisis. This is a powerful message designed to increase self-confidence and foster independence.

Communication before, during, and after a crisis is paramount for reducing panic and promoting resiliency. This communication should be culturally appropriate, easy to understand, and readily accessible (Severance & Yeo, 2006). Several exemplary projects in emergency preparedness are presented in the "Workshop Report" (PHAC, 2008). St. Christopher House uses its HATS program to provide community-based, culturally sensitive, participatory education targeted at and provided by older persons. The IDEAS network (http://www.ideasnetwork.ca) is a Web-based education project on emergency preparedness and victim-focused care in Toronto. For Seniors, By Seniors in Winnipeg provides peer-support group training in preparedness. These programs set up an extended community of individuals who will work together and form support for one another in an emergency.

The Internet is another community that provides its users with disaster preparedness information. Several agencies provide this Web-based information. FEMA (http://www.fema.gov/) provides online information on disasters for families and individuals. Specifically, there is information on planning ahead and protecting family and property on the FEMA "Prepare for a Disaster" page (2009b), as well as information on how to receive assistance during a crisis on the FEMA "Apply for Assistance" page (2009a), the immediate recovery, and information on rebuilding after a disaster strikes on the FEMA "Recover and Rebuild" page (2009c). All states and U.S. territories also have Web sites dedicated to emergency preparedness. However, most of the information available online is not specific for older persons. The Ohio Valley Appalachia Regional Geriatric Education Centers (OVAR GEC) have developed a Web site (2009) specific to the care of the older patient. The Web site provides online training about emergency preparedness programs that target the needs of older persons (Johnson, et al., 2006).

Internet-based information is easily accessed by experienced computer users, young and old alike. However, older persons often do not have access to a computer or do not have adequate skills to operate one.

Computer classes at community colleges and other community-based educational programs are effective resources for older persons to acquire computer and Internet skills.

SUMMARY

Many tools designed to aid older persons in planning for as well as surviving crises and then rebuilding their lives already exist. New tools are always welcome additions to the armamentarium because of the need for appropriate cultural, ethnic, and language-specific content. Because of health literacy concerns for some older persons, particularly those of lower income, tools such as picture boards, which do not rely on written language, are helpful. The color coding of terrorist attack threat levels—with green, blue, yellow, orange, and red indicating increasing levels of threat—is an excellent example of a pictorial display, but even this does not work for color-blind individuals.

Emergency preparedness, like so many other public health programs, is a constantly evolving system of threats and responses. As our knowledge and sophistication about disasters and emergencies change, so must our tools to respond properly. Self-help tools must be easy to use by affected individuals or by informal, untrained, or minimally trained caregivers. Self-help tools should be designed in consultation with older persons. Finally, self-help tools need to be as universal as possible. The catch phrases for the creation of new self-help tools in emergency preparedness must be to stay constantly vigilant to new threats and opportunities, to involve older people in the process, and to promote their self-confidence and independence.

REFERENCES

Acierno, R., Ruggiero, K. J., Kilpatrick, D. G., Resnick, H. S., & Galea, S. (2006). Risk and protective factors for psychopathology among older versus younger adults after the 2004 Florida hurricanes. *The American Journal of Geriatric Psychiatry, 14*, 1051–1059.

Acierno, R., Ruggiero, K. J., Galea, S., Resnick, H. S., Koenen, K., Roitzsch, J., et al. (2007). Psychological sequelae resulting from the 2004 Florida hurricanes: Implications for postdisaster intervention. *American Journal of Public Health, 97*(Suppl. 1), S103–108.

Alexander, G. C., Larkin, C. L., & Wynia, M. K. (2006). Physicians' preparedness for bioterrorism and other public health priorities. *Academic Emergency Medicine, 13*(11), 1238–1241.

Arthritis Foundation. (2007). *Arthritis Foundation self-help program.* Retrieved January 6, 2009, from http://www.arthritis.org/self-help-program.php

Arsand, E., & Demiris, G. (2008). User-centered methods for designing patient-centered self-help tools. *Informatics for Health & Social Care, 33*(3), 158–169.

Bales, C., & Tumosa, N. (2009). Minimizing the impact of complex emergencies on nutrition and geriatric health: Planning for Prevention is key. In C. W. Bales & C. S. Ritchie (Eds.), *Handbook of clinical nutrition and aging* (2nd ed., pp. 635–654). New York: Humana Press.

Barakat, L. A., Quentzel, H. L., Jernigan, J. A., Kirschke, D. L., Griffith, K., Spear, S. M., et al. (2002). Anthrax Bioterrorism Investigation Team. Fatal inhalational anthrax in a 94-year-old Connecticut woman. *The Journal of the American Medical Association, 287*(7), 898–900.

Bartos, B. J., Cleary, M. E., Kleinbeck, C., Petzinger, R. A., Sokol-McKay, D. A., Whittington, A., et al. (2008). Diabetes and disabilities: Assistive tools, services, and information. *The Diabetes Educator, 34*(4), 597–598, 600, 603–605.

Beck, A. T., Weissman, A., Lester, D., & Trexler, L. (1974). The measurement of pessimism: The hopelessness scale. *Journal of Consulting and Clinical Psychology, 42*(6), 861–865.

Bleich, A., Gelkopf, M., & Solomon, Z. (2003). Exposure to terrorism, stress-related mental health symptoms, and coping behaviors among a nationally representative sample in Israel. *The Journal of the American Medical Association, 290*(5), 612–620.

Blessman, J., Skupski, J., Jamil, M., Jamil, H., Bassett, D., Wabeke, R., et al. (2007). Barriers to at-home-preparedness in public health employees: Implications for disaster preparedness training. *Journal of Occupational and Environmental Medicine, 49*(3), 318–326.

Boscarino, J. A., Figley, C. R., & Adams, R. E. (2003). Fear of terrorism in New York after the September 11 terrorist attacks: Implications for emergency mental health and preparedness. *International Journal of Emergency Mental Health, 5*(4), 199–209.

Bradley, S. F. (1999). Prevention of influenza in long-term-care facilities. Long-Term-Care Committee of the Society for Healthcare Epidemiology of America. *Infection Control and Hospital Epidemiology, 20*(9), 629–637.

Bryant, R. A. (2006). Recovery after the tsunami: Timeline for rehabilitation. *Journal of Clinical Psychiatry, 67*(Suppl. 2), 50–55.

Bryant, R. A., & Njenga, F. G. (2006). Cultural sensitivity: Making trauma assessment and treatment plans culturally relevant. *Journal of Clinical Psychiatry, 67*(Suppl. 2), 74–79.

Carlos-Otero, J., & Njenga, F. G. (2006). Lessons in posttraumatic stress disorder from the past: Venezuela floods and Nairobi bombing. *Journal of Clinical Psychiatry, 67*(Suppl. 2), 56–63.

Carter-Pokras, O., Zambrana, R. E., Mora, S. E., & Aaby, K. A. (2007). Emergency preparedness: Knowledge and perceptions of Latin American immigrants. *Journal of Health Care for the Poor and Underserved, 18*(2), 465–481.

Castro, C., Persson, D., Bergstrom, N., & Cron, S. (2008). Surviving the storms: Emergency preparedness in Texas nursing facilities and assisted living facilities. *Journal of Gerontological Nursing, 34*(8), 9–16.

Chen, A. C., Keith, V. M., Leong, K. J., Airriess, C., Li, W., Chung, K. Y., et al. (2007). Hurricane Katrina: Prior trauma, poverty, and health among Vietnamese-American survivors. *International Nursing Review, 54*(4), 324–331.

Chung, M. C., Dennis, I., Easthope, Y., Farmer, S. & Werrett, J. (2005). Differentiating posttraumatic stress between elderly and younger residents. *Psychiatry, 68*(2), 164–173.

Chung, M. C., Werrett, J., Easthope, Y., & Farmer, S. (2004). Coping with post-traumatic stress: Young, middle-aged, and elderly comparisons. *International Journal of Geriatric Psychiatry, 19*(4), 333–343.

Connor, K. M. (2006). Assessment of resilience in the aftermath of trauma. *Journal of Clinical Psychiatry, 67*(Suppl. 2), 46–49.

Connor, K. M., Foa, E. B., & Davidson, J. R. (2006). Practical assessment and evaluation of mental health problems following a mass disaster. *Journal of Clinical Psychiatry, 67*(Suppl. 2), 26–33.

Constantine, M. G., Alleyne, V. L., Caldwell, L. D., McRae, M. B., & Suzuki, L. A. (2005). Coping responses of Asian, Black, and Latino/Latina New York City residents following the September 11, 2001 terrorist attacks against the United States. *Cultural Diversity & Ethnic Minority Psychology, 11*(4), 293–308.

Eisenman, D. P., Wold, C., Fielding, J., Long, A., Setodji, C., Hickey, S., et al. (2006). Differences in individual-level terrorism preparedness in Los Angeles County. *American Journal of Preventive Medicine, 30*(1), 1–6.

Farvolden, P., Denisoff, E., Selby, P., Bagby, R. M., & Rudy, L. (2005). Usage and longitudinal effectiveness of a Web-based self-help cognitive behavioral therapy program for panic disorder. *Journal of Medical Internet Research, 7*(1), e7.

Federal Emergency Management Agency. (2009a). *Apply for assistance.* Retrieved July 10, 2009, from http://www.fema.gov/assistance/index.shtm

Federal Emergency Management Agency. (2009b). *Prepare for a disaster.* Retrieved July 10, 2009, from http://www.fema.gov/plan/index.shtm

Federal Emergency Management Agency. (2009c). *Recover and rebuild.* Retrieved July 10, 2009, from http://www.fema.gov/rebuild/index.shtm

Finkelstein, M. S., Petkun, W. M., Freedman, M. L., & Antopol, S. C. (1983). Pneumococcal bacteremia in adults: Age-dependent differences in presentation and in outcome. *Journal of the American Geriatrics Society, 31*(1), 19–27.

Foa, E. B. (2006). Psychosocial therapy for posttraumatic stress disorder. *Journal of Clinical Psychiatry, 67*(Suppl. 2), 40–45.

Gerrard, N., Kulig, J., & Nowatzki, N. (2004). What doesn't kill you makes you stronger: Determinants of stress resiliency in rural people of Saskatchewan, Canada. *The Journal of Rural Health, 20*(1), 59–66.

Griffiths, K. M., & Christensen, H. (2007). Internet-based mental health programs: A powerful tool in the rural medical kit. *The Australian Journal of Rural Health, 15*(2), 81–87.

Helget, V., & Smith, P. W. (2002). Bioterrorism preparedness: A survey of Nebraska health care institutions. *American Journal of Infection Control, 30*(1), 46–48.

Heshka, S., Anderson, J. W., Atkinson, R. L., Greenway, F. L., Hill, J. O., Phinney, S. D., et al. (2003). Weight loss with self-help compared with a structured commercial program: A randomized trial. *The Journal of the American Medical Association, 289,* 1792–1798.

Johnson, A., Howe, J. L., McBride, M. R., Palmisano, B. R., Perweiler, E. A., Roush, R. E., et al. (2006). Bioterrorism and emergency preparedness in aging (BTEPA): HRSA-funded GEC collaboration for curricula and training. *Gerontology & Geriatrics Education, 26*(4), 63–86.

Katz, J. M., Plowden, J., Renshaw-Hoelscher, M., Lu, X., Tumpey, T. M., & Sambhara, S. (2004). Immunity to influenza: The challenges of protecting an aging population. *Immunologic Research, 29*(1–3), 113–124.

Kowarsky, A., & Glazier, S. (1997). Development of skills for coping with arthritis: An innovative group approach. *Arthritis Care and Research, 10*(2), 121–127.

Lating, J. M., & Bono, S. F. (2008). Crisis intervention and fostering resiliency. *International Journal of Emergency Mental Health, 10*(2), 87–93.

Lorig, K., Mazonson, P., & Holman, H. R. (1993). Evidence suggesting that health education for self-management in patients with chronic arthritis has sustained health benefits while reducing health care costs. *Arthritis and Rheumatism, 36*(4), 439–446.

Madjid, M., & Casscells, W. (2004). Influenza as a bioterror threat: The need for global vaccination. *Expert Opinion on Biological Therapy, 4*(3), 265–267.

Maguen, S., Papa, A., & Litz, B. T. (2008). Coping with the threat of terrorism: A review. *Anxiety, Stress, and Coping, 21*(1), 15–35.

Mallen, C. D., & Peat, G. (2008). Screening older people with musculoskeletal pain for depressive symptoms in primary care. *The British Journal of General Practice, 58*(555), 688–693.

Maltais, D., Lachance, L., Fortin, M., Lalande, G., Robichaud, S., Fortin, C., et al. (2000). Psychological and physical health of the July 1996 disaster victims: A comparative study between victims and non-victims. *Sante Mentale au Quebec, 25*(1), 116–137.

Manwaring, J. L., Bryson, S. W., Goldschmidt, A. B., Winzelberg, A. J., Luce, K. H., Cunning, D., et al. (2008). Do adherence variables predict outcome in an online program for the prevention of eating disorders? *Journal of Consulting and Clinical Psychology, 76*(2), 341–346.

Morens, D. M., Folkers, G. K., & Fauci, A. S. (2004). The challenge of emerging and re-emerging infectious diseases. *Nature, 430*(6996), 242–249.

Nucifora Jr., F., Langlieb, A. M., Siegal, E., Everly Jr., G. S., & Kaminsky, M. (2007). Building resistance, resilience, and recovery in the wake of school and workplace violence. *Disaster Medicine and Public Health Preparedness, 1*(Suppl. 1), S33–37.

National Center for Health Statistics. (2008). *Older Americans 2008: Key indicators of well being.* Retrieved January 9, 2009, from http://www.agingstats.gov/agingstatsdot net/Main_Site/Data/Data_2008.aspx

The Ohio Valley Appalachia Regional Geriatric Education Centers. (2009). *Bioterrorism and emergency preparedness.* Retrieved July 10, 2009, from http://www.mc.uky.edu/ aging/bioterrorism_and_emergency_preparedness.html

O'Sullivan, T. L., Dow, D., Turner, M. C., Lemyre, L., Corneil, W., Krewski, D., et al. (2008). Disaster and emergency management: Canadian nurses' perceptions of preparedness on hospital front lines. *Prehospital and Disaster Medicine, 23*(3), 11–18.

Pandya, S. (2001). *Nursing homes fact sheet.* Retrieved January 4, 2009, from http://www. aarp.org/research/longtermcare/nursinghomes/aresearch-import-669-FS10R.html

Pettman, T. L., Misan, G. M., Owen, K., Warren, K., Coates, A. M., & Buckley, J. D. (2008). Self-management for obesity and cardio-metabolic fitness: Description and evaluation of the lifestyle modification program of a randomised controlled trial. *The International Journal of Behavioral Nutrition and Physical Activity, 27,* 53.

Public Health Agency of Canada. (2008). *Workshop report.* Second International Workshop on Seniors and Emergency Preparedness, Winnipeg, Manitoba. Retrieved January 8, 2009, from http://www.phac-aspc.gc.ca/seniors-aines/alt_formats/pdf/pubs/emergency-urgence-eng.pdf

Ross, K. L., & Bing, C. M. (2007). Emergency management: Expanding the disaster plan. *Home Healthcare Nurse, 25*(6), 370–377.

Salcioğlu, E., & Başoğlu, M. (2008). Psychological effects of earthquakes in children: Prospects for brief behavioral treatment. *World Journal of Pediatrics, 4*(3), 165–172.

Salerno, J. A., & Nagy, C. (2002). Terrorism and aging. *The Journals of Gerontology Series A. Biological Sciences and Medical Sciences, 57*(9), M552–554.

Saliba, D., Elliott, M., Rubenstein, L. Z., Solomon, D. H., Young, R. T., Kamberg, C. J., et al. (2001). The vulnerable elders survey: A tool for identifying vulnerable older people in the community. *Journal of the American Geriatric Society, 49*(12), 1691–1699.

Severance, J., & Yeo, G. (2006). Ethnogeriatric education: A collaborative project of Geriatric Education Centers. *Gerontology & Geriatrics Education, 26*(4), 87–99.

Shiu-Thornton, S., Balabis, J., Senturia, K., Tamayo, A., & Oberle, M. (2007). Disaster preparedness for limited English proficient communities: Medical interpreters as cultural brokers and gatekeepers. *Public Health Reports, 122*(4), 466–71.

Solana, R., & Mariani, E. (2000). NK and NK/T cells in human senescence. *Vaccine, 18*(16), 1613–1620.

Somasundaram, D. J., & van de Put, W. A. (2006). Management of trauma in special populations after a disaster. *Journal of Clinical Psychiatry, 67*(Suppl. 2), 64–73.

Spillman, B. C., & Black, K. J. (2005, November). *Staying the course: Trends in family caregiving*. AARP Public Policy Research Institute and the Urban Institute (Research Report Pub. ID 2005–17), pp. 1–40. Retrieved January 5, 2009, from http://www.aarp.org/research/housing-mobility/caregiving/

Tumosa, N. (Ed.). (2004). Emergency preparedness. *Aging Successfully, 26*(3), 1–24.

U.S. Census Bureau. (2009). *Population 65 years and over in the United States, 2005–2007 American Community Survey 3-year estimates* (Table S0103). Retrieved January 5, 2009, from http://factfinder.census.gov/servlet/STTable?_bm=y&-geo_id=01000US&hqr_name=ACS_2007_3YR_G00_S0103&-ds_name=ACS_2007_3YR_G00_

U.S. Department of Veterans Affairs. (2009). *2009 Salute to Our Veterans calendar.* Retrieved January 15, 2009, from www.myhealth.va.gov

Valente, S. M., & Saunders, J. (2005). Screening for depression and suicide: Self-report instruments that work. *Journal of Psychosocial Nursing and Mental Health Services, 43*(11), 22–31.

Vederhus, K. J., & Kristensen, O. (2006). High effectiveness of self-help programs after drug addiction therapy. *BMC Psychiatry, 6,* 35.

Vial of LIFE Project. (2006). Retrieved January 1, 2009, from http://www.vialoflife.com/

Wenger, N. S., Solomon, D. H., Roth, C. P., MacLean, C. H., Saliba, D., Kamberg, C. J., et al. (2003). The quality of medical care provided to vulnerable community-dwelling older patients. *Annals of Internal Medicine, 139*(9), 740–747.

Williams, P. D., Piamjariyakul, U., Ducey, K., Badura, J., Boltz, K. D., Olberding, K., et al. (2006). Cancer treatment, symptom monitoring, and self-care in adults: Pilot study. *Cancer Nursing, 29*(5), 347–355.

Zimmerman, M., Ruggero, C. J., Chelminski, I., Young, D., Posternak, M. A., Friedman, M., et al. (2006). Developing brief scales for use in clinical practice: The reliability and validity of single-item self-report measures of depression symptom severity, psychosocial impairment due to depression, and quality of life. *Journal of Clinical Psychiatry,* *67*(10), 1536–1541.

Zung, W. W., Richards, C. B., & Short, M. J. (1965). Self-rating depression scale in an out-patient clinic: Further validation of the SDS. *Archives of General Psychiatry, 13*(6), 508–515.

9

Volunteers: Who Are They and What Are Their Roles?

NORA O'BRIEN-SURIC

RESPONDING TO DISASTERS REQUIRES COMMUNITY INVOLVEMENT

When disasters occur, the entire community is affected. Therefore, it is the responsibility of community leaders to guarantee everyone receives the assistance they need in order to survive and that no person is left behind. This requires a large corps of trained people, including, and perhaps especially, volunteers. First responders are trained to mobilize instantly when a disaster strikes, but as we witnessed during the September 11, 2001, terrorist attacks and Hurricane Katrina, first responders cannot meet the overwhelming demands subsequent to catastrophic events. Therefore, it is incumbent on community leaders to develop emergency preparedness plans that include others in the community who can supplement the services of the first responders. A corps of trained volunteers can provide the services that are part of the specific responsibilities of first responders.

In addition to trained volunteers, communities also need to consider the value of and make arrangements for spontaneous volunteers, who will undoubtedly emerge when a disaster strikes and can also provide much-needed assistance.

Disasters will happen, whether they are man-made or natural; having an emergency plan for the disaster as it occurs and to assist in the aftermath and rebuilding of the community's ability to care for its citizens is critical. Volunteers can and should play a role. In many other countries, volunteers are integral to the delivery of health and social services during and after emergencies (Padraig, 2008). Community level interventions foster community competence and ownership of problems and solutions and help strengthen and sustain the community after the disaster (Somasundaram, Asukai, & Murthy, 2003).

This chapter explores the need for volunteers in community emergency preparedness: which types of people tend to volunteer, recruiting and training volunteers, the benefits of reaching out to older adults as volunteers, and using volunteers to assist older people in particular during emergencies.

To the extent possible, this chapter references evidence-based practice in utilizing volunteers during emergencies. However, the literature review conducted for this chapter did not result in extensive research on evidence-based practice. Current research indicates evidence-based practice is not the norm in some areas of emergency management (Perry & Lindell, 2003; Ronan & Johnson, 2005).

PREPARING FOR DISASTERS

Little is known about a community's level of preparedness to meet the basic needs of its citizens immediately following a disaster, yet the health and safety of the community following a disaster depends on that level of preparedness (Adams & Canclini, 2008). Communities benefit enormously—before, during, and following a disaster—by investing the time and resources to develop an emergency plan involving as many community resources as possible. It will make the community more resilient while providing a sense of control to those involved in the emergency planning and a sense of security for the residents. Community resilience emerges from four primary sets of adaptive capacities: economic development, social capital, information and communication, and community competence, which together provide a strategy for disaster readiness (Norris, Stevens, Pfefferbaum, Wyche, & Pfefferbaum, 2008). These four elements were echoed throughout the literature review that informed this chapter. Developing a community emergency plan by using volunteers will tap into the social capital of the community as well as develop community competence. The basic idea of social capital is that individuals invest, access, and use resources embedded in social networks to gain returns (Norris, et al.). In the case of emergency preparedness, communities that tap into their social capital will reap the returns of a dedicated group of individuals working toward the good of the community while satisfying their own need to contribute and reap personal rewards. Equivalently, by having volunteers from the community assist during disasters, people will look to those similar to them for appropriate behaviors and will thereby expedite necessary procedures, such as evacuation (Norris et al.). Also essential is ensuring that emergency plans are culturally viable; recruiting volunteers from various neighborhoods will ensure that the interventions will be tailored to the cultural and community context.

COMMUNITIES NEED LEADERS PRIOR TO A DISASTER

The first step in developing a community emergency plan that includes volunteers is to identify the leaders. Leadership is key; in order to be prepared, the community must have leaders who believe a disaster could actually occur (Gibson & Hayunga, 2006). In all communities, there are formal and informal leaders. Identifying these leaders in the community and in preexisting organizations, networks, and communal relationships, and recruiting them as volunteers during a crisis, is key to rapidly mobilizing emergency and ongoing support services (Norris, et al., 2008). Engaging leaders to work within their communities to develop emergency plans will ensure that the leaders and community members are more committed to executing the plan. A main finding from the hazards research literature is that effective leadership appears vital to people's commitment to the process in terms of structuring tasks and communicating clearly (Ronan & Johnson, 2005). Therefore, identifying and nurturing community leaders is an investment in building community resilience and social capital. Findings indicate the first steps toward helping a community become more aware of the need for change, such as engaging a community in developing an emergency plan, involve just one person or a small group of people who will champion the idea and move it forward within the community (Ronan & Johnson). One example of leadership recruitment and training aimed at bringing a community together to develop an emergency plan was undertaken by the New York City Office of Emergency Management when they contracted with the Empowerment Institute to conduct a pilot program called All Together Now. The

Empowerment Institute employs experts in community-based behavior change and disaster preparedness. During the 2-year pilot project, they trained 3,800 New Yorkers living in 40 buildings and blocks throughout the five boroughs to develop disaster-resilient communities at the building and block level. Among other issues of leadership skill building, these leaders were trained in emergency necessities such as forming teams of neighbors to support one another in taking actions and serving as a support system in an emergency, identifying and helping older persons and the disabled in their buildings or on their blocks to prepare and create evacuation plans, and creating building or block committees to sustain these developments (Empowerment Institute, 2009). The All Together Now project was unique in that it included training in assisting older persons and the disabled in the community. This is an important aspect of emergency preparedness that was missing during the September 11, 2001, terrorist attacks and hurricanes Katrina and Rita, and it will be discussed further in the following sections.

COMMUNITY VOLUNTEERS AND DISASTERS

Community members are often the first to respond to a local disaster and therefore should be prepared to act while waiting for the assistance of formal organizations (Glass, 2001). Community members will also have a better understanding of their own community and the needs of fellow neighbors. Therefore, an effective disaster plan should include knowledgeable community leaders who will be more alert to areas of vulnerability, including specific populations at greater risk (Glass). These leaders and local agencies should collaborate with the emergency organizations—such as the local chapter of the American Red Cross and community emergency response teams—to produce valuable synergy in promoting community preparedness for disaster (Glass). The more a community is prepared, including collaborating with formal emergency organizations, the better the community will respond during and after a disaster. Studies have shown when relief organizations do not work together and do not collaborate with community organizations, cracks in the disaster service delivery network result. When an effective service delivery system provides a complete set of services and linkages, such cracks will not appear (Gillespie & Murty, 1994). The health and safety of communities following disasters depends on the ability of residents and local agencies to be disaster ready (Adams & Canclini, 2008).

RECRUITING VOLUNTEERS TO ASSIST IN EMERGENCIES

In order to encourage people to volunteer in emergencies, it is important to recruit and train the leaders and then the volunteers. The emphasis for recruiting volunteers to participate in community preparedness should be on empowerment—focusing on their and the community's strengths, mobilizing the community's capabilities, and helping the community become self-sufficient following a disaster. Being part of and identifying with a community affects whether and for how long individuals choose to volunteer (Dovidio, Piliavin, Schroeder, & Penner, 2006).

Once leaders are recruited and trained, the next step is to engage other community volunteers in emergency preparedness. The challenge is to convince well-meaning people that the first step in providing effective assistance to others during a disaster is to become personally prepared (Glass, 2001). As the All Together Now program showed, leaders and volunteers need to understand the basic concepts of disasters, the disaster the particular community is likely to face, and the potential dangers related to such disasters (Glass). All volunteers are trained to first prepare an emergency plan for themselves and their families. The research available demonstrated that responses are more effective with good planning and preparedness at the household level (Ronan & Johnson, 2005). Not only will volunteers then have a better understanding of planning for emergencies, but also having their own plan in place will provide them a sense of security and control and will allow them to focus on assisting others during a disaster.

Engaging the community in developing an emergency plan by identifying leaders and recruiting volunteers creates a great opportunity for the public to become aware of the community's emergency needs; it also allows people to feel they can make a real difference before, during, and after a disaster (Skinner, 2008).

VOLUNTEER INCENTIVES

The key themes from the literature review on volunteering incentives were individual motives, personal connections to organizations and causes, and side benefits arising from volunteering (Padraig, 2008). The desire to feel valued and useful and the desire to feel vital and physically active were the two most commonly cited reasons for individual volunteering

(Kerkman, 2003). One study identified six motives for volunteering: to express values related to altruistic and humanitarian concern for others, to acquire new learning experiences and/or use otherwise unused skills, to strengthen social relations or engage in behaviors favored by important others, to gain career-related benefits, to reduce negative feelings about oneself or address personal problems, and to grow and develop psychologically (Dovidio, et al., 2006). Another study identified three similar motives for volunteering: the need for achievement, affiliation, and sense of power (Rouse & Clawson, 1992).

Ellis (2001) found that many people have a strong desire to volunteer, especially during and following a disaster, because they respond to a crisis with the need to *do something*. Ellis states that other studies also found that volunteers needed to be engaged in constructive and communal behavior for their own mental health, as an outlet for rage, and to overcome a sense of powerlessness; their self-protecting actions manifested as altruistic behavior such as searching for survivors, feeding rescuers, and providing solace to grieving relatives. People also reported that they like to volunteer because it gives them satisfaction and personal fulfillment to help others and know they are making a difference (Adler, 2004).

Another incentive for volunteering is the desire to feel needed and useful, and having a purpose in life is a key to longevity. A growing body of social science research has explored the benefits of volunteering on volunteers with surprising results. The benefits of volunteering go well beyond just making the participants feel better about themselves; in fact, it helps them stay healthy and may even prolong their lives (Adler, 2004). By providing volunteer roles in emergency preparedness, community leaders can tap into these personal reasons to volunteer—from creating a means to overcome a sense of powerlessness to creating opportunities for volunteers to feel better about themselves (Ellis, 2001).

WHO VOLUNTEERS?

The decision to volunteer, like many other social behaviors, is often strongly influenced by the actions of other people (Dovidio, et al., 2006). However, extraordinary events of historic proportions can also create conditions that make volunteering more likely (Dovidio, et al.). There was a two- to three-fold increase in volunteerism in the weeks following September 11, 2001, compared to the same time period in 2000 (Dovidio, et al.). One study found that people with certain personality dispositions, such as empathy, become spontaneous volunteers following a crisis (Dovidio, et al.).

Rouse and Clawson (1992) found that the majority (85%) of adult organization volunteers were retired and over age 65 and that almost three fourths of volunteers working with youth and 60% of older volunteers were married. The adult organizations had nearly equal percentages of male (49%) and female (51%) volunteers; almost all volunteers were parents (Rouse & Clawson). Teenagers were more likely to volunteer if their parents were also volunteers (Dovidio, et al., 2006).

In the United States, members of ethnic minorities are less likely to volunteer than are European Americans, although the percentage of African Americans who reported volunteering showed a dramatic increase in a recent survey (Dovidio, et al., 2006). However, when factors such as education, income, and other socioeconomic factors are statistically controlled, racial/ethnic differences largely disappear (Dovidio, et al.).

Another social institution consistently associated with volunteerism is organized religion. A recent study suggests this relationship cuts across racial and ethnic groups (Dovidio, et al., 2006).

Survey responses indicated that both volunteers working with youth and adult organization volunteers consider training desirable (Rouse & Clawson, 1992).

TRAINING EMERGENCY VOLUNTEERS

People in the community are untapped resources simply waiting to be developed (Kerkman, 2003). Volunteers are a valuable resource when they are trained, assigned, and supervised within established emergency management systems (Points of Light Foundation & Volunteer Center National Network, 2002b). Volunteers can be successful participants in emergency management systems when they are flexible, self-sufficient, aware of risks, and willing to be coordinated by emergency management experts (Points of Light Foundation & Volunteer Center National Network, 2002b). Community leaders need to develop such volunteers by providing training, assigning specific roles, planning for follow-up and retention, and creating resources for emotional support during and after a disaster. Ideally, volunteers should be affiliated with an established organization and trained for specific disaster response activities. In April 2002, United Postal Service (UPS), the Points of Light Foundation and

Volunteer Center National Network, and FEMA convened a National Leadership Forum on Disaster Volunteerism. It was evident from the discussions that there was a need for tools, training, and resources to implement recommendations for volunteers at the local level (Points of Light Foundation & Volunteer Center National Network, 2002a). Subsequently, National Voluntary Organizations Active in Disaster (VOAD) established a national volunteer management committee to develop concepts of operation to guide planning for and managing volunteers during all phases of emergency management (Points of Light Foundation & Volunteer Center National Network, 2002b). The committee also developed concepts for planning for and managing unaffiliated volunteers, who can sometimes be underutilized or problematic.

PLANNING FOR SPONTANEOUS VOLUNTEERS

It is important to plan for spontaneous volunteers. These volunteers are eager to respond and contribute to the community's recovery but usually lack the training to be effective in these roles (Points of Light Foundation & Volunteer Center National Network, 2002b). Despite a strong desire to help, volunteers who arrive at a disaster site can actually impede rescue and recovery efforts if they are unaffiliated and untrained in disaster operations (Points of Light Foundation & Volunteer Center National Network, 2002b). Organizations that connect people with charities that need volunteers said they saw increases in calls and emails from potential volunteers following major disasters such as the September 11, 2001, terrorist attack and Hurricane Katrina (Wilhelm, 2002). "Robert Putnam, author of *Bowling Alone: The Collapse and Revival of American Community*, states Americans' sense of civic responsibility runs particularly strong following major disasters" (Wilhelm, 2002, p. 28). In New York City following the September 11, 2001, terrorist attacks, a record number of people signed up with the American Red Cross to volunteer. However, most were turned away because the Red Cross had received as many volunteers as it could handle, yet other organizations desperately needed volunteers (O'Brien, 2003.). At that time, there was no clearinghouse that could have taken calls from organizations and matched volunteers according to skills and experience. However, since then, the Lower Manhattan Development Association in New York City has developed a volunteer registry. Some online sites such as VolunteerMatch.org have made a special effort to respond quickly to emergency situations with a long-term view (Ellis, 2001).

All clearinghouses for emergency volunteers should conduct a brief interview regarding the volunteers' skills, experience, and availability (Center for Volunteer and Nonprofit Leadership of Marin County, 1999). Additionally, businesses, service clubs, and congregations should be enlisted to develop plans for volunteers to help meet immediate and long-term recovery needs in the community (Center for Volunteer and Nonprofit Leadership of Marin County).

OLDER PEOPLE AS VOLUNTEERS

Older people can be valuable volunteers as they may have specific capabilities rarely utilized in preparedness, relief, and rehabilitation programs (HelpAge International, 2007). Older people can and do play important roles within their communities in times of disasters when provided with opportunities to do so. Marc Freedman, president of Civic Ventures, a nonprofit group in San Francisco that seeks to engage older Americans in civic service, has found that retired people, because they are living and staying healthier longer, are looking for more active volunteering roles (Kerkman, 2003). A number of studies have shown that older adults who volunteer tend to be happier as a group and claim to enjoy a better quality of life (Adler, 2004). There is also evidence that older volunteers are not just happier but are also physically healthier than nonvolunteers (Adler).

The key to recruiting older people as volunteers is to develop a variety of opportunities that will appeal to them (Kerkman, 2003). One study found that a number of perspectives appealed to older adult volunteers including community capacity building, civic participation and engagement, social integration, skills development, and successful aging (Glasgow, 2008). Older adult volunteers were more motivated by achievement and affiliation than by power; therefore, it is important that volunteer coordinators consider a different, more work-oriented management style to help older adults feel a greater sense of achievement and structure in their volunteer positions (Rouse & Clawson, 1992).

Sources to recruit older volunteers include senior centers, churches, and fraternal organizations such as the Kiwanis and Rotary Clubs. Other organizations that can be tapped for older volunteers are the local chapters of the Retired and Senior Volunteer Program (RSVP), which is administered by Senior Corps and has local branches nationwide. Also, retired doctors, nurses, social workers, psychologists, and other health professionals make excellent volunteers (Wilhelm, 2002). Building community capacity through older persons' associations enhances the resilience of communities in the event of a disaster (HelpAge International, 2007).

While older volunteers may bring with them physical or other limitations, there are roles they can fill before, during, and after disasters (Kerkman, 2003). One of the advantages of older people as volunteers is that many have experienced traumatic events earlier in their life and, having survived, are better able to provide comfort, security, and reassurance to younger people (O'Brien, 2003). Evidence suggests that some older people may be more resilient than younger people in emergencies because they can draw on broad life experiences (Public Health Agency of Canada, 2008). Older volunteers can exude a resilience and stability needed during and following a traumatic event. Volunteering in disaster situations provides opportunities for older adults to share their experience, wisdom, and skills (Rouse & Clawson, 1992).

Older people should also be involved in the planning stages of emergency preparedness. Some research suggests there may be discrepancies between older people's perception of their needs and the perceptions of aid and relief organizations (Public Health Agency of Canada, 2008). Older people, especially retired professionals, can be instrumental in developing emergency management procedures for locating seniors in emergencies and disasters, identifying the most vulnerable, assessing and addressing individual and community needs, and participating in postemergency impact assessments and evaluations (Public Health Agency of Canada).

ALL EMERGENCY PLANS MUST INCLUDE ASSISTING OLDER AND DISABLED PEOPLE

There is a critical need to increase awareness and strengthen public education about older people and emergency preparedness—from prevention through preparedness and response to recovery. Older people are "invisible" to relief workers or emergency personnel (Gibson & Hayunga, 2006). HelpAge International, the world's largest global relief organization focusing on older people, reported their research that relief organizations often fail to see or understand the needs and contributions of older people during disasters (Gibson & Hayunga). The study also found that older people fight a losing a battle in the competition for resources; in the chaos of emergencies, older people are physically less able to struggle for food or travel far to find relief. Additionally, the findings showed there is an almost universal lack of consultation from older community members in developing emergency plans (Gibson & Hayunga).

Having older people assist with community preparedness would help emergency workers gain a better understanding of the physical, social, environmental, and economic factors contributing to the vulnerability of older people (Public Health Agency of Canada, 2008). Disasters can be particularly traumatic for older persons, especially those with serious physical, cognitive, or psychosocial problems (Rosenkoetter, Covan, Cobb, Bunting, & Weinrich, 2007). Poor health not only affects older persons' ability to evacuate but also increases their risk for illness-related complications during and after a disaster (Rosenkoetter, et al.). A key finding from the Harris Interactive survey conducted for AARP in November 2005 indicated that about 13 million people over age 50 say they would require help to evacuate (Gibson & Hayunga, 2006). Yet until recently, emergency organizations did not have specific plans to accommodate older people during and after disasters.

One finding in the study conducted by the International Longevity Center–USA following the September 11, 2001, terrorist attacks was that first responder organizations—such as the Office of Emergency Management, the American Red Cross, and FEMA—did not have specific plans to identify, evacuate, and provide services to older and disabled people during emergencies (O'Brien, 2003). Older people have specific needs—related to health, nutrition, and access to essential services—that are seldom given due consideration in disaster response programs (Help-Age International, 2007). Because older persons have unique needs, modifying disaster responses to meet those specific needs is essential (Rosenkoetter, et al., 2007).

Several studies have indicated that special populations have unique needs that must continue to be met during and after disasters (Glass, 2001). Recent disasters such as hurricanes Katrina and Rita reemphasized the need for effective preparedness for older persons (Rosenkoetter, et al., 2007). Yet older people are generally excluded from emergency planning and programs. Engaging older people in emergency planning will help ensure their distinct needs are identified and integrated into assessment and planning (Public Health Agency of Canada, 2008).

Although emergency organizations, such as the American Red Cross, now have materials and plans for dealing with older and disabled people during emergencies, a next important step is volunteers trained to work with vulnerable people to doubly ensure their specific needs will be met during a crisis. The materials that have recently become available can be useful tools for training volunteers.

One study found that older people know very little about how to protect themselves during emergencies (Rosenkoetter, et al., 2007). There is a tremendous need for public education about emergency preparedness. More must be done to reach older persons and persons with disabilities (Gibson & Hayunga, 2006). If older persons do not know how to prepare, if they are unable to do so, or if they do not know they should be preparing, then by definition they are at risk (Rosenkoetter, et al.). The findings suggest communication that adequately and accurately informs older people of approaching disasters is critical (Rosenkoetter, et al.). Accurate and timely predisaster information is especially important and should include developing and tailoring messages to influence older people (Public Health Agency of Canada, 2008). Officials could promote public acceptance by explaining how decisions are made, what emergency measures need to be taken, and where older adults can access information (Rosenkoetter, et al.). It is particularly important that older people are involved in these discussions and decisions, advising on how best to reach older people in emergency situations and how older people want to receive such messages (Public Health Agency of Canada). Volunteers could then be recruited to create and distribute educational information at senior centers, religious and congregate meal sites, and where low-income older adults are known to cluster.

Communities need to maintain *special needs registries* to assist older adults, especially those with physical and mental illnesses or disabilities, with medical and transfer needs in the event of a disaster and encourage residents to plan ahead as well as to know where they can go and how to get there (Rosenkoetter, et al., 2007). As governments are invariably overextended in times of emergency, and humanitarian and other relief agencies are under-resourced, communities have an important role in maintaining links between older people and disaster recovery services (Public Health Agency of Canada, 2008). More emergency preparedness planning is needed at the community level. Engaging neighborhood leaders and block wardens is an effective way to keep vulnerable persons from slipping through the cracks (Gibson & Hayunga, 2006).

VOLUNTEERS PROVIDING AND RECEIVING MENTAL HEALTH SERVICES

An important area of consideration is providing mental health services to survivors as well as to volunteers following a disaster. The ability of social supports to protect mental health has been demonstrated repeatedly (Somasundaram et al., 2005). Because disasters affect entire networks, the need for mental health support may simply exceed its availability as support networks become saturated (Somasundaram et al.). Therefore, it is necessary to recruit social workers and psychologists to provide such services and to ensure there will be enough professional volunteers ready to mobilize when a disaster strikes.

Volunteers may also need mental health counseling. Even though volunteers should receive training prior to a disaster, it is difficult to truly understand how one will react when a crisis actually happens. Disasters create an emotional experience and intense environment that is challenging for some individuals, and so it is necessary to plan for mental health assistance for volunteers (Novotncy, 2008). As the weeks pass after a disaster, many generous professional and volunteer helpers will still be on the front lines. Unfortunately, during a crisis the emotional and physical needs of those who help others are often forgotten (Center for Volunteer and Nonprofit Leadership of Marin County, 1999).

The initially heightened level of helping and concern seldom lasts for the full length of the recovery process (Somasundaram et al., 2005). Perhaps the most important lesson learned from the research is that the stress precipitated by catastrophic disasters is often long lasting (Somasundaram et al.). Thus, the response to a disaster must include ongoing attention to the psychological aspects of the event as part of the overall emergency response (Somasundaram et al.).

When communities devise emergency plans, it is essential to ensure there is a cadre of volunteer therapists who can provide mental health services to the residents as well as to professionals and volunteers during and after the crisis.

VOLUNTEERS AND POSTDISASTER WORK

The aftermath of a disaster may be when volunteers can be most useful. Helping behavior and community cohesion are abundant initially, but they do not last, and certain resources will not be available after the impact of a disaster (Norris, et al., 2008). The failure of relief organizations to work together results in cracks in the postdisaster service delivery network (Gillespie & Murty, 1994). Community leaders and volunteers can fill in the cracks by holding meetings where residents can brainstorm about rebuilding the community (Domosundaram, et al., 2005). Planning and community collaborations are essential to ensure a community works together on getting back on its feet. This not only helps them come to terms with the reality of loss but also helps them identify and discuss local problems and initiate collective action toward common goals (Ronan & Johnson, 2005). Encouraging community cohesiveness in this way contributes to the healing process of both individuals and the larger community.

Developing a community emergency plan by engaging leaders, recruiting and training local volunteers, and including older people in the process will help build community resilience in advance of disaster, which will serve residents well during and after a crisis. Disaster readiness is about social change (Norris, et al., 2008).

In summary, volunteering is part of the American can-do spirit. The social change needed to create a corps of volunteers requires initiatives sparked by the government and nurtured by natural community leaders. The Peace Corps and Teach for America are but two examples of the success of creating a corps of volunteers for a specific purpose. Developing a similar program to assist in disasters will benefit everyone.

REFERENCES

Adams, L. M., & Canclini, S. B. (2008). Disaster readiness: A community–university partnership. *Online Journal in Issues in Nursing, 13*(3).

Adler, R. (2004, July–August). The volunteer factor. *Aging Today, 25*(44). Retrieved September 7, 2009, from http://www.civicventures.org/publications/articles/the_volunteer_factor.cfm

Center for Volunteer and Non-Profit Leadership of Marin County. (1999). *Building our community: Disaster preparedness.* Retrieved September 7, 2008, from http://www.cvnl.org/community/disaster_prep.html

Dovidio, J. F., Piliavin, J. A., Schroeder, D. A., & Penner, L. A, (2006). *The social psychology of prosocial behavior.* Mahwah, NJ: Lawrence Erlbaum Associates.

Ellis, S. J. (2001, October). *A volunteerism perspective on the days after the 11th of September.* Retrieved October 20, 2008, from http://www.energizeinc.com/hot/01oct.html

Empowerment Institute. (2009). *All together now: Neighbors helping neighbors create a resilient New York City.* Retrieved September 7, 2009, from www.empowermen tinstitute.net/atn/

Gibson, M. J., & Hayunga, M. (2006, May). *We can do better: Lessons learned for protecting older persons in disasters* [Brochure]. Washington, DC: AARP Public Institute.

Gillespie, D., & Murty, S. (1994). Cracks in a post disaster service delivery network. *American Journal of Community Psychology, 22,* 639–660.

Glasgow, N. (2008, July 31). *Older people as volunteers: Motivations, contexts, opportunities and challenges.* Paper presented at the annual meeting of the American Sociological Association, Sheraton Boston and the Boston Marriott Copley Place, Boston, MA. Retrieved January 11, 2009, from http://www.allacademic.com/meta/p242908_index.html

Glass, T. A. (2001). Understanding public response to disasters. *Public Health Reports, 116,* S69–73. Retrieved January 11, 2009, from http://www.pubmedcentral.nih.gov/picrender.fcgi?artid=1497258&blobtype=pd

HelpAge International. (2007). *Older peoples associations in community disaster risk reduction, a resource book on good practice.* Retrieved September 7, 2009, from http://www.helpage.org/Resources/Manuals#R5ZH

Kerkman, L. (2003, September). Tips for recruiting and managing older volunteers. *The Chronicle of Philanthropy.* Retrieved January 10, 2009, from http://philanthropy.com/jobs/2003/10/08/20031024–636748.htm

Norris, F. H., Stevens, S. P., Pfefferbaum, B., Wyche, K. F., & Pfefferbaum, R. L. (2008). Community resilience as a metaphor, theory, set of capacities, and strategy for disaster readiness. *American Journal of Community Psychology, 41,* 127–150.

Novotney, A. (2008). Postgrad growth area: Disaster mental health [Electronic version]. *Grad PSYCH, 6*(1). Retrieved September 7, 2009, from http://gradpsych.apags.org/jan08/postgrad.html

O'Brien, N. (2003, Spring). *Emergency preparedness for older people* [Issue Brief Spring 2003]. New York: International Longevity Center-USA.

Padraig, M. (2008). The give and take of volunteering: Motives, benefits, and personal connections among Irish volunteers. *Voluntas, 19*(2), 125–139.

Perry, R. W., & Lindell, M. K. (2003). Preparedness for emergency response: Guidelines for the emergency planning process. *Disasters, 27,* 336–350.

Points of Light Foundation, & Volunteer Center National Network. (2002a). *Preventing a disaster within the disaster: The effective use and management of unaffiliated volunteers.* Washington, DC: Author. Retrieved January 11, 2009, from http://www.pointsoflight.org/disaster/disaster.cfm

Points of Light Foundation, & Volunteer Center National Network (2002b.). *Managing spontaneous volunteers in times of disaster: The synergy of structure and good intentions.* Retrieved January 11, 2009, from http://www.pointsoflight.org/downloads/pdf/programs/disaster/brochure.pdf

Public Health Agency of Canada. (2008). *Building a global framework to address the needs and contributions of older people in emergencies* (Cat. No. HP 25–5/2008E-PDF). Ottawa, Ontario: Author. Retrieved January 11, 2009, from http://www.phac-aspc.gc.ca/seniors-aines/pubs/global_framework/pdfs/UN_GlobalFwk08_eng PDF_web.pdf

Ronan, K. R., & Johnson, D. M. (2005). *Promoting community resilience in disasters: The role for schools, youth, and families* (2nd ed.). New York: Springer Publishing.

Rosenkoetter, M. M., Covan, E. K., Cobb, B. K., Bunting, S., & Weinrich, M. (2007). Populations at risk across the lifespan: Empirical studies—Perceptions of older adults regarding evacuation in the event of a natural disaster. *Public Health Nursing, 24*(2), 160–168.

Rouse, S. B., & Clawson, B. (1992). Motives and incentives of older adult volunteers. *Journal of Extension, 30*(3), 1–10.

Skinner, R. (2008, September 12). *CPTV special underscores need for emergency services volunteers* [6:00 AM posting]. Message posted to http://citizencorps.blogspot.com/2008/09/cptv-special-underscores-need-for.html

Somasundaram, D., Norris, F. H., Asukai, N., & Murthy, R. S. (2003). Natural and technological disasters. In B. L. Green, M. J. Friedman, J. T. V. M. de Jong, S. D. Solomon, T. M. Keane, J. A. Fairbank, et al. (Eds.), *Trauma interventions in war and peace: Prevention, practice, and policy* (pp. 291–318). New York: Kluwer Academic/Plenim.

Wilhelm, I. (2002). Turning good will into action. *The Chronicle of Philanthropy, 14*(16), 27–29.

Clinical Response to the Needs of Older Persons During Disasters

10

Psychosocial and Pharmacological Interventions for Older Persons in Disasters

DOUGLAS M. SANDERS AND MARK R. NATHANSON

While the growing body of research has shed light onto the likely seque-lae of the response of older adults in disasters, a critical central theme has emerged—there is no typical response. In fact, the growing body of literature has diverged from formulaic methods of assessment and treat-ment for this population. While the research literature does yield com-mon domains that an effective clinician should be oriented to and address in his or her work, this work should cede to individualization, context, and nuance of experience. The goal of this chapter is to integrate the other chapters' reviews of the major domains of symptoms experienced by older persons in disasters and to identify mediating and buffering factors that promote resilience and quality of life. The authors also outline interven-tions that integrate and are sensitive to both common symptoms and id-iosyncratic responses to disaster. The emphasis will be on how both these categories of symptoms can change and must therefore be assessed dy-namically through time. Ultimately, this chapter guides clinicians in the decision-making processes that promote comprehensive and individual-ized developmental assessment. Accordingly, this assessment process can lead to the development of effective, evidence-informed, eclectic inter-ventions that help people cope with disaster and foster personal resilience. Interventions discussed include both psychosocial and pharmacological approaches and how these treatments may be combined for optimally effective intervention.

COMPREHENSIVE, INDIVIDUALIZED ASSESSMENT

As discussed in previous chapters, the growing research literature on responses to disaster has not only delineated the *normal* reactions of individuals, including older adults, but also has underlined the dynamic quality of symptom presentation over time. While there is often considerable overlap of pre-, during-, and postdisaster responses, clinicians need to refrain from static assessment processes that deem a person to be *handling it well* in an early stage and assume this managed response will continue. Krause (2004), in fact, indicated it may take years for disaster-related clinical symptoms to dissipate and suggests that researchers and clinicians take an extended longitudinal view of a person's response to disaster. In addition, previous exposure to traumatic events and premorbid psychiatric/cognitive/medical status symptoms may buffer or exacerbate the presentation of these symptoms.

The complexity of this assessment process requires a strategy that considers all aspects of a person's functioning and continually reassesses these modalities over time. While Lazarus (1981) emphasizes the use of seven such modes of functioning, this chapter will include *spirituality,* or the *existential domain,* as the eighth sphere as the literature points to the prominence of this area in understanding an older person's response to disaster. Similarly, attention must be given to the central role of choice and choosing (Gurland & Gurland, 2008a, 2008b) in maintaining an older person's quality of life during disasters, including Banerjee's additional subdomains within choice and choosing: empowerment, respect, and identity (Banerjee, et al., 2009). Overall, the effective clinician will evaluate an individual across all spheres of their experience, including the behavioral, affective, cognitive, sensory, imagery, interpersonal, physiological, and spiritual-existential domains. While the following tables comprehensively delineate symptoms as they may be experienced across the time continuum of disaster, the interaction of these symptoms needs to be assessed; this holistic orientation best captures a person's experience and will lead to more obvious and specifically indicated treatments. Additionally, it is imperative that clinicians realize that assumed resiliency and recovery from many of these symptoms is the expected baseline. The normalization of what might otherwise wrongly be viewed as clinical symptoms is paramount to a person's wellness postdisaster.

It is imperative that the disaster mental health clinician is aware of the individual's baseline functioning prior to the traumatic event in order to understand the interaction of pre-event, event, and post-event contributions to an individual's response to disaster. The latter interaction may not only provide the clinician with a tool for comprehensive assessment but also may lead to very specific intervention strategies that incorporate pre-event functioning. Table 10.1 provides a guide for assessing eight specific modalities a clinician should investigate. Examples provided within each domain are not meant to be all-inclusive but can prompt the clinician's queries and reveal more relevant information. Ultimately, these areas should not be viewed as isolated categories but as domains of experience that continually interact. It should also be noted that older disaster victims may not be able to provide much of this information. In such instances, the clinician should determine the availability of a key informant to provide as much information as possible. Family members, community-based and facility staff, peers, clergy, and others may be useful during the assessment process.

All these domains greatly affect an individual's ultimate response to a disaster as well as how he or she may respond to varying intervention strategies. Even without the devastation of a disaster, effective treatment should consider these clinical areas—the experience of a disaster only makes the need to do so more acute. The potential interactions between disaster and these baseline modalities of experience are noteworthy. How does disaster differentially affect the individual with a very structured, compulsive daily routine? How might disaster influence a dependent personality-disordered individual's already intense interpersonal affect? Is a disaster-caused injury aggravating existing chronic pain? Mix in a preexisting cognitive impairment made worse by disaster and you have a compulsive, affectively intense and labile, medically compromised person in physical pain who is confused, disoriented, and without familial and social support due to a long history of interpersonal instability and conflict. While this hypothetical patient may be dizzying clinically, it likely underestimates the complexity of most people, where the individual nuance of a person's past, present, and disaster experience create truly unique presentations. This complexity is intensified in older persons. In addition, while this example highlights clinical problem areas and their interaction, strengths can be assessed in each modality and their interactions observed and utilized to foster positive coping responses to disaster. Might

Table 10.1

PRE-DISASTER/BASELINE DOMAINS OF COMPREHENSIVE ASSESSMENT

BEHAVIORAL	AFFECTIVE	SENSORY	IMAGERY	COGNITIVE	INTERPERSONAL	PHYSIOLOGICAL	SPIRITUAL
Independent living skills/ Capacity for autonomy ***	Overall emotional functioning and lability ***	Perceptual capacities across hearing, vision, and other senses ***	Self-image, including image of self-efficacy ***	Overall cognitive status/ Relatedness ***	Level of social and familial support ***	Medical issues/ Medications/ Medical history ***	Religious beliefs ***
Average, overall activity level ***	Specification of affective quality and intensity ***	Pain associated with medical conditions ***	Dynamic image of self-in-aging process ***	Presence of dementia ***	Social self-image ***	Ongoing medical assessment ***	Existential place in life ***
Time spent in specific activities, including leisure, and their effects on other modalities ***	Pre-existing mood disorder or vulnerability ***	Overall sensitivity/ Orientation to sensation	Self-perception of self-efficacy ***	Specific memory problems ***	Professional/staff supports ***	Assessment of aging-related health variables ***	Retrospective and defined purpose and meaning ***
Routine or rituals that structured the individual's daily life	Emotional self-image		Pre-existing coping imagery ***	Processing speed difficulties ***	Outgoing? Dependent? Assertive?	Specific medical issues known to be exacerbated by disaster, such as hypertension	Perceived major accomplishments and achievements and perceived "legacy"
			"Narrative" imagery of "life's high-lights"	Attitude toward world, self, others, and aging process			

a dependent personality be more open to supportive help offered by a clinician than someone with greater autonomy?

Following in Table 10.2 is a list of symptoms commonly experienced by individuals as immediate responses to disaster. Symptoms that are particularly common or noteworthy in older populations are well represented. As you review Table 10.2, consider what interventions would be appropriate for each specific symptom as well as for symptom clusters. What interventions would be inappropriate or too far ahead of where a client is? It is important to recognize if a disoriented client is currently capable of answering the existential why questions of disaster: Why did this disaster happen? Why so much pain and loss? What does the confused, misinformed individual need? Does an individual consumed by pain attend to, or are they even oriented toward, basic hygiene and self-care? Does a person who just lost a loved one need detached reassurance that everything will be okay or quiet support that respects their loss?

As you read these questions, grounded, realistic, and helpful thoughts will come to mind as to how you might help individuals in these circumstances. This, indeed, is a primary governing principle of much of disaster mental health care—to provide very basic help to an individual given their most acute needs at a specific moment in time. Basic reorientation to time, place, and person, accurate information provision; quick referral (escorting) to medical help; connection with supportive emotional loved ones or pets; and nonverbally engaging (being with) a grieving person are considered to be potentially on-target mental health interventions for the aforementioned dispositions. Ultimately, the comprehensive and efficient intervention approaches are often best informed by practical assessment.

For every symptom indicated in Table 10.2, there are direct and indirect interventions the creative and flexible clinician can formulate. Intervention strategies, however, become more complicated when considering the potential multifaceted and interactive nature of issues across each of these modalities. Obviously indicated calming or distraction-based techniques, for example, are not likely to be effective with an older person who views these particular activities and everything in general as pointless. The interaction of these domains, in what Lazarus (1981) describes as the establishment of a *firing order*, should also be undertaken. Consider the following example of treating social withdrawal. A person's desire for isolation may be caused by intense fear and terror, which, on close examination, may be sporadically elicited by repetitive and intrusive imagery of

Table 10.2

DURING-DISASTER SYMPTOM DOMAINS AND COMPREHENSIVE ASSESSMENT

BEHAVIORAL	AFFECTIVE	SENSORY	IMAGERY	COGNITIVE	INTERPERSONAL	PHYSIOLOGICAL	SPIRITUAL
Skills/capacity for self-regulation, not attending to basic self-care ***	Intense, erratic emotional lability; feeling overwhelmed ***	Sensory/perceptual overload/Aggravated impairment of capacities across hearing, vision, and other senses ***	Frightening, intrusive, and repetitive imagery of disaster ***	Impaired cognitive status and disorientation ***	Loss of social and familial support due to death/injury ***	Disaster-caused injury ***	"Primitive" questioning of religious beliefs/Question of "why" ***
Agitation or decreased over-all activity level ***	Emotional numbing ***	Pain associated with disaster-induced injury, or disaster-aggravated medical conditions ***	Images of self-inadequacy to cope or help others ***	Confusion, aggravated by lack of clear, valid information ***	Social and familial self-images radically altered ***	Trauma/stress induced medical complications ***	Sense that "everything has been lost" ***
Withdrawal and isolation ***	Painful loss of people and possessions ***	Sensory dis-orientation (delirium)	Images of death (self and others)	Inability to focus; and easily distracted ***	Relocation induced social withdrawal and isolation	Aggravation of existing medical issues ***	Pervasive "pointlessness"
Routine disruption/Lack of governing structure life	Rage, terror, fear, guilt, ***			Aggravation of pre-existing memory problems ***		No access to medical/psychiatric medications ***	
	Aggravation of pre-existing mood problems			Altered basic attitudes toward world, self, others, and perceived lack of security and safety		Aggravation of the above with aging-related health varables ***	
						Increased hypertension and related complications	

the disaster. In this example, the root or proximal cause of withdrawal is highly specific to imagery. The best management of this symptom interaction may be to target the provocative imagery with high clinical priority and offer competing imagery to the suffering person (Lazarus).

RESILIENCY AND DISASTER MENTAL HEALTH

Assessment should also include a basic review of those factors that might buffer the aforementioned effects of disaster. Many resiliency factors have been identified in the literature. While the previous section focused on symptoms often present in the wake of disaster, more recently much research has focused on factors that mediate the expression of these symptoms and that best predict resilience in the older population postdisaster. The major factors that can potentially promote resilience, and that the clinician needs to promote, include the following:

- Degree of disaster-event exposure, both static and ongoing
- Perceived family support
- Perceived community-based support
- Socioeconomic status/education level
- Culture
- Male gender
- Perceived nondiscrimination
- Evidence of pre-disaster psychiatric history
- Symbolic meaning applied to the disaster event

(Acierno, Ruggiero, Kilpatrick, Resnick, & Galea, 2006; Bolin & Klenow, 1988; Krause, 1987; Lawson & Thomas, 2007; Melick & Logue, 1985; Norris, et al., 2002; Norris, Friedman, & Watson, 2002; Seplaki, Goldman, Weinstein, & Lin, 2006; Ticchurst, Webster, Carr, and Lewin, 1996; Watanabe, Okumura, Chiu, & Wakai, 2004; Weems, et al., 2007).

Interventions flowing from the assessment of resilience factors include the following: limiting exposure to disaster, increasing actual or perceived levels of familial and community-based support, ensuring equal distribution of services to recipients without discrimination, and helping an individual attempt to frame their experience in adaptive ways. Formal intervention models have been developed and utilized effectively using resiliency as a framework, such as Green and Graham's (2006) Resiliency-Enhancing Model (REM). Clearly, these factors, as we will review in the following intervention section, set the context for how to best help older persons in a disaster.

INDIVIDUALIZED, DYNAMIC, AND RESILIENCY-BASED INTERVENTION APPROACHES

What clinical intervention and support should be provided during and following a disaster is, perhaps, the greatest ongoing controversy in the disaster mental health intervention literature. Questions that remain to be answered conclusively include the following: What intervention strategies are most effective and at what time? Are there potential deleterious implications of particular interventions? How much structure, following protocol, versus individualization should interventions possess?

Just as symptoms need to be evaluated in time context relative to a disaster, treatment interventions must also be temporally sensitive. Interventions during the midst or within the immediate unfolding of a disaster would obviously differ greatly from interventions for an individual still suffering from sequelae 6 months postdisaster. Accordingly, this section not only integrates the previous sections of clinical assessment strategies and factors promoting resilience, but it identifies how interventions would typically be employed over time to older victims of disaster. The remainder of this chapter will review and summarize both psychosocial and pharmacological intervention strategies in the during, immediate, and longer term follow-up stages of recovery from disaster.

EVIDENCED-INFORMED, DURING-DISASTER INTERVENTIONS

During-disaster interventions are driven by a basic pragmatism that guides helpers to first promote and protect safety, increase comfort, decrease pain and discomfort—both physical and psychological—and provide an environment that promotes inner security. In a publication dedicated to providing clinical guidance to disaster mental health clinicians that incorporates *evidenced-informed* practices, which is necessary due to the dearth of internally valid studies that would illuminate *evidence-based* practice, Hobfoll and colleagues (2007) outlined the hierarchical progression of how intervention strategies should unfold in response to disaster. In addition, these target areas are also consistent with the consensus reached in the

"Mental Health and Mass Violence Review" offered by a panel of leading researchers and practitioners in the 2007 publication titled *Evidence-Based Early Psychological Intervention for Victims/Survivors of Mass Violence: A Workshop to Reach Consensus on Best Practices* (National Institute of Mental Health [NIMH], 2002). The reader should note this document not only as a clinical resource but also as a remarkable attempt to integrate a very wide, diverse, and heterogeneous body of literature. Specifically, the authors recommend the following equivalent of a disaster *hierarchy of needs,* which should guide clinical assessment and intervention relevant to an individual's current most pressing issues:

1. Foster sense of safety: Promoting an actual and nurturing a perceived sense of safety is the first line of intervention for the disaster mental health clinician. This involves mitigating ongoing actual threats of a disaster and reducing harm due to indirect affects of disaster. An example of the latter would be not having access to necessary medical care. Obviously, until personal safety and a sense of security are established, all other intervention efforts would not only be misguided but also ineffectual. The provision of safety, or at the minimum fostering a sense of it, may be complicated by clinical issues presented by older persons.

2. Facilitate personal calming: Even after a threat has been reduced to a manageable level, individuals often have great difficulty reducing their heightened physiological response to a disaster. This inability to calm oneself may elicit internal cues that bodily indicate it is not safe yet, thus perpetuating a cycle of hyper-vigilance and further duress. This early maladaptive response is not only extremely uncomfortable, but its endurance may predict poor psychiatric prognosis. Very basic helping techniques like deep breathing and distraction-based efforts may help calm individuals who are at risk from having more permanent disaster-related symptoms develop. Basic group activities that encourage light recreational or productively helpful activity may quell an over-stimulated nervous system.

3. Develop sense of personal/self and community efficacy to cope or overcome: While basic coping skills may be taught at this early stage to help manage acute symptoms of distress, a person, and more collectively a community of people, must believe in their capacity to *get through* their experiences and feel better as a result of their efforts. If coping strategies are viewed as useless or

ineffective, or are perceived to be beyond one's ability to implement, the probability of people exercising them is low. Beliefs such as "I can make it" or "We can get through it together" may precede any specific intervention that would, indeed, help someone manage intense emotions during crisis. At the community level, disaster by definition can overwhelm a community and give individuals the maladaptive thoughts that "Everything has been destroyed" and "We can never recover." While a clinician indicating that everything is going to be all right may be perceived as disrespectful and likely invalidating, temperate and modulated thinking at the individual and community level should be encouraged as it *sets the stage* and enables active coping efforts to be engaged.

4. Promote connectedness: Not feeling alone in personal, family, and community contexts is a critical factor that can reduce an individual's current emotional duress and, in addition, may improve his or her future prognosis. It is important to note that high levels of perceived social and familial support are a significant factor underlying personal resilience in the wake of disaster. Group-oriented helping behavior or activity may not only help promote calming but may also promote connectedness.

5. Installation of hope: During a disaster, when all may seem lost, it is often the basic sense of hope that keeps people going. If all of the pain, suffering, and loss experienced by an individual during a disaster are compounded by a growing sense that things will only get worse, it may disable an individual's ability to benefit from supportive help. Disasters can destroy temporal context, and distorting a person's cognitive sense of time can be quite debilitating. The collective hope of a community must also be nurtured by the disaster mental health clinician.

Given these symptoms and the very basic needs of individuals after disasters, it is consistent that treatment should focus on a progression of interventions to help a person establish a basic sense of safety, provide skills that enable them to self-calm, promote interpersonal connection, and, ultimately, lead an individual or group to feel they can manage and get through it. During the early phase of disaster response, a collection of very individualized interventions that promote all four of these elements has become known as providing "Psychological First Aid," or PFA (NIMH, 2002, p.24). PFA, as described in the NIMH "Mental Health and Mass Violence Review," is a set of strategies focused on reducing the immediate impact of disaster-related stress (NIMH, p. 24). Hobfoll and colleagues' (2007) hierarchical focus for effective intervention also applies to the next phase of disaster response.

POSTDISASTER SYMPTOM DOMAINS AND COMPREHENSIVE ASSESSMENT

Table 10.3 lists symptoms commonly experienced by older individuals in response to disaster after the immediate threat posed by the disaster has waned. While many symptoms may persist from a person's during-disaster response, new symptoms typical of this stage may also appear. While there is considerable overlap in these symptoms, this provides the first opportunity for clinicians to begin to assess those individuals who may need a greater level of clinical care than that provided by baseline disaster outreach interventions. The clinician should look for the first signs of possible acute stress disorder (ASD) and possible PTSD-related symptoms, which would emerge and be diagnosed at least 6 months post-event. While PFA-type interventions may still be helpful for many of the listed symptoms, more formal intervention—such as more traditional psychotherapy and pharmacological interventions—may be indicated.

LONGER TERM POSTDISASTER SYMPTOMS AND THEIR ASSESSMENT

Table 10.4 lists symptoms experienced by individuals who have ongoing deleterious responses to disaster long after a disaster and its immediate effects have subsided. While it is rare for people to experience this persistence of symptoms from their during- and immediate postdisaster response, lingering chronic symptoms may arise, particularly if untreated at an early stage. The focus of assessment here is ASD and PTSD symptoms and their treatment. Table 10.4 assembles the symptoms of ASD and PTSD into an analogous multimodal chart form.

Viewing these symptom areas as interactive, as opposed to isolated events, leads to more precise and effective treatment indications. While the following interventions are broken down into basic psychotherapeutic categories, the effects of interventions, like symptoms, are interactive. For example, a synergistic result of behavioral interventions affecting a

Table 10.3

POSTDISASTER SYMPTOM DOMAINS AND COMPREHENSIVE ASSESSMENT

BEHAVIORAL	AFFECTIVE	SENSORY	IMAGERY	COGNITIVE	INTERPERSONAL	PHYSIOLOGICAL	SPIRITUAL
Skills/capacity for self-regulation, not attending to basic self-care ***	Less intense but still erratic emotions ***	Sensory/perceptual overload; Aggravated ***	Frightening, intrusive, and repetitive imagery of disaster ***	Impaired cognitive status and disorientation ***	Loss of social and familial support due to death/injury ***	Disaster-caused injury ***	"Deeper" questioning of religious beliefs ***
Agitation or decreased overall activity level ***	Cued mood lability ***	Impairment of capacities across hearing, vision, and other senses ***	Imagery based on "re-exposure" to disaster-associated stimuli ***	Confusion, aggravated by lack of clear, valid information ***	Social and familial self-images radically altered ***	Trauma/stress induced medical complications ***	Question of why leading to anger and disappointment ***
Withdrawal and isolation ***	Breakthrough emotions vascillating with periodic numbing ***	Pain associated with disaster-induced injury or disaster-aggravated medical conditions ***	Imagery cued by visual, affective, or other environmental triggers ***	Inability to focus; easily distracted ***	Relocation induced social withdrawal and isolation	Exacerbated medical issues evolving to chronic status ***	More grounded appraisal of the magnitude of loss ***
Routine disruption/Lack of governing structure life	Cued, painful loss of people and possessions ***		Images of self-inadequacy to cope or help others ***	Aggravation of pre-existing memory problems ***		Limited access to or desire for engagement in medical/psychiatric medications ***	"Pointlessness" of the event
	Rage, terror, fear, guilt ***	Sensory disorientation (delirum)	Images of death (self and others)	Altered, basic attitudes toward world, self, others, and perceived lack of security and safety		Cued hyperarousal and associated cardiovascular problems ***	
	Aggravation of pre-existing mood problems					Aggravation of the above with aging-related health variables	

Table 10.4

LONGER-TERM-DISASTER SYMPTOMS OF ASD AND PTSD

BEHAVIORAL	AFFECTIVE	SENSORY	IMAGERY	COGNITIVE	INTERPERSONAL	PHYSIOLOGICAL	SPIRITUAL
Skills/capacity for self-regulation, not attending to basic self-care	Less intense, but still erratic emotions	Sensory/perceptual overload;	Frightening, intrusive, and repetitive imagery of disaster based on "re-exposure" to disaster-associated stimuli	Ongoing, impaired cognitive status and disorientation	Loss of social and familial support due to death/injury	Disaster-caused injury	"Deeper" questioning of religious beliefs
Agitation or decreased overall activity level	Cued mood lability	Aggravated impairment of capacities across hearing, vision, and other senses	Imagery cued by visual, affective, or other environmental triggers	Faulty assumptions based on misinformation that generate excessive fear and hopelessness	Social and familial self-images radically altered	Trauma/stress induced medical complications	Question of why leading to anger and disappointment
Withdrawal and isolation	Breakthrough emotions vascillating with periodic numbing	Pain associated with disaster-induced injury, or disaster-aggravated medical conditions	Images of self-inadequacy to cope or help others	Inability to focus; easily distracted	Relocation induced social withdrawal and isolation	Exacerbated medical issues evolving to chronic status	More grounded appraisal of the magnitude of loss
Routine disruption/Lack of governing structure life	Cued, painful loss of people and possessions	Sensory disorientation (delirium)	Images of death (self and others)	Ongoing, aggravation of pre-existing memory problems		Limited access to or desire for engagement in medical/psychiatric medications	"Pointlessness" of the event
	Rage, terror, fear, guilt			Altered, basic attitudes toward world, self, others, and perceived lack of security and safety		Cued hyperarousal and associated cardiovascular problems	
	Aggravation of pre-existing mood problems					Aggravation of the above with aging-related health variables	

person's cognition and subsequent affect is to be expected and facilitated by the disaster mental health clinician.

Behavioral Interventions

Behavioral interventions are well suited for disaster mental health clinical work as they tend to be very basic and focused on symptom reduction and environmental factors that may trigger or maintain problematic issues. Included in this intervention category would be distraction-based interventions; basic coping skill instruction, including deep breathing and relaxation training; and more sophisticated functional analyses of problematic or symptomatic behavior. The latter technique involves a review of the potential environmental triggers that may elicit symptoms; self-monitoring of the severity of symptoms, sometimes formally measured by a subjective unit of distress scale (SUDS); and careful attention to and notation of those activities that may decrease distress. Avoiding triggering circumstances, employing techniques that reduce distress, and reinforcing or encouraging coping or recovery behavior are all interventions within the behavioral model of intervention.

Cognitive Interventions

Cognitive interventions are principally focused on adopting thinking that promotes adjustment and wellness. While Beck (1995) and Ellis (2001) have formal, structured methods of helping people change their thoughts and attitudes, these methods would need to be adapted to disaster mental health. The adaptations, while retaining the core principles of the model, would likely focus on the disputation of irrational thinking related to recovery, encouraging a resiliency-focused attitude, and encouraging adaptive rational restructuring of the disaster event itself.

Interpersonally Based Interventions

Interpersonally oriented interventions focus on promoting connectedness at many levels and may include fostering relations between the affected person and their family, staff who work at their agency, clergy, pets, or, more directly, with the disaster mental health clinician. Many disaster survivors often recount the grounding experience of connection with others during times of crises as paramount to their early and prolonged recovery. As such, this domain should never be underemphasized. In addition, interventions in this category are also very likely to focus on and process or memorialize personal/familial/social loss.

Imagery-Based Interventions

Imagery-based interventions can be helpful in not only reducing current distress, but they may also be used to facilitate the acquisition of coping skills. An example of the former would be focusing on imagery that promotes relaxation and serves as a means of promoting calm and a sense of safety. This can also supplant disaster-related, repetitive, and intrusive imagery. Future-based imagery can also help restore the temporal sense often lost in disaster and help individuals restore hope. Coping imagery encourages patients to see themselves as strong and resilient and may, more specifically, encourage them to imagine using coping techniques as taught by a disaster mental health clinician.

Psychodynamic and Existential Models

While this model category is extremely broad and should be utilized only if the client directs or leads the intervention toward these clinical issues, it is an area identified as being paramount to many individuals' recovery. This area of intervention, it should be noted, is more specifically likely to be a focus for older persons as existential issues become more acute in later years, and age-related existential anxiety may strongly interact with the experience of disaster. This model, overall, can help place the disaster within a personalized, narrative frame; help individuals attempt to make some meaning or sense of the event; or help an individual begin to incorporate this experience into their larger sense of having a purposeful and meaningful life. It should be noted that some of the aforementioned intervention paths may actually *increase* distress, and they should only be used when the person is ready to process the material. These clinical areas, however, remain influential in most people's prognosis and should, at the very least, be incorporated into the assessment/treatment process.

PSYCHOPHARMACOLOGY AND TREATMENT OF PTSD AND PSYCHOPATHOLOGIC SYNDROMES IN THE GERIATRIC POPULATION

The use of psychotropic medications in older victims of disasters and those who have current symptoms and signs of ASD or PTSD requires careful administration and titration of doses for all categories, including antidepressant medications, anxiolytics, hypnotics, and, when required, antipsychotics. The general approach to medication in older persons is to start at the lowest dose possible and increase slowly based on the individual's clinical response and side effects. Normal aging is associated with the slowed metabolism of all medications in the kidney and liver, and, since most psychotropic medications are metabolized this way, dosage adjustment needs to be considered (Flint, 2004). A general principle is to choose the psychotropic agent with the shortest half-life to avoid the accumulation of the medication and its active metabolites in the client. For example, when choosing a benzodiazepine for an older person, we would use lorazepam, which is not metabolized by the liver, rather than the long-acting diazepam, which, with its active metabolites, accumulates for several days.

As discussed in this chapter, the use of all psychotropic medications should be considered only in those clients whose symptoms so overwhelm their functionality that psychotherapy alone cannot be implemented or would best be augmented by medication. Psychotropic medications should not be used in the acute stage of a disaster when emotional supports and psychological comfort often suffice. Situational anxiety and depression of a mild to moderate degree of symptom severity will respond over a brief time to the nonmedication strategies discussed in this chapter. Therefore, the question arises as to when one should consider referral to a psychiatrist for a trial of medication.

Again, we should examine the degree and intensity of symptoms, the impairment of vegetative functioning, and the overall level of distress in our client. A risk-benefit analysis must determine if a medication trial outweighs the risks of potential side effects. All psychotropic medications will increase the risk of falls, gait disturbance, sedation, mental confusion, sensory impairment, and physical symptoms such as lowering the blood pressure (hypotension), disturbing dryness of the mouth, and constipation. The older client is often reluctant to take any medication for psychological distress and might feel it would be a character weakness to do so. The literature on research for the treatment of PTSD in the older person with pharmacologic agents is sparse as limited studies specifically test agents in older persons' population (Mohamed & Rosenheck, 2008). On the other hand, if the client has signs of severe depression with suicidal intent, delusional thinking, and overwhelming anxiety, including dread and panic that disable their activities, then medication would appear to be indicated.

If a medication trial is initiated, the clinician should titrate the dose to an effective level and monitor the client on a regular weekly basis until symptom relief has been attained. In an acute disaster, we might consider the short-term use of a benzodiazepine with a short half-life, such as lora-zepam, in the client with overwhelming fear, dread, and panic symptoms that are not responsive to psychological support. The choice of medication, as previously noted, should be based on the degrees of distress, the current and chronic medical problems of the client, the total amount of medications they are taking, and other risk factors for falls, such as sedation and confusion. Sedatives such as barbiturates, meprobamate, and diazepam should be avoided due to their accumulation in the body.

The client with a prior history of PTSD who was asymptomatic but then experienced another trauma is at risk for a recurrence. If warranted, a trial of a selective serotonin reuptake inhibitor (SSRI), the pharmacologic treatment of choice for anxiety and panic, should be initiated, which will also be effective in improving symptoms of depression. SSRIs are considered the first-line pharmacological treatment for PTSD. However, even when treated with this class of drugs, response rates rarely exceed 60% and less than 20–30% of patients achieve full remission (Schoenfeld, Marmar, & Neylan, 2004). Agents such as citalopram and escitalopram have a relative benign side effect profile in the older client and can be initiated at an initial dose of 5–10 mg per day. Sertraline in younger adults was effective in the PTSD clusters of avoidance and arousal but not in symptoms of re-experiencing the events (Brady, Pearlstein, & Asnis, 2000).

At this time, there are six SSRIs currently available on the world market: sertraline, paroxetine, fluoxetine, fluvoxamine, citalopram, and escitalopram. Although only the first two have FDA approval for PTSD treatment, the others are also commonly used for this purpose. Although double-blind trials do not exist, evidence from open trials suggests that fluvoxamine and escitalopram may also be helpful for PTSD (Davidson, Weisler, Malik, & Tupler, 1998; Robert, Hamner, Ulmer, Lorberbaum, & Durkalski, 2006). Other agents for mitigating depression in older persons, including SSRI and serotonin-norepinephrine reuptake inhibitor (SNRI) medications, are better tolerated in the older population than tricyclic antidepressants and cause fewer cardiovascular side effects. Trazodone has some benefit for nighttime calming and sedation and is used widely as an adjunctive treatment for depression-associated insomnia.

Nightmares and chronic insomnia can be extremely debilitating. Prazosin, an alpha-1 adrenergic blocking agent, has been used with some success for this purpose and appears to improve these symptoms without causing significant orthostatic hypotension (Peskind, Bonner, Hoff, & Raskind, 2003). Hypnotics are commonly used in the treatment of insomnia; hypnotic use among older adults is more prevalent than with younger adults. Unfortunately, the use of hypnotics is not well studied in the geriatric population, and the medication benefit is usually not impressive. Insomnia in older adults is usually treated with benzodiazepines, nonbenzodiazepines, and other agents such as trazodone, valerian, and melatonin. Using appropriately selected agents and therapy initiated with a low dose and careful monitoring of the patient could minimize common unwanted side effects (Tariq & Pulisetty, 2008). Based on the limited data available on older adults, zopiclone, zolpidem, zaleplon, eszopiclone, and ramelteon represent modestly effective and generally well-tolerated treatments for insomnia (Dolder, Nelson, & McKinsey, 2007). There is no indication for the use of any hypnotics in the long-term treatment of PTSD. Also, there is no specific recommendation for pharmacotherapy to prevent PTSD.

Antipsychotic medications should be considered in the presence of severe anxiety and psychosis, including delusions and hallucinations, and in the reactivation of an underlying chronic comorbid disorder, such as schizophrenia or bipolar mania, during a trauma. Risperidone is the medication with the strongest empirical support as an alternative treatment of PTSD, particularly as an augmentation strategy, although there is little evidence for improvement in avoidance and emotional numbing. Risperidone can be an effective adjunctive treatment in cases where patients do not fully respond to SSRIs.

Table 10.5 summarizes data from nongeriatric studies presented by Berger and colleagues (2009) in a thorough review of alternative agents to antidepressants in the treatment of ASD and PTSD.

EFFECTIVE, INDIVIDUALIZED, AND INTEGRATIVE INTERVENTION STRATEGIES

This chapter attempts to clinically frame the dynamics of an older person's response to disaster over time and to outline treatment indications that follow from the assessment process. It is hoped the reader is impressed by the complexity of the interaction between advanced age, disaster, and idiosyncratic factors involving a person's response to disaster as well as their response to the disaster mental health interventions provided. Overall, the disaster mental health clinician should be guided by comprehensive assessment, which spans the behavioral, affect, sensory, imagery, cognitive, interpersonal, physiological, and spiritual/existential modalities. In addi-

Table 10.5

POSSIBLE BENEFITS OF SELECT PSYCHOTROPIC MEDICATIONS AND THEIR COMMON DOSAGE RANGE IN YOUNG ADULTS

CLASS OF DRUGS	AGENT	DOSAGE RANGE (YOUNG ADULTS)	POSSIBLE BENEFIT
Antidepressant	**SSRI:** citalopram, sertraline, paroxetine, escitalopram, fluvoxamine, fluoxetine		First-line treatments for global PTSD symptom clusters
	SNRI: venlafaxine	25–150 mg/day	Positive clinical response except for hyperarousal
	Trazodone	25–100 mg bedtime	Insomnia and comorbid depression, hyperarousal
Benzodiazepines			
	Alprazolam, lorazepam	0.5–2 mg/day	Short-term treatment of anxiety and panic symptoms and during antidepressant titration to clinical effectiveness
Antipsychotics			
	Risperidcne	1–4 mg/day	Treatment of PTSD with psychosis and reduction of nightmares; adjunctive therapy to SSRIs
	Olanzapine	5–10 mg/day	Short-term reduction in arousal symptoms, insomnia
	Quetiapine	25–300 mg/day	Adjunctive therapy, improvement of sleep quality, reduction of vivid dreams and nightmares

(Continued)

Table 10.5

POSSIBLE BENEFITS OF SELECT PSYCHOTROPIC MEDICATIONS AND THEIR COMMON DOSAGE RANGE IN YOUNG ADULTS (*Continued*)

CLASS OF DRUGS	AGENT	DOSAGE RANGE (YOUNG ADULTS)	POSSIBLE BENEFIT
Anticonvulsants			
	Valproic acid	500–1500 mg/day	Improvement in hyperarousal and avoidance clusters
	Lamotrigine	Mean 380 mg/day	Improvement in hyperarousal and avoidance clusters
	Carbamazepine	300–1200 mg/day	Improvement in impulsivity and aggression
	Topiramate	Mean 150 mg/day	Improvement in reexperiencing symptoms
Adrenergic Inhibitors			
	Prazosin	Mean 13 mg/day	Reduction of arousal symptoms, vivid nightmares, and insomnia
	Propranolol	120–160 mg/day	Improvement in hyperarousal and re-experiencing symptoms

tion, these domains should not be viewed in static isolation but as dynamic realms of human experience that are affected by both aging and the experience of disaster. Combined with a basic pragmatism and collaborative orientation toward the client, this clinical frame and its application will likely help older persons successfully recover from disaster, restore normalcy, and attain higher levels of subjective well-being.

REFERENCES

Acierno, R., Ruggiero, K. J., Kilpatrick, D.G., Resnick, H. S., & Galea, S. (2006). Risk and protective factors for psychopathology among older versus younger adults after the 2004 Florida hurricanes. *American Journal of Geriatric Psychiatry, 14*(12), 1051–1059.

Banerjee, S., Willis, R., Graham, N., & Gurland, B. J. (2009). The Stroud/ADL Dementia Quality Framework: A cross-national population-level framework for assessing the quality of life impacts of services and policies for people with dementia and their family carers. *International Journal of Geriatric Psychiatry, 25,* 26–32.

Beck, J. S. (1995). *Cognitive therapy: Basics and beyond.* New York: The Guilford Press.

Berger, W., Mendlowicz, M., Marques-Portella, C., Kinrys, G., Fontenelle, L., Marmar, C., et al. (2009). Pharmacologic alternatives to antidepressants in post traumatic stress disorder: A systematic review. *Progress in Neuro-Psychopharmacology & Biological Psychiatry, 33,* 169–180.

Bolin, R., & Klenow, D. (1988). Older people in disaster: A comparison of black and white victims. *International Journal of Aging and Human Development, 26*(1), 29–33.

Brady, K., Pearlstein, T., & Asnis, G. (2000). Efficacy and safety of sertraline treatment of PTSD. *Journal of the American Medical Association, 14,* 1837–1844.

Davidson, J. R., Weisler, R. H., Malik, M., & Tupler, L. A. (1998). Fluvoxamine in civilians with posttraumatic stress disorder. *Journal of Clinical Psychopharmacology, 18,* 93–95.

Dolder, C., Nelson, M., & McKinsey, J. (2007). Use of non-benzodiazepine hypnotics in the elderly: Are all agents the same? *CNS Drugs, 21*(5), 389–405.

Ellis, A. E. (2001). *New directions for rational emotive behavior therapy: Overcoming destructive beliefs, feelings, and behavior.* Amherst, New York: Prometheus Books.

Flint, A. J. (2004). Anxiety disorders. In J. Sadavoy, L. F. Jarvik, & C. T. Grossberg (Eds.), *Comprehensive textbook of geriatric psychiatry* (3rd ed., pp. 687–699). New York: Norton.

Greene, R. R., & Graham, S. A. (2006). Care needs for older adults following a traumatic or disastrous event. *Journal of Human Behavior in the Environment, 14*(1–2), 201–219.

Gurland, B. J., & Gurland, R. V. (2008a). The choices, choosing model of quality of life: Description and rationale. *International Journal of Geriatric Psychiatry, 24,* 90–95.

Gurland, B. J., & Gurland, R. V. (2008b). The choices, choosing model of quality of life: Linkages to a science base. *International Journal of Geriatric Psychiatry, 24,* 84–89.

Hobfoll, S. E., Watson, P., Bell, C. C., Bryant, R. A., Brymer, M. J., Friedman, M. J., et al. (2007). Five essential elements of immediate and mid-term mass trauma intervention: Empirical evidence. *Psychiatry, 70*(4), 283 415.

Krause, N. (2004). Lifetime trauma, emotional support, and life satisfaction among older adults. *Gerontologist, 44,* 615–623.

Krause, N. (1987). Exploring the impact of a natural disaster on the health and psychological well-being of older adults. *Journal of Human Stress, 13*(2), 61–69.

Lawson, E. J., & Thomas, C. (2007). Wading in the waters: Spirituality and older Black Katrina survivors. *Journal of Health Care for the Poor and Underserved, 18,* 341–354.

Lazarus, A. A. (1981). *The practice of multimodal therapy.* Baltimore, MD: Johns Hopkins University Press.

Melick, M., & Logue, J. (1985). The effect of disaster on the health and well-being of older women. *International Journal of Aging and Human Development, 21*(1), 27–38.

Mohamed, S., & Rosenheck, R. A. (2008). Pharmacotherapy of PTSD in VA: Diagnostic and symptom-guided drug selection. *Journal of Clinical Psychiatry, 69,* 959–965.

National Institute of Mental Health. (2002). *Mental health and mass violence: Evidence-based early psychological intervention for victims/survivors of mass violence. A workshop to reach consensus on best practices* (NIH Pub. No. 02-5138). Washington, DC: U.S. Government Printing Office.

Norris, F. H., Friedman, M. J., Watson, P. J., Byrne, C. M., Diaz, E., & Kaniasty, K. (2002). 60,000 disaster victims speak: Part I. An empirical review of the literature, 1981–2001. *Psychiatry, 65*(3), 207–239.

Norris, F. H., Friedman, M. J., & Watson, P. J. (2002). 60,000 Disaster victims speak: Part II. Summary and implications of the disaster mental health research. *Psychiatry, 65*(3), 240–260.

Peskind, E., Bonner, L., Hoff, D., & Raskind, M. (2003). Prazosin reduces trauma-related nightmares in older men with chronic PTSD. *Journal of Geriatric Psychiatry and Neurology, 16,* 165–171.

Robert, S., Hamner, M., Ulmer, H., Lorberbaum, J., & Durkalski, V. L. (2006). Open-label trial of escitalopram in the treatment of post traumatic stress disorder. *Journal of Clinical Psychiatry, 67,* 1522–1526.

Schoenfeld, F., Marmar, C., & Neylan, H. (2004). Current concepts in pharmacotherapy for post traumatic stress disorder. *Psychiatric Services, 55,* 519–531.

Seplaki, C., Goldman, N., Weinstein, M., & Lin, Y. (2006) Before and after the 1999 Chi-Chi earthquake: Traumatic events and depressive symptoms in an older population. *Social Science and Medicine, 62*(12), 3121–3132.

Tariq, S. H., & Pulisetty, S. (2008). Pharmacotherapy for insomnia. *Clinics in Geriatric Medicine, 24,* 93–105.

Ticehurst, S., Webster, R., Carr, V., & Lewin, T. (1996). The psychosocial impact of an earthquake on the elderly. *International Journal of Geriatric Psychiatry, 11*(11), 943–951.

Watanabe, C., Okumura, J., Chiu, T. Y., & Wakai, S. (2004). Social support and depressive symptoms among displaced older adults following the 1999 Taiwan earthquake. *Journal of Traumatic Stress, 17*(1), 63–67.

Weems, C. F., Watts, S. E., Marsee, M. A., Taylor, L. K., Costa, N. M., Cannon, M. F., et al. (2007). The psychosocial impact of Hurricane Katrina: Contextual differences in psychological symptoms, social support, and discrimination. *Behaviour Research and Therapy, 45,* 2295–2306.

11

Case Management for Older Persons in Disasters

MICHAEL B. FRIEDMAN AND KIMBERLY A. WILLIAMS

In the aftermath of a major disaster, most people experience emotional distress, some people experience an exacerbation of an existing mental disorder, and a few people develop new mental disorders, such as depression or PTSD. Contrary to common expectation, older adults often weather a disaster better than younger people. Frequently, they have had experiences that have prepared them to deal with difficult events and, therefore, may be more resilient than expected. In fact, older adults can be an important source of comfort and support to those experiencing significant emotional distress (Brown, 2007). However, older adults with mental disabilities—such as dementia, schizophrenia, major depressive disorder, anxiety disorders, substance abuse problems, and/or PTSD—are a particularly vulnerable population (Kessler, 1999).

An adequate response to the mental health needs of older people in the aftermath of a disaster must, of course, include concrete services such as a safe place to live, food, clothing, money for necessities, reunification with family, and so forth. But it also must include mental health services such as mental health education, brief counseling, and treatment for those with either ongoing mental disorders or atypically severe emotional reactions to the disaster. These services are provided by various types of mental health professionals and paraprofessionals, including psychiatrists, psychologists, clinical social workers, psychiatric nurses, and case managers. This chapter provides an overview of the critical role of case management in helping older adults with mental disorders or troubling emotional reactions in the aftermath of a disaster.

There are four underlying assumptions for this chapter.

1. Most older persons are not disabled—either mentally or physically (Geriatric Mental Health Alliance of New York, 2007). Many are highly resilient, have survived difficult times in the past, and have developed coping skills that many younger people have not developed.
2. Needs for services and supports vary depending on whether the older adult is disabled, has a history of serious mental illness, has a severe psychological reaction to a disaster, or is having a *normal* difficult emotional reaction to a disaster (Brown, 2007).
3. Needs also vary depending on where the older adult lives—independently in the community, with caregiving family, in senior housing, in special needs housing, in a nursing home, and so forth (Brown, 2007).
4. Disasters unfold in stages:
   a. Preparing for the disaster
   b. Coping with the immediate crisis
   c. Reconstructing day-to-day life for self, family, and community
   d. Dealing with long-term mental and substance use disorders

WHAT IS CASE MANAGEMENT?

There are many definitions and models of case management (Naleppa, 2006; Roberts-DeGennaro, 2008; Rose & Moore, 1995; Rosen & Teeson, 2001; Vanderplasschen, Wolf, Rapp, & Broekaert, 2007).

Sometimes the term *case management* is used, particularly by social workers, to distinguish providing services to address the concrete needs of clients for shelter, food, clothing, income, and so forth from providing clinical social work services that often include some form of psychotherapy.

At other times, case management is used to refer to a combination of activities that include concrete services as well as linkages to services and supports and coordination of care.

It is important to note that most discussions of case management assume on ongoing relationship between case manager and client. But sometimes, case management is provided on a one-shot basis. For example, in the aftermath of a disaster, a case manager may be temporarily available to help an individual or family to meet their basic needs as quickly as possible and to develop a plan to meet their longer term needs later on. That case manager often is not available for ongoing interaction and assistance.

Despite the variety of definitions and models, there are several core functions of case management even when provided on a one-time basis:

- Assessment and screening
- Case planning
- Addressing concrete needs, especially helping establish eligibility for and linkages to shelter, cash relief, medical care, and so forth
- Seeking and linking to services and benefits
- Providing mental health education
- Providing emotional support

Ongoing case management also may include the following:

- Following up to be sure linkages are successful
- Reaching out to clients who have not connected with services to which they were referred and/or who have not stayed in contact with the case manager
- Negotiating on behalf of the client
- Coordinating services and supports
- Providing crisis response
- Providing ongoing emotional support
- Taking overall responsibility for helping the client meet his or her needs

THE EFFECTIVENESS OF CASE MANAGEMENT

A ProQuest search revealed no studies regarding the effectiveness of case management with older persons experiencing emotional distress or mental or substance use disorders in the aftermath of a disaster. However, there has been considerable research about the effectiveness of case management (Rosen & Teesson, 2001; Smith & Newton, 2007; Vanderplass-chen, et al., 2007). Unfortunately, this research is of limited value for the purposes of this chapter because of the highly varied meanings of case management; because the populations studied—people with severe, long-term mental illness and people with severe substance use disorders—are not typical of the population needing help after a disaster; and because different studies have looked at different outcomes ranging from clinical improvement to stabilized housing.

In addition, research findings have varied considerably. For example, according to Smith and Newton (2007), two Cochrane systematic reviews in the 1990s focusing on case management for severe mental disorders were published. The first review found little evidence for benefits of case management with regard to clinically significant improvement, social functioning, or quality of life (Marshall & Lockwood, 1998). The second review showed more positive outcomes generally, especially for assertive community treatment (Marshall, Gray, Lockwood, & Green, 1998). This study concluded that the question of whether case management works is too imprecise to be answered and that each type of case management needs to be assessed separately. It is important to note, as well, that the Cochrane reviews focused on people with severe long-term mental disorders. Thus, their findings have very limited applicability to people who need emotional help in the aftermath of a disaster—most of whom do not have a severe, let alone a long-term, mental disorder.

The effectiveness of several different complex interventions to help frail older persons remain in the community has been studied recently. A meta-analysis indicates that addressing multiple dimensions of need in frail older persons produces better outcomes with regard to community tenure and quality of life than standard care, even though it does not appear to increase life expectancy (Beswick, et al., 2008). Complex interventions generally include case management in one form or another. Thus, these studies suggest that case management is a useful component of efforts to improve the quality of life of frail older persons.

In the absence of definitive studies regarding the effectiveness of case management with older persons with complex needs, it is not possible to identify evidence-based approaches. However, based on experience and anecdotal evidence, it is reasonably clear that it is simply not possible to help older persons experiencing dislocation and emotional distress in the aftermath of a disaster without providing services that fall within one or another of the many definitions of case management.

THE POPULATION IN NEED

Most older persons do not need special assistance regarding mental health in the aftermath of a disaster. The assumption that they do reflects our society's inherent ageism. In fact, many older persons are more resilient and better able to cope with disasters than are younger people (Brown, 2007).

However, many older persons do need special attention to their mental health. These can be categorized in the following ways:

1. On the basis of their psychological history and current psychological needs, including whether they were receiving mental health services prior to the disaster
2. On the basis of where they live

The role and availability of case management varies depending on these factors.

Psychological History and Need

Some older persons have significant mental problems prior to a disaster for which they may or may not have been getting treatment, including the following:

- Dementia (usually Alzheimer's disease)
- Long-term psychiatric disabilities such as schizophrenia or treatment-refractory affective disorders
- Recent disorders resulting in ongoing mental disability
- Long-term or recent mental disorders interfering with social functioning but not severely disabling
- Lifelong or late-life substance use problems, especially overuse of alcohol and prescription and over-the-counter medications
- Emotional difficulty managing the developmental transition to old age

Some older persons experience psychological difficulties in the aftermath of a disaster, including the exacerbation of mild mental problems that have existed, often untreated, for years, including the following:

- Acute psychosis
- Anxiety states
- Depressed mood or diagnosable minor or major depression
- PTSD
- Difficult-to-manage stress reactions

- Increased substance abuse, especially alcohol abuse
- Normal emotional turmoil

Residential Status

The need for, and nature and availability of, case management services varies depending on where people live, what supports and services are there, and whether case management is built in or not.

Community-Dwelling Older Persons

Most older persons live independently in the community in their own homes.

Although upwards of 30% of older persons live alone, this is not a problem for many because they have significant personal relationships and engage in satisfying activities—vocational, communal, recreational, and social. Some, however, live in *social isolation* without relatives or friends with whom they have regular contact. Disasters pose serious problems for those who are socially isolated.

Many, probably most, older persons who live independently in the community get no special assistance in the home other than ordinary domestic help or minor support from family.

However, quite a number of older persons—a higher and higher percentage as they age—are disabled to some degree and need, and sometimes get, support in the home, mostly from family caregivers with whom they often live. Often family caregivers can themselves benefit from supportive care because they are at high risk for depression, anxiety disorders, and physical illness.

Older persons may also get help in the home from personal care workers, home health workers, case managers from the aging services or mental health systems, or elder care managers. Sometimes, disabled older persons get mental health treatment in their homes.

Naturally Occurring Retirement Communities (NORCs)

Many older persons live independently in apartment buildings or neighborhoods in which a majority of residents are older persons. Some of these communities have supportive service programs (NORC-SSPs), which can include case management as well as health services and volunteer, recreational, and social activities.

Older Persons in Special Housing

A relatively small proportion of older persons live in settings that special-ize in serving people with mental or physical disabilities or who are older and need some degree of assistance. In some cases, such as community residences for people with mental illness or mental retardation, older per-sons have lived in these settings much of their lives. In other cases, older persons have chosen, or been forced, to move to these settings. Older per-sons live in the following settings:

■ Senior housing, which provides apartments for independent living but often includes on-site social and/or medical services; many of these housing complexes are subsidized by governmental entities

■ Supportive housing, which is designed for people with low incomes, histories of homelessness, or serious illnesses or disabilities such as HIV/AIDS or mental illness

■ Mental health housing, which is funded and overseen by the men-tal health system and includes supervised group residences, apart-ments with visiting case management, and single-room occupancy dwellings with on-site supports

■ Housing for people with mental retardation or developmental dis-abilities, which includes intermediate care facilities, community residences, and supported apartments

■ Residences for older persons with substance abuse disorders

■ Residences for people who cannot live independently but do not qualify for nursing home care, which provide a place to sleep, meals, and very limited case management services often combined with on-site or nearby mental and physical health services

■ Nursing homes, which provide skilled nursing care 24 hours per day, 7 days per week usually in institutional settings but some-times in smaller, more homelike facilities using a *greenhouse*[1] or similar model

CASE MANAGEMENT ROLES IN DIFFERENT STAGES OF RESPONSE

Preparatory Stage

The stage of preparing for disasters is divided into two parts—the period of preparing for disasters generally and the period of preparing after it is known, or is strongly believed, that a disaster will strike soon, such as when a hurricane is on the way.

General Preparation

Every community should have a disaster plan that includes identifying and assigning responsibility for helping vulnerable older persons in the community. This plan should include outreach to warn these individuals and save them if necessary. It should also include shelter, food, medical care, and so forth. It is particularly important to have a plan to retrieve or replace critical medications. The plan should also include identifying older persons with current mental problems and anticipating that some older persons will develop mental health problems. Cadres of people need to be trained to provide intervention in disasters and should include people trained in case management. Necessary skills include engagement, assessment, triage, how to develop a service plan, knowledge about resources and how to access them, negotiation on behalf of clients, and how to provide mental health education and emotional support. Connection to case management services and case management services themselves should be available via telephone and Internet as well as face-to-face.

In addition, service programs, whether community based or residential, should have specific plans for how to help the people for whom they are providing services. Responsible case managers should be designated for those who do not currently have case managers, and case managers should be trained and prepared to do assessments, to develop service plans, to provide concrete services, to link to services and benefits, and to provide emotional support. A backup plan is also needed because some assigned case managers will be directly affected by the disaster and will not be available to help their clients.

It is important not to assume that older persons who need help will welcome it. Help may be rejected for any number of reasons such as fear of where one will be taken, suspiciousness sometimes of paranoid proportions, desire for stability, or desire to stay with one's pets or with the important material things accumulated over a lifetime such as family photographs. Disaster planning needs to anticipate such problems.

Preparation for a Specific, Anticipated Disaster

Once a disaster is anticipated, the people who are expected to provide services, including case managers, need to be mobilized, reminded of their responsibilities, and asked to begin the process of preparing those for whom they are responsible for during the disaster. This often will include outreach, making an effort to persuade those who are living independently to take appropriate precautions, providing them with transportation to safe places, assuring they have adequate provisions if remaining in their homes, providing emotional support if they need it, and so forth.

Similar arrangements need to be set in motion for those who live in special residential settings.

Crisis Stage

Disaster Response Centers

In the aftermath of severe disasters—when people lose their homes and electricity and telephone service may be disconnected, leaving them without food to eat, clean and dry clothing, and so forth—much of the immediate response will be provided in service centers and temporary shelters operated by the Red Cross; other not-for-profit organizations; or local, state, or federal governments. Crisis teams will be assembled in these settings, and one of the central functions of these teams is helping people get what they need to survive and begin to reconstruct their lives—case management by any other name. For everyone whose life has been disrupted by a disaster, recovering stability is a critical need. This is particularly true for people with pre-existing mental conditions such as dementia, schizophrenia, serious depression, or mental retardation, who tend to become extremely anxious and confused when their routines are disrupted.

The job of the case manager in these settings includes the following:

- Rapid assessment
- Triage
- Arranging immediate services
- Determining eligibility for services and benefits
- Providing information and referral
- Providing immediate linkage to needed services
- Assisting to get information about missing family members and facilitating family reunification
- Providing emotional support
- Providing education for parents and grandparents about how to manage their own and their families' emotional distress.

It is generally believed to be important to combine emotional support services with the provision of concrete services rather than to refer people to a mental health professional in a separate part of the emergency response center or shelter. In general, people do not want and do not need to have separate psychological services during the phase of immediate crisis. What is important to them is getting their lives together. Treatment can wait.

The exception is those people exhibiting severe psychological symptoms, some of whom will need immediate outpatient treatment or to be hospitalized. One of the key roles of case managers is to determine who needs treatment and who can wait until a later phase. When treatment is necessary, case managers need to not just make a referral but also provide a real linkage to assure those who need treatment get it. This is often easier to arrange for people who need inpatient care than for those who need outpatient care. Those who provide mental health treatment in the community may have had their services disrupted, and many of them may have become the temporary case managers helping manage the immediate crisis. In some communities, telephonic and Internet services are available to connect people to the care they need.

Older Persons Who Remain at Home

Many older persons who are adversely affected by disasters will not go to disaster relief centers or shelters. They will remain in their own homes unless it becomes absolutely impossible, even at the risk of their own lives. For these people, outreach is critical. Case managers need to be available to go into their homes as soon as possible. Arrangements also have to be made for animal companions. The preceding section describes the function of case managers.

Older Persons in Special Housing

Hopefully, residential settings for older persons are adequately prepared to protect and meet the basic needs of their residents. The case management role in these facilities is essentially the same as that described earlier. However, all too frequently plans break down. Improvisation becomes necessary—an important skill of case managers in these kinds of situations.

Reconstruction Stage

Community-Dwelling Older Persons

Once survival and basic safety are assured, the stage of immediate crisis response phases into the stage of reconstructing lives and includes the following steps:

- Returning to, and often rebuilding, existing housing or arranging for new permanent housing
- Establishing a stable, temporary, or permanent source of income through income maintenance programs, work, or a legal settlement
- Re-establishing family relationships if families have been separated
- Reconnecting or establishing new ties with a community

These needs apply as much to community-dwelling older persons as to younger people because older persons need to re-establish relationships and satisfying activities. In addition, older persons are often concerned about the well-being of younger family members, including their children and grandchildren. Often they want to know how to help.

For this reason, as well as because they may have difficult emotional reactions themselves, mental health education and brief counseling can be very useful for older persons who were not receiving mental health services prior to the disaster and who do not need mental health treatment postdisaster.

Case managers, if they are available, can help older persons during this stage to achieve all the goals noted previously. In addition, they can be extremely helpful in assessing the need for more intensive mental health services, providing or linking older persons to information and referral services, linking them to needed services, following up to assure they get the services they need, coordinating care, and arranging affordable treatment or financial help to cover the costs of treatment. For example, after September 11, 2001, and after Hurricane Katrina, the Red Cross funded mental health benefits programs through which treatment could be provided at no cost to the patient.

For older persons who were receiving mental health services prior to the disaster, it is important their service providers provide a case management function focused on assuring the concrete needs of their clients that were created by the disaster are adequately addressed. Treatment without attention to achieving some stability will probably be far less effective than treatment with case management supports as needed.

Older Persons in Special Housing

The key need for older persons in special housing is to reattain the stability they had before the disaster. Case managers in these facilities need to focus, therefore, on the issues noted earlier. However, often their caseloads are so large that it is extremely difficult for them to adequately provide the kinds of case management services described in this chapter.

Long-Term Mental and Substance Use Disorders

After the phase of reconstruction, when life has stabilized for almost all people adversely affected by the disaster, some people, including some older persons, continue to have mental or substance use disorders related to the experience of the disaster. Some of these people had clinically significant disorders prior to the disaster that were exacerbated by the experience. Others developed disorders in the aftermath of the disaster. Some were receiving care and treatment prior to the disaster; some began treatment after the disaster. Others were not and continue to not be in treatment.

Case managers can help those who are not in treatment and who deny their need for treatment by offering valued concrete services. If properly trained, they can identify those who have clinically significant mental or substance use disorders and provide mental health education and emotional support; they may be able to persuade their patients to seek diagnosis and treatment.

For those who are in treatment, case managers can provide the full range of services typical of case management including help with concrete needs, access and linkage to needed services and benefits, service coordination, crisis intervention, and so forth.

For older persons with co-occurring mental and physical conditions, case managers can play a vital role by assuring their clients follow up on treatment regimens and lifestyle changes such as smoking cessation, diet, and exercise, which can be essential to improving and maintaining physical and mental health.

WHO PROVIDES CASE MANAGEMENT?

During disasters, FEMA, state and local emergency services, the Red Cross, and other disaster-oriented not-for-profit providers share primary responsibility for organizing disaster relief. Public health, mental health, substance abuse, and aging services systems are also involved in the provision of vital services, including case management. In addition, the private sector plays an important role during disasters through employee-assistance programs, managed behavioral health care, and elder care management.

In each system, case management is conceptualized differently, and the capability and capacity of their case managers vary.

Disaster response organizations have short-term responsibilities. Although they sometimes mount or pay for fairly sophisticated case management services that include responses to ordinary mental health needs, these services are time-limited and are not designed for people who need mental health or substance abuse treatment. They are therefore of limited value to people—older or younger—with long-term mental health needs.

In the health and mental health systems, case managers tend to have very large caseloads and serve administrative functions for home-based service providers and residential services rather than provide the kind of case management functions described in this chapter. Unfortunately, public health and mental health systems throughout the United States pay little attention to the needs of older persons. As a result, case managers, even those who are mental health professionals, are generally not trained or skilled regarding the mental health and substance use problems of older persons.

Employer-based mental health services such as employee-assistance programs and managed behavioral health organizations usually attempt to be helpful to employees and their families during a disaster. Employee-assistance programs are designed to help people to identify their needs and get access to needed services. During a disaster, they and managed behavioral health organizations (MBHOs) sometimes also offer debriefing services, mental health education, and enhanced access to outpatient mental health treatment services. These services can be useful to older persons in the workforce and to those who are being cared for by family members in the workforce. But they are not essentially designed to serve this population.

Elder care management is a service generally available only to those who can afford to pay for it. Some not-for-profit organizations provide these services on a sliding scale. Case managers for older persons are expected to visit people in their homes and work to help them remain in their homes. They are expected to take a high degree of responsibility for their clients, help them get access to the services and benefits they need, and attempt to coordinate services. They usually have some knowledge about physical health care, but generally they are not trained or skilled in identifying or dealing with people with mental or substance use disorders.

Elder care managers generally take full responsibility for aiding older persons with disabilities. In essence, they substitute for family caregivers to the extent to which this is possible. During a disaster, elder care managers should take responsibility for providing the full range of case management services described in this chapter.

POLICY CONSIDERATIONS

The roles of case management for older persons with mental and substance abuse problems during a disaster that have been described in this chapter are, unfortunately, most often unfulfilled. Disaster plans, to the extent to which they exist at all for people with mental illness, tend to neglect older persons; plans for older persons tend to neglect mental and substance use disorders. In addition, there is a critical shortage of personnel prepared to provide case management or other services for older persons with mental or substance abuse disorders. In general, the underlying missions and visions of the service systems through which case management is provided are too limited to give priority to building a cadre of people prepared to provide case management services for older persons with mental health problems in the aftermath of a disaster.

Addressing these shortfalls requires a major reconceptualization of disaster services and of the aging, mental health, and health services systems, which currently neglect the mental health and substance use problems of older persons not only in disasters but also in their day-to-day functioning.

In addition, given the lack of literature in this area, there is a great need for research on the most effective models of case management for older persons in disasters.

NOTE

1. The greenhouse model is a nursing home model that alters the physical environment, the staffing model, and the philosophy of care to make nursing home life more

home-like. The homes have, at most, 10 older adults, each with private rooms and bathrooms and a shared communal space.

REFERENCES

Beswick, A. D., Rees, K., Dieppe, P., Ayis, S., Gooberman-Hill, R., Horwood, J., et al. (2008). Complex interventions to improve physical function and maintain independent living in elderly people: A systematic review and meta-analysis. *The Lancet, 371*(9614), 725–736.

Brown, L. (2007). Issues in mental health care for older adults after disasters. *Generations, 31*(4), 21–27.

Geriatric Mental Health Alliance of New York. (2007). *Geriatric mental health policy: A briefing book.* Retrieved January 15, 2009, from http://mhaofnyc.org/gmhany/ GMHPolicyBriefingBook12_2008.pdf

Kessler, R., Sonnega, A., Bromet, E., Hughes, M., Nelson, C. B., & Breslau, N. (1999). Epidemiological risk factors for trauma and PTSD. In R. Yehuda (Ed.), *Risk factors for posttraumatic stress disorders* (pp. 23–60). Washington, DC: American Psychiatric Press.

Marshall, M., Gray, A., Lockwood, A., & Green, R. (1998). Case management for people with severe mental disorders. *Cochrane Database of Systematic Reviews, 2* (Art. No. CD000050).

Marshall, M., & Lockwood, A. (1998). Assertive community treatment for people with severe mental disorders. *Cochrane Database of Systematic Reviews, 2* (Art. No. CD001089).

Naleppa, M. J. (2006). Case management services. In B. Berkman (Ed.), *Handbook of social work in health and aging* (pp. 521–528). New York: Oxford University Press.

Roberts-DeGennaro, M. (2008). Case management. In T. Mizrahi & L. E. Davis (Eds.), *Encyclopedia of social work: Vol. 1* (20th ed., pp. 341–347). Washington, DC: NASW Press.

Rose, S. M., & Moore, V. L. (1995). Case management. In R. L. Edwards & J. G. Hopps (Eds.), *Encyclopedia of social work* (19th ed., pp. 335–340). Washington, DC: NASW Press.

Rosen, A., & Teesson, M. (2001). Does case management work? The evidence and the abuse of evidence-based medicine. *Australian and New Zealand Journal of Psychiatry, 35,* 731–746.

Smith, L., & Newton, R. (2007). Systematic review of case management. *Australian and New Zealand Journal of Psychiatry, 41,* 2–9.

Vanderplasschen, W., Wolf, J., Rapp, R. C., & Broekaert, E. (2007). Effectiveness of different models of case management for substance-abusing populations. *Journal of Psychoactive Drugs, 39*(1), 81–95.

12

Complementary and Alternative Approaches

LUCIA McBEE, CONCETTA M. TOMAINO, RICHARD MANDELBAUM, THERESE M. MIERSWA, AND ANDREA SHERMAN

COMPLEMENTARY AND ALTERNATIVE MEDICINE (CAM)

The ability to cope with disaster is mediated by internal and external resources. For many older persons, the aging process has provided abundant experience in coping with life challenges. Norris and colleagues (2002) reviewed research on disasters and concluded that when middle-aged adults were differentiated from older adults, in every American sample middle-aged adults were almost consistently more affected by disasters than older adults. While older persons may have some disadvantages due to their physical and cognitive disabilities, they often have experienced loss, pain, disruption, and disability and may have developed effective coping skills already.

One example of these coping skills is the increased use of CAM by older persons for symptomatic relief of multiple chronic conditions (Montalto, Bhargava, & Hong, 2006). In this chapter, we review a number of CAM skills designed to enhance the ability of older adults and their caregivers to respond to disaster, internally and externally. The National Center for Complementary and Alternative Medicine, or NCCAM (National Institute of Health, 2009), defines CAM as treatments that are not part of contemporary conventional medicine. Complementary interventions

213

are used *in conjunction* with conventional medicine, and alternative interventions are used *in place* of conventional interventions. While often described as *new age,* CAM modalities include healing practices that have been used for over 3,000 years such as acupuncture, meditation, rituals, prayer, and herbs. CAM modalities tend to be holistic—for example, viewing mind, body, and spirit as intrinsically connected.

There is an extensive range of treatments under the CAM rubric. In a 2005 survey, the Institute of Medicine listed 100 CAM therapies, practices, and systems. The National Institutes of Health's Complementary and Alternative Medicine Program categorizes CAM models and interventions as the following:

- Alternative medical systems
- Mind/body interventions
- Biologically based therapies
- Manipulative and body-based methods
- Energy therapies

Alternative medical systems fundamentally differ from the diagnose-and-treat model of Western medicine. Ancient alternative systems include Indian Ayurvedic medicine, traditional Chinese medicine, and homeopathy. *Mind/body interventions* incorporate meditation, prayer, and cognitive and creative therapies. *Biologically based therapies* use herbs, vitamins, and food. *Manipulative therapies* comprise massage and chiropractic medicine. *Energy therapies* include Reiki, chi gong, and magnetic fields (National Institutes of Health, 2009).

As it targets symptom relief, CAM is especially appropriate for older persons and those with chronic conditions. Four out of 10 U.S. adults have used at least one form of CAM in the past 12 months according to a 2007 study released by the NCCAM division of the National Institutes of Health (Barnes, Bloom, & Nahin, 2008). In a 2000 study of 848 adults over age 50, nearly 70% of the respondents used at least one CAM modality, with 44% reporting using curative CAM and 58% reporting using preventive/curative CAM (Montalto, Bhargava, & Hong, 2006). In a large survey, researchers found that 88% of those over 65 years old used CAM (Ness, Cirillo, Weir, Nisly, & Wallace, 2005). In another survey, it was noted that individuals age 40–64 had the highest rates of CAM use (Tindle, Davis, Phillips, & Eisenberg, 2005). CAM services are generally low risk, low cost, and appeal to culturally diverse populations. Targeting symptom relief and using a holistic approach, these modalities address the multifaceted conditions and losses confronting older persons. CAM also may identify and strengthen spiritual resources, especially important for some facing illness, loss, and death.

This chapter includes descriptions of mindfulness, yoga, meditation, rituals, spirituality, creative arts therapies, and herbal medicine. It is not intended to be an all-inclusive survey of CAM therapies for older persons as part of disaster preparedness. It is intended to describe the general reasons that CAM might be effective and describe in detail several specific treatments, applications, and recommendations. The application of these modalities for professional and family caregivers is equally important. Caregivers are the primary contact for older persons. If the caregiver is distressed, the older person also will be distressed. CAM modalities offer a means to heal and support both caregiver and care receiver.

MINDFULNESS-BASED APPROACHES: LEARNING TO RESPOND, NOT REACT

> Mindfulness is "paying attention in a particular way: on purpose, in the present moment, and non-judgmentally"
>
> —Kabat-Zinn, 1994, p. 4

Mind-body interventions utilize the connections among the mind, body, emotions, and spirit for healing. An individual's personal experience may have already informed much of what science is now validating—the mind and body are connected! Not only obvious connections like stress headaches or a nervous stomach, studies now connect high levels of stress with lowered levels of cortisol, affecting our immune system's ability to fight large and small diseases (Sapolsky, 2004). Of the CAM domains, mind-body medicine is the most widely used. In 2002, a U.S. national study confirmed that three mind-body relaxation techniques—imagery, biofeedback, and hypnosis—taken together were used by more than 30% of the adult population (Wolsko, Eisenberg, Davis, & Phillips, 2004).

Mindfulness skills promote an ability to *respond*, rather than *react*, to crisis. This section describes mindfulness skills and other interventions that can be implemented mindfully. Mindfulness training has been shown to reduce anxiety and strengthen immune response, offering preventative tools for both mind and body (Baer, 2006; Davidson, et al., 2003; Didonna, 2008; Kabat-Zinn, 1982; Kabat-Zinn, Lipworth, Burney, & Sellers, 1986; Kabat-Zinn, et al., 1992; Stanley, 2009). Recent preliminary studies have found that these skills can be adapted to teach older persons with physical and cognitive frailties and stress (McBee, 2008; Smith, 2004). In addition, small studies on the use of mindfulness training, to date unpublished, also demonstrate the effectiveness of mindfulness and mind-body skills following a disaster or trauma specifically to treat PTSD (Anchorena, 2009; Niles, Klunk-Gillis, & Paysnick, 2009; Saveland, 2009; Smith, 2009). Gordon, Staples, Blyta, Bytyqi, and Wilson (2008) reported that 82 high school students in Kosovo who met the criteria for PTSD as measured by the Harvard Trauma Questionnaire were offered a program using guided imagery, breathing techniques, and biofeedback as well as creative expressive therapies. The percentage of participants with symptoms indicating PTSD was significantly reduced from 100% to 18% following these interventions. The symptom reduction remained at follow-up 3 months later.

Mindfulness is a core mind-body practice. As with all mind-body practices, understanding the intellectual concepts is only one aspect. In order to teach mindfulness, the teacher must also be a practitioner. The following exercise is intended for disaster preparedness program planners or health professionals who need self-help tools to maintain optimum performance during and after disasters. The exercise can be adapted easily for use with older persons; their caregivers; volunteers; professionals and ancillary support staff; and others pre-, during-, and postdisaster.

Try this:

> Find a quiet space where you will not be interrupted for the next few minutes. Sit or lie comfortably in a position that you can hold without moving. Also, make sure you can breathe comfortably. Make sure your chest and belly are open, and if your clothing is tight around the waist, loosen it. Close your eyes if it is comfortable for you, otherwise, find a spot on the floor, wall, or ceiling to gaze at. Keep this gaze soft and steady, focusing internally. Notice your breath. Is it fast or slow, even or ragged, deep or shallow? Stay with each breath. In and out, notice the pauses between the in and the out, the exhalation and the inhalation. Do this exercise for 1–3 minutes. Has your mind wandered? At times, our mind may pull us away to events in the past or the future. At times, physical sensations may distract us, or emotions arise. When this happens, and you become aware of it, simply take note and return your attention to your breath. (McBee, 2008, p. 17)

In mindfulness meditation, the practitioner maintains an open awareness, acceptance, and even curiosity of whatever may arise. Mindfulness is a mind-body intervention that incorporates formal and informal practices. Formal practice sets aside established periods for meditation, walking, and yoga. Informal practice includes everything else—eating, sleeping, working, and playing can all be done with awareness.

Acquiring mindfulness skills is the result of cultivation and practice implemented over time as a preventative measure. Programs such as Mindfulness-Based Elder Care (McBee, 2008) are excellent resources for both older persons and caregivers. Skills that lead to increased resilience offer a disaster prophylactic for older persons and caregivers.

Administrators, staff, and professional and family caregivers also benefit from mindfulness training (McBee, 2008). An ability to be calm, present, compassionate, knowledgeable, and decisive, and to communicate these states verbally and nonverbally, is important to leadership, especially during a crisis. Stress is contagious, but a calm presence is also contagious.

Following a disaster, aromatherapy, hand massage, creative therapies, and humor may be excellent tools for reducing stress and anxiety. Aromatherapy promotes healing and well-being by using pure essential oils from plants. Our sense of smell is linked to the limbic brain, connecting directly to memory and emotion. Essential oils have been found to evoke common responses and symptomatic relief from a variety of conditions. Lavender is the most all-purpose essential oil and would be a simple, effective tool for reducing the distress associated with crises and disaster.[1] (See the "Use of Herbal Medicine" section for a more complete discussion on essential oils and lavender.)

Hand massage is also an excellent tool that may calm not only the person receiving the massage but also the person giving the massage. For older persons, a very gentle slow massage is best, with careful attention to skin, circulation, and other conditions.

Creative therapies and humor may offer tools for coping with meaning and healing in a disaster. Music, art, poetry, and drama are common responses to tragedy, and even older persons with extreme cognitive and physical frailties can access their creative nature. In a poetry group for older persons with physical disabilities, older persons used prewritten words on large pieces of cardboard similar to magnetic poetry to evoke memory and feelings. In the feelings art group on a dementia unit, older persons with dementia participated in art projects designed to evoke feelings and memories (Bober, McClellan, McBee, & Westreich, 2002). Creative modalities are also discussed in the "Music Therapy and Other Creative Arts Programs" section.

The use of humor during a crisis may seem like an oxymoron, and yet laughter can be profoundly healing and connecting (DeWitt Brandler, 2007). Again, it may also be a way to connect with older persons who are confused and frail. In the midst of a stressful situation, a good laugh together connects us all. It offers not only mental but also physical relief by allowing us to breathe deeply and massage our internal organs. Laughter is also contagious.

The mindful use of all these skills may form a first aid kit for disaster preparedness. Mindfulness groups help older persons and caregivers cope with daily stressors and inoculate them from the stress of a disaster. Other CAM modalities may be useful during a crisis or in the aftermath. In the hours following the World Trade Center disaster, some older persons were evacuated from nearby residences and senior centers. One anecdotal report describes the use of humor to cope with the stress of these moments (DeWitt Brandler, 2007; Mariano, Sherman, & Sherman, 2007). Mindfulness is not so much what we do but how we do it. The most important tool we bring to older persons is our complete presence in each moment.

GENERAL OVERVIEW OF CREATIVE ARTS THERAPY APPROACHES

All creative arts therapies provide services to a broad population including children, adolescents, adults, older adults, groups, and families. The difference is the medium used to assess and facilitate the therapeutic process. Treatment may be directed at mental health problems including anxiety, depression, and other mental and emotional problems and disorders; addictions; family and relationship issues; abuse and domestic violence; social and emotional difficulties related to disability and illness; physical, cognitive, and neurological problems; or psychosocial difficulties related to medical illness. Such problems may have preceded the disaster or trauma or may have developed as a result of the traumatic experience of disaster. Creative arts therapy programs are found in a number of settings including home care, skilled nursing homes, subacute care, clinics, hospitals, public and community agencies, educational institutions, businesses, wellness centers, and private practices.

Creative arts therapies encompass a large and varied group of therapies. This section describes a wide variety of specific creative arts therapies and focuses on music therapy most comprehensively as one example of the application of creative therapies for older adults coping with trauma or disaster. It deserves mention here that in all cases, creative arts therapies should be directed by trained therapists.

Music therapy is the systematic use of music within a developing relationship between a professional music therapist and client to restore, maintain, and/or improve physical, emotional, psychosocial, and neurological function (American Music Therapy Association, 2009).

Art therapy is based on the belief that the creative process involved in artistic self-expression helps people resolve conflicts and problems, develop interpersonal skills, manage behavior, reduce stress, increase self-esteem and self-awareness, and achieve insight (American Art Therapy Association, 2009). Collage therapy has been used with older persons for stress management related to disasters (Mariano, Sherman, & Sherman, 2007).

Dance/movement therapy is the psychotherapeutic use of movement as a process to further the emotional, social, cognitive, and physical integration of the individual (American Dance Therapy Association, 2009).

Poetry and journaling therapy and bibliotherapy are used synonymously to describe the intentional use of poetry and other forms of literature for healing and personal growth (National Association of Creative Arts Therapies, 2009).

Drama therapy is the intentional use of drama and/or theater processes to achieve therapeutic goals (National Association for Drama Therapy, 2009).

Psychodrama is one of the earliest of the arts therapies and was developed as an action-oriented alternative to classical psychoanalysis (American Society of Group Psychotherapy and Psychodrama, 2009).

Reaching Older Persons With Dementia Through Music

Music is a powerful tool for reaching those for whom words no longer effectively convey meaning, particularly those with communication impairment as commonly found in older persons with dementia. This is especially true during times of communal stress such as disasters. Clinical studies in music therapy have demonstrated that the use of familiar songs has a positive therapeutic influence on associative memory recall as well as mood in persons with dementia (Clair, 1996; Cocconetti, Fionda, Zannino, Ettore, & Margialino, 1999; Sacks & Tomaino, 1991; Schulkind, Hennis, & Rubin, 1999; Tomaino, 1998a, 1998b). Because of the strong associations attributed to songs or particular harmonies, music can be used to affect mood states. Listening to pleasing music can result in enhanced mood and reduced discomfort or pain (Blood, Zatorre, Bermudez, & Evans, 1999). Music can also serve to relax the older person through slow rhythmic patterns, which entrain slower breathing patterns and result in a calming effect similar to techniques used in meditation and yoga. In general, music can be used therapeutically to promote attention, physical activity, relaxation, self-awareness, learning, communication, self-expression, creativity, social interaction, and personal development.

There are both active and passive music therapy techniques that can be used in disaster preparedness. Passive music listening such as using prerecorded music via CD or MP3 player can provide a comforting environment, mask environmental sounds, induce rest and sleep, reduce perception of pain, stimulate imagery and reminiscence, facilitate conversation, and provide spiritual comfort.

Active music making, facilitated by a credentialed music therapist, can include vocal/breathing exercises, musically assisted exercises, musically assisted meditation and relaxation, drumming, song writing, and improvisation. In addition, active music making can enhance self-expression, provide an emotional outlet in a protective environment, provide opportunities to interact with others, decrease the perception of pain, increase the duration of physical activity, decrease agitation, and decrease withdrawal.

How Can Caregivers / Care Providers Use Music Therapeutically?

Care providers and caregivers should start to create music listening programs for the older persons they care for before cognitive impairment makes it impossible to determine the individual's preferred music. If the individual cannot be engaged in choosing the music, there are some ways to determine what types of music may be most appropriate. First, consider music that has been part of rituals and special occasions with which the individual is most familiar. These include hymns; spirituals; holiday songs; songs from special events, such as weddings, family gatherings, and vacations; ethnic music, and so forth. Second, consider the genre of music (pop, jazz, classical, opera, etc.) in which the individual had shown a previous interest. Third, consider music for different purposes such as music for relaxation, reminiscence, or increased physical exercise. Provide lightweight headphones so the individual is immersed in the music. This will consequently block out environmental sounds that may cause stress or fear. Remember that sudden noises, particularly after an emergency or disaster, will stimulate a fight-or-flight response that can exacerbate agitation or withdrawal.

Where to Find a Therapist

Creative arts therapies address multiple therapeutic needs through the medium of art-based activities and interventions. Such therapies play an important role in the treatment of individuals when verbal approaches alone are not effective. It is especially true in the area of adult trauma, where an individual's impaired cognition may impede his or her ability to understand and respond to a sudden change in environment or otherwise normal circumstances. Most creative arts therapy associations maintain a national roster where you can locate a therapist in your area.

THE USE OF HERBAL MEDICINE TO PROMOTE AND PROTECT THE MENTAL HEALTH OF GERIATRIC PATIENTS DURING DISASTERS

Herbal Remedies as a Gateway to Mental Health

The growing field of zoopharmacognosy[2] demonstrates that we have evolved as a species that uses plants as medicine. Mental health is ultimately an expression of relationships: with ourselves, with other people, and with the world around us. Using medicinal plants can be part of returning to a more interactive, natural, and healthy relationship with our world, particularly in promoting good mental health.

In disasters, the sympathetic nervous response, which is expressed as fight or flight, will most likely be stimulated to an unnatural degree. In the general population, this fight-or-flight response can serve a crucial biological role as the increased alertness and adrenal activity may be needed to deal with the urgent situation. However, an older patient dependent on caregivers for basic tasks will derive little benefit from being in a stimulated, sympathetic state during an emergency or disaster. The situation will need to be controlled when the duration of the excited state is excessive or leads to anxiety or panic or is experienced by a debilitated or frail patient. Furthermore, the adrenal stress response can trigger a cascade of secondary physical effects including hypertension, elevated blood glucose levels, tachycardia, suppressed immune response, and impaired digestion. Therefore, the mental and emotional reaction to a disaster, significant and challenging enough on its own, can snowball into a much more serious and complex medical emergency if uncontrolled in a frail older person.

In the most obvious sense, physical discomfort or pain can have a profound impact on mental health and vice versa, increasing the multitude of challenges faced in coping with disaster. It is important for the practitioner to keep in mind that strong emotional responses to a disaster—including shock, depression, anger, sadness, or confusion—in many cases should be considered *normal*. Ironically, it is the older person who experiences none of these emotions who should cause the most worry for family, friends, and health care providers. However, it is crucial that caregivers have enough tools available to be able to control the situation in the short-term as older persons who experience debilitating mental or emotional stress during a crisis can endanger themselves and others. As any practitioner knows, remedies are effective to varying degrees with different persons, often for unidentifiable reasons. A facility that has the widest range of modalities and therapies to prepare for a disaster will be at an advantage.

One crucial aspect to including herbal medicines and other holistic approaches in disaster preparedness is to incorporate them into practice in the health care facility *before* disaster strikes and, in fact, independent of disaster preparedness. The reasons for this are twofold: (1) many of the most profound effects of herbs are long-term and preventive in nature, meaning that their use can mitigate the negative impact a disaster can have on the mental health of patients, and (2) doing so allows both older patients and caregivers to become comfortable and familiar with the use of herbs. Attempting to incorporate new modalities in the stressful and fast-paced context of a disaster scenario is neither realistic nor recommended.

The benefits of medicinal plants as aromatherapy should also be seriously considered both in long-term-care settings as well as in acute situations such as disaster response. Despite their gentleness, essential oils should never be used in direct contact with skin or mucus membranes and should be used only by experienced practitioners. Smell is the sense most directly linked to cerebral function, and aromatherapy—literally breathing in the myriad chemicals that make up a plant—has multiple and proven benefits in promoting mental and emotional balance. Aromatherapy has the advantage of portability, fast patient response time, and a general gentleness, as well as a reduced likelihood of adverse reactions or interactions, although this risk is already low with the gentle botanicals that appear in the list of herbal medicines that ends this section. These are crucial points for work in a disaster setting, where emotional and mental disturbances may be exacerbated and can impinge on the safety of others to a higher degree than under normal circumstances. Essential oils have the added advantage of potential incorporation into massage oils for use by massage therapists.

Herbs as Modulators—Nervines and Adaptogens

So what does it mean to use herbs holistically? It means the medicinal activity of herbs must be viewed more broadly than simply as replacements for pharmaceutical activity. Plants and herbs are a complex blend of dozens of constituents, many of which interact both within the plant itself and in the human body after ingestion.[3] In some cases, one chemical constituent can potentiate another, thereby increasing a specific physiological effect. In other cases, one constituent will buffer another, reducing the potential for adverse effects or extending the time frame for its metabolism. In still other cases, complex chemical interactions can have less obvious or synergistic effects, creating medicinal usages not present in any one of the individual constituents. The most distinct advantage that botanical remedies have over conventional approaches in a disaster is in their ability to modulate or aid the body and mind in reestablishing normal, balanced, physiological, and psychological functioning. This modulating activity is best illustrated by herbs activity as *nervines, adaptogens,* and *immunomodulators*—all of which are pertinent to mental health and disaster preparedness.

Of particular usefulness in the area of mental health are herbs that act as nervines and adaptogens. As Winston and Maimes (2007, p. 206) wrote, "Nervines are nerve tonics, that is, calming herbs that are mildly relaxing without the overtly suppressant effects of sedatives." Some nervines act as trophorestoratives, restoring energy and vitality to an autonomic nervous system overstimulated and exhausted by a disaster. Adaptogens are gentle, nonspecific tonics that serve to reestablish the general adaptive capacity of a properly functioning autonomic nervous system that may be compromised in a disaster. For the purposes of disaster preparation, adaptogens are most effective when their use begins prior to or in the early stages of a stressful incident.

Examples of Useful Medicinal Plants for Promoting Improved Mental Health

Many herbal remedies have value in a disaster. Some significant ones are listed in this section. Herbs that can also be used as essential oils in aromatherapy are noted. This list is not intended to be exhaustive and merely offers some of the herbs that have been used in holistic approaches to health. It is not to be used as a practitioner's guide to the use of medicinal plants in disaster preparedness. In all cases, practitioners should consult a credentialed herbalist when developing a program for using herbal medicine for older persons in disasters. The American Herbalists Guide (2009) provides a comprehensive digest of information on herbal remedies.

- **Ashwagandha,** sometimes referred to as the *ginseng of India,* is indicated for people who are run-down or depleted and at the same time suffer from anxiety, nervousness, and insomnia. Ashwagandha has a long history of use as a sleep aid and in higher doses has a mild sedative quality.
- **Chamomile** is useful in cases of mild anxiety and insomnia and has the added advantage of being anti-inflammatory, spasmolytic, and calming to the gastrointestinal tract. It is helpful in treating stress-related gastrointestinal symptoms and can also be used as an essential oil in aromatherapy.
- **Ginseng** is perhaps the most well-known medicinal herb and may have special utility in a disaster. Ginseng is indicated for fatigue, weakness, overexertion, shock, shortness of breath, and feeble pulse. Ginseng calms the mind and consciousness and along with licorice is useful in cases of adrenal exhaustion. One potential drawback for some older persons is the stimulating effect of ginseng, which can sometimes exacerbate anxiety or insomnia. Better options for such patients include American ginseng, eleuthero, or ashwagandha.
- **Lavender** is very useful for cases of insomnia and anxiety, both acute and chronic. Like rosemary, lavender is useful for improving clarity of thought, memory, concentration, and cognitive function in general. Lavender is also useful for tension headaches, dyspepsia, and sluggish digestion, and can be used topically for burns, cuts, and bacterial and fungal infections. Lavender is perhaps the most widely used essential oil and is an important aromatherapeutic remedy.
- **Lemon balm** calms the nerves, elevates the mood, and relaxes tension. It is useful for stress, anxiety, irritability, mild to moderate depression, gastrointestinal complaints, and dyspepsia. Lemon balm essential oil is very useful in aromatherapy and shows positive results in treating dementia in preliminary clinical trials (Akhondzadch, ct al., 2003; Ballard, O'Brien, Reichelt, & Perry, 2002).
- **Licorice** has marked mood-elevating effects, helps to restore homeostasis, and is useful for dry irritated coughs, wheezing, asthma, and pertussis.
- **Reishi** and other medicinal mushrooms have been shown to exhibit wide-ranging immunomodulating activity, making reishi useful for

autoimmune conditions as well as immune deficiencies. It can be quite important in building resistance to infection in older patients with low resistance, especially if used as a tonic prior to a disaster. Reishi is a gentle, widely appropriate, yet effective remedy for treating anxiety, insomnia, mania, mild to moderate depression, poor memory, and impaired cognitive function. It has a very low potential for adverse effects.

- **Rosemary** is a potent antioxidant and cognitive enhancer and is recommended as a remedy for poor memory, a confused state of mind, depression, and melancholy. Rosemary has the added advantage of being an effective essential oil.
- **Sacred basil** is an adaptogen, a nervine, and a cognitive stimulant and is used to elevate mood; combat depression, anger, and irritability; and increase concentration, cerebral function, and memory. It is an essential oil.
- **Skullcap** is a calming nervine that not only calms and soothes the mind but also helps restore vitality in patients depleted from fatigue and adrenal exhaustion. Skullcap is also useful for tics and spasms and is especially useful where stress or emotional imbalance lead to or exacerbate muscular tension.
- **St. John's wort** has a proven track record as an effective remedy for mild to moderate depression; for nerve-related pain and discomfort such as sciatica, peripheral neuropathy, and other neuralgias; and as a vulnerary, promoting the healing of tissue from wounds, burns, and other injuries. St. John's wort should not be combined with pharmaceutical antidepressants.
- **Valerian** is a useful remedy for insomnia, anxiety, and for mild to moderate depression.

Special Considerations: Safety, Contraindications, and Herb-Drug Interactions

Certain factors must be considered for geriatric patients when determining the appropriateness of a particular remedy: specific dosage, frequency, and duration of herbal use. These factors include the potential for low body weight and frailty, hypoacidity and slow absorption rate, reduced renal function, reduced liver metabolism, and, perhaps most importantly, the increased likelihood of multiple medical conditions and drug use. In all cases, practitioners should consult a qualified herbalist when developing a disaster preparedness plan that includes the use of medicinal plants.

The potential for adverse reactions from the use of herbal remedies is vastly lower than with pharmaceuticals, and most reactions that do occur are minor in nature. That being said, herbs can be used inappropriately and, as a result, can potentially exacerbate or worsen a condition or cause new ones. The more complicated the health status of the patient, including his or her use of multiple pharmaceuticals, the more caution a responsible herbal practitioner should exercise.

- With regard to herb-drug interactions, it is important to keep in mind that most problems occur from easily preventable mistakes that would be manifest from a clear understanding of the herb's activity. One such example might be administering licorice to a patient on hypotensive drugs. While a full discussion of the subject is beyond the scope of this chapter, it is incumbent on the practitioner to be well versed in the potential adverse effects and interactions of every remedy that may be used by the older person whether pharmaceutical, herbal, or other. Herb-drug combinations more likely to cause problems are ones in which the herb and drug are known to have either a similar or potentiating activity or a countervailing or antagonistic activity.
- Herbs with a marked effect on hepatic, gastrointestinal, or renal function are more likely to affect the bioavailability and metabolism of drugs taken concomitantly.
- More caution should be exercised when combining herbs or drugs that have a narrow therapeutic index or a known propensity to provoke adverse reactions.
- A more conservative approach is required for frail or debilitated patients, patients with known sensitivities or allergies to drugs or foods, and patients on multiple drugs.
- Always consult a credentialed herbalist practitioner; proceed with caution, and use fewer and milder herbs; and begin with lower doses and build up gradually.

Conclusion

Herbal remedies can play an important role in both preparing for and dealing with a disaster. In such cases, drugs may be in short supply or may not be adequate on their own; water supplies may be tainted, exposure to toxins increased, and greater stress levels may exacerbate many underlying conditions. Existing mental health conditions may be heightened, and in some cases previously unmanifested symptoms and conditions may arise. One of the advantages of herbal medicine over recently introduced drugs, or even many supplements for that matter, is that there exists a tremendous amount of empirical knowledge based on centuries of clinical use by trained practitioners. More and more reliable scientific data on medicinal plants are becoming available in the medical literature. While a simple use of gentle herbs is accessible to all, a more complex or serious condition calls for an expert in the field of herbal medicine just as in any other modality or specialization. Facilities wishing to put together a toolkit of herbal and aromatherapy remedies and to train staff in their proper usage should work in consultation with a qualified herbalist if it is not possible to have an herbalist on staff. A qualified herbalist can also consult on subject matter generally not well understood by conventional practitioners but crucial to the effective use of herbal medicine, such as herbal product quality. Most communities have at least one such qualified practitioner. The American Herbalists Guild (2009) is an excellent resource for identifying well-qualified practitioners.

SPIRITUAL CARE

Spirituality

Spirituality is a relationship with a God, an other being, or a connection to an energy that keeps one centered (Moberg, 2002). Many older persons who report a spiritual connection have better physical and mental health than their peers (Mackenzie, Rajagopal, Meibohm, & Lavizzo-Mourey, 2000; Shaw, Joseph, & Linley, 2005). Disaster survivors who call upon their spirituality increase their resiliency and ability to regain control of their lives (Farley, 2007). The spiritual beliefs of disaster survivors allow them to comprehend and integrate what has happened within the broader context of life's journey (Koenig, 2006). Decker (1993) noted that even when trauma has caused psychological distress, there is a search for spiritual meaning following a disaster.

Eighty-five percent of older adults state that religion and spirituality are important in their lives, and 95% of the adult population use prayer as a form of spiritual expression (Lewis, 2001). Banerjee et al. (2009) emphasize four distinct subdomains within his choice and choosing model, which has been adapted from the work of Gurland and his associates

(Gurland & Gurland, 2008a, 2008b; Gurland, Gurland, Mitty, & Toner, 2009). The subdomains are the following: empowerment, respect, identity and spirituality (Banerjee et al., p. 30).

The term *spirituality*, however, has very little meaning for cohorts born prior to 1935 (Simmons, 2005). Their primary experience is with denominational or cultural religious rituals aimed at strengthening their faith in a God. When a disaster occurs, they turn to the clergy and other members of their religious affiliation (Kilijanek & Drabek, 1979).

Those born a decade later were introduced to broader concepts of spirituality during their formative years in the 1960s (Simmons, 2005). For these older persons, spirituality is felt and experienced in a number of ways. For some it is a transcendental experience with a higher being. For others it is a communal experience with nature. For still others it may be that feeling of oneness with other human beings who are working for the greater good of all. But like the aforementioned older age cohort, spirituality also may be tied to a religious tradition or belief system.

Ethnic Variations

Sue, Arredondo, and McDavis (1992) addressed the importance of cultural competencies in counseling. Their work has relevance for professionals working in disaster relief and specifically in the area of spirituality. They caution professionals to be attentive to their own beliefs, which may bias their ability to effectively provide multicultural (and in this instance multispiritual) support. Furthermore, they emphasize the need for professionals to understand the culture of the population they are assisting and to utilize that knowledge when choosing interventions.

The New York Disaster Interfaith Services, or NYDIS (Harding, 2007), reaffirms the importance of developing cultural competencies. A lengthy chapter in the manual for clergy and spiritual caregivers focuses on the ongoing process of developing cultural competency and its importance in providing spiritual care during disasters.[4] A brief review of the typical spirituality patterns of multicultural populations comprising some of the largest ethnic or cultural groups in the United States offers an example of the wide diversity of spirituality with which professionals must contend.

There is no better example of spiritual nuances than the over 500 native North American tribes. While most if not all emphasize a relationship with nature, each has its own particular spiritual practices. The commonly held belief is that nature and animals have special spiritual power that can strengthen humans. The spirituality of native North Americans is intertwined intimately with ancestors, whose spirits reside within the living and are the basis for an individual's growth in wisdom (Institute of Spirituality and Aging, n.d.).

For many African Americans, spirituality includes both traditional religious practices, such as Bible reading, as well as a sense of the divine passed down by word of mouth. Some Black spirituality has roots in various African tribal rituals that have become intermingled with songs and storytelling from slavery (Institute of Spirituality and Aging, n.d.). Older African Americans utilize prayer, forgiveness, helping others, and other private spiritual practices to relieve their concerns and stress during difficult times (Lee & Sharpe, 2007).

Asian Americans are one of the fastest growing ethnic groups. Yet the paucity of studies on the spirituality of the 43 Asian subethnic groups makes it difficult to generalize about their spiritual practices within this brief review. However, Lee (2007) reported that older foreign-born Chinese and Koreans who reside in the United States participate in religious events of various types and have daily spiritual experiences that give them emotional support.

Puerto Rican spiritualism is called *espiritismo*. It is a combination of Christian, African, and South American spiritual and religious practices (Baez & Hernandez, 2001; Rivera, 2005) that prides itself on keeping a balance among all these influences. Those who practice *espiritismo* use herbs for purification and communication with incarnate spirits.

The majority of Mexican Americans, the second fastest growing ethnic population in the United States, practice fairly traditional Christian spirituality. However, Aztec rituals that connect individuals with the spirits or saints may be imbedded within that tradition. Most of these rituals involve incense, pilgrimages, herbs, limpias, sacrifices, and establishing shrines to key saintly spirits. With the sacrifice is a request for favor or protection (Lujan & Campbell, 2006).

Spirituality's Relationship to Disasters

Older Black survivors of Hurricane Katrina called upon spirituality to help them rebound from the effects of the disaster (Lawson & Thomas, 2007). Most of them relied upon their belief that a higher power, referred to as God, was listening to their prayers and pleas for help. Many perceived the possibility of miracles and identified moments in their rescue that provided hope (Lawson & Thomas). Spiritual and inspirational readings provided a tool for many of this cohort to regain control of their situation. Daily reading was a task that could provide both comfort and courage. The active role that many of the survivors played in helping others is supported by the literature as one way in which their spirituality was expressed (Mackenzie, et al., 2000; Smith, Pargament, Brant, & Oliver, 2000).

Some African American Katrina survivors who were interviewed after the hurricane reported asking God for forgiveness. Forgiveness and reconciliation allow people to move into a place of greater emotional strength. However, when there is a perception that God has not granted forgiveness, one's spirituality can be jolted, and psychological stress frequently occurs (Connor, Davidson, & Lee, 2003; Exline, Yali, & Lobel, 1999; Falsetti, Resick, & Davis, 2003; Maton, 1989; Monahan & Lurie, 2007: Schuster, et al., 2001; Sigmund, 2003). Restoring the spiritual connection becomes the healing goal.

After the 1966 Topeka tornado, several older persons bemoaned the loss of their gardens and the trees that had been growing in their neighborhood rather than the material loss of their possessions (Kilijanek & Drabek, 1979). Victims of a major flood in the Midwest in the summer of 1993, who had an established religious propensity prior to the disaster, said their beliefs brought a sense of strength and coping both right after the flood and 6 months later (Smith, et al., 2000).

Seniors participating in focus groups in New York after the September 11, 2001, terrorist attacks reflected on how they had relied on their spirituality for strength (Schuster, et al., 2001). Other participants noted that the disaster had precipitated a questioning of their beliefs (Mohahan & Lurie, 2007).

Spiritual Tools for Older Persons in Disasters

Numerous studies have demonstrated the importance of identifying how people utilize their strengths and exhibit resiliency during disasters, although there are only a handful of studies that have focused directly on older persons and their use of spirituality during disasters (Lawson & Thomas, 2007; Monahan & Lurie, 2007; Tyiska, 2008, as cited in Roberts & Ashley, 2008). Similarly, there are only a small number of evidence-based practices in spirituality that have been developed specifically for older persons. However, the literature can provide some guidance for professionals developing disaster response strategies and tools for working with older persons.

The initial task of mental health professionals during or postdisaster is to *normalize* the event for the older persons by the following (Greene & Graham, 2006, p. 206):

- Setting a positive tone
- Listening to their stories
- Finding positive aspects of their experiences
- Reminding them of past successes with adversity
- Indicating that help is on the way
- Giving encouragement

It is important that professionals who work with older persons during disasters be attuned to the spiritual propensity of this population and help older persons retrieve these strengths as they remember their prior experiences of coping with stress and adversity. It is not uncommon for those who have been traumatized by disaster to express or feel one or more of the following (Taylor, 2008):

- Anger with God (or a higher being) or religious leaders
- Distance from God or sudden need to turn to God
- Withdrawal from established religious institutions or uncharacteristic involvement
- Questioning of one's beliefs
- Emptiness with spiritual or religious practices and rituals
- Belief that God does not care or is not in control
- Belief that we have failed God

Those who are connected to a particular religious tradition will be best helped spiritually if they feel attention is paid to helping them meet their religious requirements. These include, but are not limited to, the following (Roberts & Ashley, 2008, p. xviii):

- Access to religious worship
- Access to sacred scripture and (religious) texts
- Access to food that meets a person's religious needs
- A multifaith sacred space that can be used for meditation and prayer
- Appropriate, timely, religious care of the dead

Identifying God images can be one assessment factor in deciding whether or not to use spirituality in counseling. Those with a view of God as reachable and visible in others and themselves and who allow themselves to yield control to God typically have positive coping abilities and lessened feelings of anxiety (Aten, et al., 2008). Identifying disaster survivors' images of God could allow for social interaction and support among those with similar God images (Aten, et al.).

Spiritual direction and counsel provided by the clergy are important during all phases of a disaster (Greene & Graham, 2006; Roberts & Ashley, 2008). In the United States, clergy have been involved formally in postdisaster spiritual care since the enactment of the Aviation Disaster Assistance Act of 1996. The role of the clergy is not to convert but to be attentive and comforting to emotional needs that disaster victims and recovery workers may have as a result of the disaster (Davidowitz-Farkas & Hutchinson-Hall, 2005; Roberts & Ashley). Some of the ways clergy can assist during disasters are listed in Table 12.1.

Two programs developed for veterans that make use of spirituality also could be adapted for older persons. Chaplain William P. Mahedy has initiated a program called the Spiritual Bootcamp for Combat Veterans. The program incorporates the Alcoholics Anonymous model to move veterans who experience feelings of helplessness to a place of reliance on a greater spiritual being (Sigmund, 2003). The Posttraumatic Stress Disorder Residential Rehabilitation Program (PRRP) at Dayton VA Medical utilizes a spirituality group that focuses on forgiveness and acceptance as tools for letting go and releasing anger for those with symptoms of PTSD (Sigmund).

The prayer wheel, which originated from the Buddhist tradition and is illustrated in Figure 12.1, is a nondenominational way of interactive prayer adapted for use with older persons (Rajagopal, MacKenzie, Bailey, & Lavizzo-Mourey, 2002; Rossiter-Thornton, 2000). It has been found to be effective for relieving symptoms of subsyndromal anxiety in a small sample and could be used with groups of older adults following a disaster.

Each component takes 5 minutes to complete. Participants choose either a private or public response to each of the eight portions of the wheel as directed by the particular component. This technique may empower older persons and help restore some control over their life situations (Rajagopal, et al., 2002; Rossiter-Thornton, 2000).

The Spiritual Practices Web site provides an ongoing interdenominational and nonreligious set of spiritual practices based upon 37 key spiritual words. The practices include quotations, videos, books, art, music, and inspirational synopses that one can use with a group for reflection and discussion or for individual reflection (Brussat & Brussat, 2008). The prac-

Table 12.1

KEY PRINCIPLES OF DISASTER SPIRITUAL CARE

1. Basic needs come first. Particularly in the immediate hours and days after a disaster, before helping with the spiritual needs of those affected, assess that the person you were working with is not hungry, has access to and has taken any medications that he or she normally requires, and has a safe place to sleep. Most people are unable to focus on spiritual issues when their basic physical needs are in doubt.
2. Do no harm.
3. Each person you work with is unquie and holy.
4. Do not proselytize, evangelize, exploit, or take advantage of those affected by a disaster, and don't allow others to do so.
5. Respect the spiritual, religious, and cultural diversity of those you are working with—ask questions about things you do not understand.
6. Presence—meet the person you are working with wherever they may be in their spiritual and religious life. Accept them as they are and where they are.
7. Help victims and survivors tell their stories.
8. Be aware of confidentiality.
9. Make neither promises nor anything that even sounds like a promise.
10. Grief, both short- and long-term, looks different in different cultures and religions—ask before you assume.
11. Be sensitive to language barriers. Remember that it is often difficult to express yourself effectively in a second language. If possible, provide spiritual care in the person's native language by finding a spiritual care provider who speaks that language. Allow the person or family you are working with to choose their own translator. Ideally, do not use children as interpreters, though it is sometimes necessary to do so.
12. Remember when working with immigrants that both legal and illegal immigrants often fear or distrust the government due to their life circumstances.
13. Practice active listening—listen with your ears, eyes, and heart. Do far less talking than you do listening. Never respond with, "I know how you feel," or "You think that is bad, let me tell you my story."

Excerpt is from *Disaster Spiritual Care: Practical Clergy Responses to Community, Regional, and National Tragedy* by Stephen B. Roberts and Willard W. C. Ashley, 2008, Woodstock, VT: Skylight Paths Publishing. Copyright © 2008 by Skylight Paths Publishing, http://www.skylightpaths.com. Reprinted with permission.

tices have been tested with nursing home and assisted-living residents and have been found to be useful and effective for sparking spiritual practices with older persons. Although they have not been tested with disaster victims, the practices recommended for faith, hope, compassion, meaning,

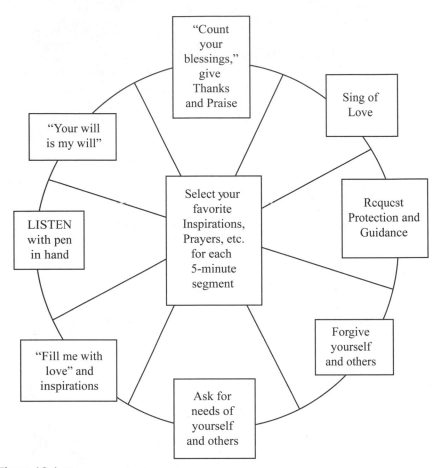

Figure 12.1 The prayer wheel.
From "The Effectiveness of a Spiritually-Based Intervention to Alleviate Subsyndromal Anxiety and Minor Depression Among Older Adults," by D. Rajagopal, E. MacKenzie, C. Bailey, and R. Lavizzo-Mourey, 2002, *Journal of Religion and Health, 41,* pp. 153–166. Copyright © 2002 by Springer Netherlands. Reproduced with permission.

and forgiveness might be useful immediately after a disaster, while topics such as joy, imagination, and vision would have a place in later months following a disaster crisis.

Sharing meals is another spiritual ritual that can bring focus to older disaster victims. Gathering to eat and beginning the meal with a poem or reflection about the disaster, or remembering those who have been affected dramatically by the disaster, acknowledges the current situation. At the same time, there is normalization through participation in a routine activity such as meal sharing. Posting pictures and mementos helped many victims of September 11, 2001, ensure their loved ones were immediately honored and not forgotten.

Disaster victims will have their own suggestions of rituals or spiritual practices that can help them cope with postdisaster life changes. The professionals' job is to listen to their pleas for support, help them regain touch with their spirituality, and help find avenues of expression for those who rely upon spirituality for strength during crisis.

Self-Help and Spiritual Skills Building

Providing spiritual care (like mental health counseling) can be extremely draining on spiritual caregivers and responding professionals during times of disaster. Studies have found that many clergy who respond to disasters develop compassion fatigue (Lutheran Disaster Response of New York, 2008; Roberts, Flannelly, Weaver, & Figley, 2003). Spiritual caregivers also become traumatized themselves from the experiences or distress of the older persons for whom they are attempting to provide care. Mindfulness strategies (McBee, 2008) that are critical to providing strong spiritual care may be compromised as professionals decompensate. Paying attention to the developing signs of physical and mental exhaustion will strengthen the spiritual caregivers' resiliency and ability to continue providing services. Resources accessed through New York Disaster Interfaith Services can assist clergy and spiritual caregivers who require support and respite. Roberts and colleagues determined in their research that consistent debriefing and discussion about feelings, concerns, and issues resulted in lower rates of compassion fatigue and burnout.

Spiritual care during disasters requires a special set of skills that includes an understanding of public versus personal trauma as well as whether the required intervention is spiritual care, counseling, or a mental health referral (Davidowitz-Farkas & Hutchison-Hall, 2005). New York Disaster Interfaith Services (Harding, 2007) provides training and has developed a list of emotional, behavioral, cognitive, physical, and spiritual symptoms that manifest throughout the different stressful stages of disaster and postdisaster. These outward signs can be cues for determining the most appropriate spiritual and mental health response.

RITUALS FOR DISASTER PREPAREDNESS AND RESPONSE

Ritual is one of the oldest forms of human activity. The word *ritual*, which has an Indo-European derivation and is associated with rite, means "to fit together" (*Encarta World English Dictionary,* 2009). We use this translation of the term because we are *fitting together* the changes that occur within a person during a transitional experience. Ritual is an activity that weaves the metaphysical with the physical to bring meaning to one's life. Ritual is especially valuable at times of disaster and crisis, when healing rituals can provide comfort and restoration both during the immediacy of the disaster and later, when commemorating the tragedy. As noted by Myerhoff (1978), rites of passage in later life can minimize the existential uncertainty and anxiety of growing older and of transition. For older persons and their caregivers, ritual can play a significant role in restoring wellness and overall health and well-being, especially during and after a disaster.

Neuroscience reveals that human beings are *hardwired* to engage in ritual. Neurobiologists D'Aquili and Laughlin (1996) explain the connection between myth and ritual. They argue that given the structure of the brain, human beings construct myths to explain their world and exhibit these explanations through ceremonial ritual. This condition was evident during and after September 11, 2001, by the spontaneous expressions of grief that occurred. Within hours of the disaster, people came together randomly and in official community gatherings to share flags, photographs, flowers, toys, and candles.

Ritual has a transformative healing power that can restore wholeness, healing, and hope after disaster. It is particularly valuable for older persons and their caregivers, who may be facing psychosocial issues of aging coupled with the familiar disaster issues of anxiety, fear, depression, trauma, and stress. Through ritual, the needs of the older person can be met on an individual level and within the community. One of ritual's powerful aspects is that it functions as a frame. By focusing on a slice of reality, ritual gives reality definition and attributes it with a special meaning. In so doing, it becomes a way to symbolically link events and changes with meaning and integration.

The word *ritual*, often used synonymously with the word *ceremony*, evokes a variety of images and associations. There are religious, secular, everyday, social, and civic rituals, all of which may be relevant during times of disaster. An example of a religious disaster ritual is a memorial service for those who have died. Silent processions or candlelight parades are examples of secular disaster rituals. Everyday rituals may include a moment of reflection with your morning coffee or tea or a daily walk for renewal. Social rituals might include organizing a series of suppers at the local library where families can gather, civic leaders and local mental health care workers can participate, and resources and support can be shared. Civic disaster rituals include parades and anniversary commemorations.

It is important to distinguish between ritual and habit. Ritual is an act that is value added and imbued with meaning and conscious intention via the senses and symbols. The sensory and symbolic experience of ritual integrates theatrical elements such as storytelling, dance, music, performance, singing, and oral reading.

Benefits and Types of Rituals for Disaster

As developed by Transitional Keys (Sherman & Weiner, 2004), there are rituals of loss, turning point, and celebration. The benefits of rituals include the following:

1. Relief and comfort in times of anxiety
2. Integration and healing in times of loss
3. Order and clarity in times of change
4. Continuity and community during times of crisis

Rituals that are particularly valuable at times of disaster include rituals of loss and grief, hope and resolution, relief for first responders and health care providers, commemoration and anniversaries, and renewal and self-care. The anniversary of a disaster or traumatic event can provide an opportunity to move toward emotional healing from anger, lack of meaning, sadness, and despair.

The Ritual Toolkit

The toolkit provides the necessary elements to develop and perform rituals in a variety of settings and situations. Objects may include stones, colored cloth, a bowl of water, bread, a vase with flowers, candles, oils, shells, personal photographs, bubbles, a ball, affirmations, pine cones, candies, and music.

A ritual toolkit consists of objects selected for their symbolic meaning and things to stimulate the senses and memory. Though the items in the ritual toolkit may be ordinary, they endow a simple activity with meaning. When developing your own ritual toolkit, consider the culture and needs of the participants and the variety of rituals that will be conducted. Activities using the toolkit include blessings to build community, toasts for renewal, ripping cloth to symbolize grief, releasing negativity through burning, using affirmations to enhance positive well-being, lighting a candle to symbolize hope, and replanting trees for the future.

For example, the following describes a ritual that uses objects from one of Transitional Keys' TULKITS™[5] (Sherman & Weiner, 2004).

Ritual of the Stones

This is a ritual of replenishment to reconnect with individual and collective sources of strength, courage, and compassion—all of which are essential in caring for older adults and a team of caregivers through times of disaster. This ritual can be done with older adults or staff.

- *Objects from the Tulkit:* Small stones of any description—including glass, plastic, natural, opaque, or translucent—that are placed in a bowl or small basket.
- *Activity:* The leader guides everyone in taking a few full breaths, reminding them to inhale and exhale. Once everyone is centered, the leader asks the participants to acknowledge the immediate chaos surrounding them or to think about a challenging time in their lives. The leader then asks the participants to identify what qualities brought them through the difficulty.
- *Facilitation:* The leader asks something such as, "Think of something that has helped you through a difficult time. What gave you strength? Was it friendship, humor, faith, or something else?"
  - The leader passes around the basket of stones. Each participant is directed to handle all the stones while thinking of what gave them strength. While imbuing the stones with that quality, each person is asked to state a quality from which they derived strength that they would like to share with the group. For instance, someone might say, "I share with you the strength of friendship," and others might note love, or beauty, or faith.
  - The basket returns to the leader, who then acknowledges that all of the stones have been transformed and as a result embody all the qualities that have touched them. The leader might continue the ritual by saying something such as, "These stones now have all the strength of our group. We can all share in each other's strength." The basket is then passed around the circle a second time, and everyone takes a stone.

Self-Care

During the aftermath of a disaster, it is imperative that health care providers and caregivers to older persons practice self-care to replenish their minds, bodies, and spirit. Care of the self is a fundamental component to maintaining and nourishing the caregiver/care receiver relationship. Ritual is an excellent tool for self-care. It can be as simple as ritualizing everyday activities such as consciously washing one's hands and saying "I wash away stress" or using positive affirmations such as "When I laugh I embrace my power" or "I take the time to notice and appreciate beauty" to improve the quality of everyday life. Affirmation cards can be placed on a desk or taped to a mirror and changed to continually inspire and restore.

Another self-care tool is to use the healing power of music. For example, humming, singing, clapping, and playing instruments can restore joy and overall well-being. Musical *baths* can be taken during the course of the day through humming after a particularly difficult interaction with a client, listening to the radio or a CD, and releasing stress through playing an instrument or belting out a song on the way home from work.

CONCLUSION

There is an ongoing need for ritual, even in contemporary life, for the well-being of individuals as well as communities. In times of disaster, rituals address a range of psychological, social, and civic needs associated with both immediate post-impact and long-term stages of disaster recovery. Rituals for disaster provide opportunities to honor the past, accept the present, and move more easily into the future. Rituals provide a framework for understanding and contextualizing disaster from which a sense of safety, community, and well-being can be rebuilt. They are medicine for the spirit!

SUMMARY

Disaster preparedness calls for multiple approaches. Older persons may be at increased risk due to pre-existing frailties. They may also bring skills from their life experiences. CAM is often helpful for symptom relief; most interventions can be used in conjunction with conventional therapies. Using modalities that are multicultural and universal, as well as increasingly accepted and researched, CAM is an important addition to conventional approaches. As this chapter illustrates, CAM covers a wide array of interventions aimed at strengthening and healing the mind, body, and spirit. Adapting these therapies, practices, and systems for older persons and their caregivers is an important next step in preparing our aging population for potential disaster.

NOTES

1. For detailed instruction on the use of aromatherapy for frail elders, see http://www.luciamcbee.com.
2. Zoopharmacognosy refers to the use of botanical medicines by animals.
3. One example is the use of St. John's wort in lieu of an SSRI.
4. The manual can be accessed from the NYDIS Web site at http://www.nydis.org/nydis/downloads/manual/Manual_NYCRL_NYDIS_Leaders_Manual.pdf.
5. *Tulkits* is a term derived from Finnish that means interpreter. Transitional Keys' TULKITS™ contain objects used to interpret symbolically the meaning of transitional events.

REFERENCES

Akhondzadeh, S., Noroozian, M., Mohammadi, M., Ohadinia, S., Jamshidi, A. H., & Khani, M. (2003). Melissa officinalis extract in the treatment of patients with mild to moderate Alzheimer's disease: A double blind, randomized, placebo controlled trial. *Journal of Neurology, Neurosurgery, & Psychiatry, 74*(7), 863–866.

American Art Therapy Association. (2009). *About art therapy.* Retrieved August 25, 2009, from www.arttherapy.org/aboutart.htm

American Dance Therapy Association. (2009). *About us: Who we are.* Retrieved August 25, 2009, from www.adta.org/about/who.cfm

American Herbalists Guild. (2009). *Find an herbalist.* Retrieved September 9, 2009, from http://www.americanherbalistsguild.com/fundamentals

American Music Therapy Association. (2009). *What is music therapy?* Retrieved September 9, 2009, from www.musictherapy.org

American Society of Group Psychotherapy and Psychodrama. (2009). Retrieved August 26, 2009, from www.asgpp.org/pdrama1.htm

Anchorena, M. N. (2009, March). *Mindfulness, acceptance, and the willingness to turn toward what is: A progressive approach based on mindfulness and acceptance in working with trauma and PTSD.* Paper presented at the 7th Annual International Scientific Conference for Clinicians, Researchers, and Educators Investigating and Integrating Mindfulness in Medicine, Health Care, and Society, Worcester, MA.

Aten, J. D., Moore, M., Denney, R. M., Bayne, T., Stagg, A., Owens, S., et al. (2008). God images following Hurricane Katrina in South Mississippi: An exploratory study [Electronic version]. *Journal of Psychology and Theology, 36,* 249–257.

Baer, R. A. (Ed.). (2006). *Mindfulness-based treatment approaches: Clinician's guide to evidence base and applications.* Amsterdam: Academic.

Baez, A., & Hernandez, D. (2001). Complementary spiritual beliefs in the Latino community: The interface with psychotherapy [Electronic version]. *American Journal of Orthopsychiatry, 71,* 408–415.

Ballard, C. G., O'Brien, J. T., Reichelt, K., & Perry, E. K. (2002). Aromatherapy as a safe and effective treatment for the management of agitation in severe dementia: The results of a double-blind, placebo-controlled trial with Melissa. *Journal of Clinical Psychiatry, 63*(7), 553–558.

Banerjee, S., Willis, R., Graham, N., & Gurland, B. J. (2009). The Stroud/ADL Dementia Quality Framework: A cross-national population-level framework for assessing the quality of life impacts of services and policies for people with dementia and their family carers. *International Journal of Geriatric Psychiatry, 25,* 26–32.

Barnes, P. M., Bloom, B., & Nahin, R. L. (2008) *Complementary and alternative medicine use among adults and children: United States, 2007* (National Health Statistics Report. No. 12). U.S. Department of Health and Human Services, Center for Disease Control and Prevention, National Center for Health Statistics. Retrieved June 6, 2009, from http://nccam.nih.gov/news/2008/nhsr12.pdf

Blood, A. J., Zatorre, R. J., Bermudez, P., & Evans, A. C. (1999). Emotional responses to pleasant and unpleasant music correlate with activity in paralimbic brain regions. *Nature Neuroscience, 2*(4), 382–387.

Bober, S., McClellan, E., McBee, L., & Westreich, L. (2002). The Feelings Art Group: A vehicle for personal expression in skilled nursing home residents with dementia. *Journal of Social Work in Long-Term Care, 1*(4), 73–84.

Brussat, F., & Brussat, M. A. (2008). *Spirituality and practice: Resources for spiritual journeys.* Retrieved January 3, 2009, from http://www.spiritualityandpractice.com

Clair, A. A. (1996). *Therapeutic uses of music with older patients.* Baltimore, MD: Health Professionals Press.

Cocconetti, P., Fionda, A., Zannino, G., Ettorre, E., & Marigalino, V. (2000). Rehabilitation in Alzheimer's dementia. *Receti Progressi in Medicina, 91*(9), 450–454.

Connor, K. M., Davidson, J. R. T., & Lee, L. (2003). Spirituality, resilience, and anger in survivors of violent trauma: A community survey [Electronic version]. *Journal of Traumatic Stress, 16,* 487–494.

D'Aquili, E. G., & Laughlin, C. D. (1996). The neurobiology of myth and ritual. In R. L. Grimes (Ed.), *Readings in ritual studies* (pp. 132–135). Upper Saddle River, NJ: Prentice Hall.

Davidowitz-Farkas, Z., & Hutchison-Hall, J. (2005). Religious care in coping with terrorism [Electronic Version]. *Journal of Aggression, Maltreatment, & Trauma, 20*(2), 565–576.

Davidson, R. J., Kabat-Zinn, J., Schumacher, J., Rosenkranz, M., Muller, D., Santorelli, S. F., et al. (2003). Alterations in brain and immune function produced by mindfulness meditation. *Psychosomatic Medicine, 65,* 564–570.

Decker, L. R. (1993). The role of trauma in spiritual development [Electronic version]. *Journal of Humanistic Psychology, 33*(4), 33–46.

DeWitt Brandler, M. (2007). *Humor and healing and stress management during disasters.* Unpublished manuscript, Columbia University Stroud Center, New York.

Didonna, F. (2008). *Clinical handbook of mindfulness.* New York: Springer Publishing.

Encarta world English dictionary (North American edition). (2009). Retrieved September 10, 2009, from http://encarta.msn.com/dictionary_/Rite.html

Exline, J. J., Yali, A. M., & Lobel, M. (1999). When God disappoints: Difficulty forgiving God and its role in negative emotion [Electronic version]. *Journal of Health Psychology, 4,* 365–379.

Falsetti, S. A., Resick, P. A., & Davis, J. L. (2003). Changes in religious beliefs following trauma [Electronic version]. *Journal of Traumatic Stress, 16,* 391–398.

Farley, Y. R. (2007). Making the connection: Spirituality trauma and resiliency [Electronic version]. *Journal of Religion and Spirituality in Social Work, 26,* 1–15.

Gordon, J. S., Staples, J. K., Blyta, A., Bytyqi, M., & Wilson, A. T. (2008). Treatment of posttraumatic stress disorder in postwar Kosovar adolescents using mind-body skills groups: A randomized controlled trial. *Journal of Clinical Psychiatry, 69*(9), 1469–1476.

Greene, R. R., & Graham, S. A. (2006). Care needs of older adults following a traumatic or disastrous event [Electronic version]. *Journal of Human Behavior in the Social Environment, 14,* 201–219.

Gurland, B. J., & Gurland, R. V. (2008a). The choices, choosing model of quality of life: Description and rationale. *International Journal of Geriatric Psychiatry, 24,* 90–95.

Gurland, B. J., & Gurland, R. V. (2008b). The choices, choosing model of quality of life: Linkages to a science base. *International Journal of Geriatric Psychiatry, 24,* 84–89.

Gurland, B. J., Gurland, R. V., Mitty, E., & Toner, J. A. (2009). The choices, choosing model of quality of life: Clinical evaluation and intervention. *Journal of Interprofessional Care, 23*(2), 110–120.

Harding, S. (2007). *New York Disaster Interfaith Services manual for New York City religious leaders: Spiritual care and mental health for disaster response & recovery.* Retrieved October 12, 2009, from http://www.nydis.org/nydis/downloads/manual/Manual_NYCRL_NYDIS_Leaders_Manual.pdf

Institute for Spirituality and Aging. (n.d.). *Spirituality and aging.* Retrieved January 4, 2009, from http://cas.umkc.edu/casaw/sa/Spirituality.html

Kabat-Zinn, J. (1982). An outpatient program in behavioral medicine for chronic pain patients based on the practice of mindfulness meditation. *General Hospital Psychiatry, 4,* 33–47.

Kabat-Zinn, J. (1994). *Wherever you go, there you are: Mindfulness meditation in everyday life.* New York: Hyperion.

Kabat-Zinn, J., Lipworth, L., Burney, R., & Sellers, W. (1986). Four-year follow-up of a meditation-based program for the self-regulation of chronic pain: Treatment outcomes and compliance. *Clinical Journal of Pain, 2*(3), 159–174.

Kabat-Zinn, J., Massion, A. O., Kristeller, J., Petersen, L. G., Fletcher, K. E., Pbert, L., et al. (1992). Effectiveness of a meditation-based program in the treatment of anxiety disorders. *American Journal of Psychiatry, 149*(7), 936–943.

Kilijanek, T. S., & Drabeck, T. E. (1979). Assessing long-term impacts of a natural disaster: A focus on the elderly [Electronic version]. *The Gerontologist, 19,* 555–566.

Koenig, H. G. (2006). *In the wake of disaster: Religious responses to terrorism and catastrophe.* West Conshochoken, PA: Templeton Foundation Press.

Lawson, E. J., & Thomas, C. (2007). Wading in the waters: Spirituality and older black Katrina survivors. *Journal of Health Care for the Poor and Underserved, 18,* 341–354.

Lee, E. O. (2007). Religion and spirituality as predictors of well-being among Chinese American and Korean American older adults [Electronic version]. *Journal of Religion, Spirituality, and Aging, 19,* 77–100.

Lee, E. O., & Sharpe, T. (2007). Understanding religious/spiritual coping and support resources among African American older adults: A mixed-method approach [Electronic version]. *Journal of Religion, Spirituality, and Aging, 19,* 55–75.

Lewis, M. M. (2001). Spirituality, counseling, and elderly: An introduction to the spiritual life review [Electronic version]. *Journal of Adult Development, 8,* 231–240.

Lujan, J., & Campbell, H. (2006). The role of religion on the health practices of Mexican Americans [Electronic version]. *Journal of Religion and Health, 45,* 183–195.

Lutheran Disaster Response of New York. (2008). *Resources: Spiritual care: Pastoral support program to prevent burnout.* Retrieved October 12, 2009, from http://www.ldrny.org/Resources/Resources4.asp

Mackenzie, E. R., Rajagopal, D. E., Meibohm, M., & Lavizzo-Mourey, R. (2000). Spiritual support and psychological well-being: Older adults' perceptions of the religion and health connection [Electronic version]. *Alternative Therapies, 6,* 37–45.

Mariano, C., Sherman, A., & Sherman, D. (2007). Section 8: Disaster recovery for older adults: Holistic integrative therapies. In J. Howe, A. Sherman, & J. Toner (Eds.), *Geriatric mental health disaster and emergency preparedness curriculum* (Section 8, p. 3, Portal of Geriatric Online Education [POGOe] Product No. 18848). Retrieved September 11, 2009, from http://www.pogoe.com

Maton, K. I. (1989). The stress-buffering role of spiritual support: Cross-sectional and prospective investigations [Electronic version]. *Journal of the Scientific Study of Religion, 28,* 310–323.

McBee, L. (2008). *Mindfulness-based elder care.* New York: Springer Publishing.

Moberg, D. O. (2002). Assessing and measuring spirituality: Confronting dilemmas of universal and particular evaluative criteria [Electronic version]. *Journal of Adult Development, 9,* 47–70.

Monahan, K., & Lurie, A. (2007). Reactions of senior citizens to 9/11: Exploration and practice guidelines for social workers [Electronic version]. *Social Work in Health Care, 45,* 33–47.

Montalto, C. P., Bhargava, V., & Hong, G. S. (2006). Use of complementary and alternative medicine by older adults: An exploratory study. *Complementary Health Practice Review,* *11*(1), 27–46.

Myerhoff, B. (1978). *Number our days.* New York: Touchstone Books.

National Association of Creative Arts Therapies. (2009). *Poetry therapy.* Retrieved August 26, 2009, from http://www.nccata.org/poetry_therapy.htm

National Association for Drama Therapy. (2009). *Drama therapy with a geriatric population.* Retrieved September 9, 2009, from www.nadt.org/upload/file/factsheet_elderly.pdf

National Institute of Health, National Center for Complementary and Alternative Medicine. (2009, May 12). *What is complementary and alternative medicine?* (NCCAM Pub. No. D347). Retrieved July 28, 2009, from http://nccam.nih.gov/health/whatiscam/

Ness, J., Cirillo, D. J., Weir, D. R., Nisly, N. L., & Wallace, R. B. (2005). Use of complementary medicine in older Americans: Results from the retirement study. *The Gerontologist, 45*(4), 516–524.

Niles, B. L., Klunk-Gillis, J., & Paysnick, A. (2009, March). *Introducing mindfulness to veterans with PTSD: Results of a telehealth intervention.* Paper presented at the 7th Annual International Scientific Conference for Clinicians, Researchers, and Educators Investigating and Integrating Mindfulness in Medicine, Health Care, and Society, Worcester, MA.

Norris, F. H., Friedman, M. J., Watson, P. J., Byrne, C. M., Diax, E., & Kaniasty, K. (2002). 60,000 disaster victims speak: Part I. An empirical review of the empirical literature, 1981–2001. *Psychiatry, 65,* 207–239.

Rajagopal, D., MacKenzie, E., Bailey, C., & Lavizzo-Mourey, R. (2002). The effectiveness of a spiritually based intervention to alleviate subsyndromal anxiety and minor depression among older adults [Electronic version]. *Journal of Religion and Health, 41,* 153–166.

Rivera, E. T. (2005). Espiritismo: The flywheel of the Puerto Rican spiritual traditions [Electronic version]. *Interamerican Journal of Psychology, 39,* 295–300.

Roberts, S. B., & Ashley, W. W. C. (2008). *Disaster spiritual care: Practical clergy responses to community, regional, and national tragedy.* Woodstock, VT: Skylight Paths Publishing.

Roberts, R. S. B., Flannelly, K. J., Weaver, A. J., & Figley, C. R. (2003). Compassion fatigue among chaplains, clergy, and other respondents after September 11th. *The Journal of Nervous and Mental Disease, 191*(11), 756.

Rossiter- Thornton, J. F. (2000). Prayer in psychotherapy [Electronic Version]. *Alternative Therapies in Health and Medicine, 6,* 124–128.

Sacks, O., & Tomaino, C. (1991). Music and neurological disorder. *International Journal of Arts Medicine, 1*(1), 10–12.

Sapolsky, R. (2004). *Why zebras don't get ulcers.* New York: Henry Holt & Co.

Saveland, J. (2009, March). *Training U.S. Forest Service firefighters in mindfulness-based situational awareness.* Paper presented at the 7th Annual International Scientific Conference for Clinicians, Researchers, and Educators Investigating and Integrating Mindfulness in Medicine, Health Care, and Society, Worcester, MA.

Schulkind, M. D., Hennis, L. K., & Rubin, D. C. (1999). Music, emotion, and autobiographical memory: They're playing your song. *Memory & Cognition, 27*(6), 948–955.

Schuster, M. A., Stein, B. D., Jaycox, L. H., Collins, R. L., Marshall, G. N., Elliott, M. N., et al. (2001). A national survey of stress reactions after September 11, 2001, terrorist attacks [Electronic version]. *The New England Journal of Medicine, 345,* 1501–1508.

Shaw, A., Joseph, S., & Linley, P. A. (2005). Religion, spirituality, and posttraumatic growth: A systemic review [Electronic version]. *Mental Health, Religion, and Culture, 8,* 1–11.

Sherman, A., & Weiner, M. B. (2004). *Transitional keys, a guidebook: Rituals to improve quality of life for older adults.* New York: Transitional Keys.

Sigmund, J. A. (2003). Spirituality and trauma: The role of clergy in the treatment of posttraumatic stress disorder [Electronic version]. *Journal of Religion and Health, 42,* 221–229.

Simmons, H. C. (2005). Religion, spirituality, and aging for "the aging" themselves [Electronic version]. *Journal of Gerontological Social Work, 45,* 41–49.

Smith, A. (2004). Clinical uses of mindfulness training for older people. *Behavioral and Cognitive Psychotherapy, 32,* 423–430.

Smith, J. D. (2009, March). *The benefits and risks of MBSR with those who have posttraumatic stress disorder (PTSD): Results of a mixed methods pilot study.* Paper presented at the 7th Annual International Scientific Conference for Clinicians, Researchers, and Educators Investigating and Integrating Mindfulness in Medicine, Health Care, and Society, Worcester, MA.

Smith, B. W., Pargament, K. I., Brant, C., & Oliver, J. M. (2000). Noah revisited: Religious coping by church members and the impact of the 1993 Midwest flood [Electronic version]. *Journal of Community Psychology, 28,* 169–186.

Stanley, E. A. (2009, March). *Mindfulness-based training in a pre-deployment military context.* Paper presented at the 7th Annual International Scientific Conference for Clinicians, Researchers, and Educators Investigating and Integrating Mindfulness in Medicine, Health Care, and Society, Worcester, MA.

Sue, D. W., Arredondo, P., & McDavis, R. J. (1992). Multicultural counseling competencies and standards: A call to the profession [Electronic version]. *Journal of Multicultural Counseling and Development, 20*(2), 64–88.

Taylor, T. (2008). *Caring for our pastoral leaders and care-givers.* Retrieved October 12, 2009, from http://www.ldrny.org/Resources/materials/Taylor.pdf

Tindle, H. A., Davis, R. B., Phillips, R. S., & Eisenberg, D. M. (2005). Trends in use of complementary and alternative medicine in the U.S. 1997–2002. *Alternative Therapies in Health and Medicine, 11*(1), 42–49.

Tomaino, C. M. (1998a). *Music on their minds: A qualitative study of the effects of using familiar music to stimulate preserved memory function in persons with dementia.* Unpublished doctoral dissertation, New York University.

Tomaino, C. M. (1998b). Music and memory. In C. M. Tomaino (Ed.), *Clinical applications of music in neurologic rehabilitation* (pp. 19–27). St. Louis, MO: MMB Music.

Tyiska, C. G. (2008). Working with elderly after a disaster. In S. B. Roberts & W. W. C. Ashley, Sr. (Eds.), *Disaster spiritual care: Practical clergy responses to community, regional, and national tragedy* (pp. 297–313). Woodstock, VT: Skylight Paths Publishing.

Winston, D., & Maimes, S. (2007). *Adaptogens: Herbs for strength, stamina, and stress relief.* Rochester, VT: Healing Arts Press.

Wolsko, P. M., Eisenberg, D. M., Davis, R. B., & Phillips, R. S. (2004). Use of mind-body medical therapies: Results of a national survey. *Journal of General Internal Medicine, 19,* 43–50.

Identifying and Classifying Mental and Related Health Problems

PART IV

13

The Interdisciplinary Treatment Team as a Geriatric Mental Health Resource Prior to and During Disasters

JOHN A. TONER AND EVELYN S. MEYER

Interdisciplinary approaches to the management of health care for older persons have received a great deal of attention in the scientific literature in recent years. Much of this literature focuses on the need in all health care fields to develop efficient methods for organizing and coordinating health care as well as a framework for communication between health care professionals (Barr, Koppel, Reeves, Hammick, & Freeth, 2005; Miller, 2004; Toner, 2008; Toner, Miller, & Gurland, 1994). This need is particularly severe with regard to the mental health care of older people during disasters (Toner, Howe, & Nathanson, 2007).

Almost 10 years after the Institute of Medicine published its report on safety and medical errors in American health care (Institute of Medicine [IOM], 2001) and called for better systems for coordinating care, the Institute of Medicine (2008) issued its most recent report, which highlights the importance of the interdisciplinary treatment team in reducing medical errors, improving safety and enhancing quality of life, and caring for older persons. A recent review of evidence-based studies of new models of geriatric care, conducted by the Institute of Medicine Committee on the Future Health Care Workforce for Older Americans (IOM, 2008, p. 3.15), concluded that there is some evidence that the care provided by the interdisciplinary team demonstrates, "improved survival and quality of life, quality of care and patient satisfaction . . . some also showed lower total costs, fewer hospital admissions, physician visits, emergency department visits and x-rays." Toner (2006, p. 218) reviewed the evidence-based studies of interprofessional education and interdisciplinary team training provided by Barr and colleagues (2005) and concluded that the researchers "have succeeded in synthesizing the evidence base and in so doing have established a knowledge base related to good interprofessional education" (p. 218).

Improved quality of care has for a long time been the raison d'etre of the interdisciplinary team and teamwork. *Quality of life* is less often discussed in relation to interdisciplinary teams but may be implicit. In recent years, serious attention has been given to the ways in which quality of life should serve as a central and unifying theme in interdisciplinary teamwork in health care and specifically within geriatric interdisciplinary teamwork. Two major streams of activity are revolutionizing health care for older persons: (1) the recognition of quality of life as a field of science with its own language, methods of inquiry, and applications to clinical practice (Banerjee et al., 2009; Gurland & Gurland, 2008a, 2008b; Gurland & Katz, 2006) and (2) an increased reliance on patient-centered interdisciplinary teamwork strategies that might "relieve restrictions or distortions of the choice and choosing process imposed by aging, ill health, or a restricting environment" (Gurland, Gurland, Mitty, & Toner, 2009, p. 110), all of which are exacerbated during disasters. This is accomplished only through an understanding on the part of interdisciplinary team members that they must empower older persons to define for themselves, as much as is feasible, and for the interdisciplinary team, the appropriate methods and goals of care related to their quality of life. In cases when older persons are unable to express their needs because of communication deficits and/or cognitive decline, the interdisciplinary team must be the advocate for the older person's needs and perceived wishes. In the context of quality of life and the choice and choosing process (Gurland & Gurland, 2008a), the interdisciplinary team "offers a single protean pathway for effectively helping people to improve their quality of life through opening choices within the range of their preferences and assisting their exercise of choosing" (Gurland et al., 2009, p. 112). Clark (1995) indicated that as health care has moved from an acute illness model of care, with an emphasis on sustaining life at all costs, to a chronic disease model of care, with its focus on quality-of-life issues, conflicts between disciplines on the treatment team and communication problems among health care providers have created important challenges. While the field of interdisciplinary team collaboration has become more widely appreciated and more health care professionals have received training and experience in interdisciplinary teamwork, little is known about the best methods for building health care workers' skills in interdisciplinary teamwork. This is particularly true in geriatric mental health and especially so in the context of disasters.

OVERVIEW

A plethora of research exists regarding the health effects of disasters and emergencies on exposed individuals, particularly children and younger adults. Recently, the field of disaster research has experienced an increased interest in the health effects of disasters on older people and those who care for them (American Association for Geriatric Psychiatry [AAGP] Disaster Task Force, 2009; Herman, 1997; Reeves & Sully, 2007; Rothschild, 2006). In fact, the American Association for Geriatric Psychiatry (AAGP) recently produced a consumer brochure that focuses on mental health issues for older adults and strategies for older persons and caregivers regarding preparing for and coping with disaster (AAGP Disaster Task Force).

In chapter 6 in this volume, Sully, Wandrag, and Riddell indicate that strategies such as narrative and reflective practice techniques can be used by interdisciplinary teams to effectively prepare for disaster situations and manage team members' stress during disasters. Using such strategies can empower the interdisciplinary team to anticipate events during disasters while maintaining a client-centered focus. The authors provide a model of reflective practice that demonstrates how teams can plan for the inevitable crises that arise during disasters.

The purpose of this chapter is to describe interdisciplinary teamwork methods that have been incorporated into a model interdisciplinary team training program applied to geriatric mental health disaster preparedness. This chapter provides a summary of the interdisciplinary team process— team development, team management, and team maintenance—and strategies for team training in geriatric mental health and disaster preparedness.

Definition of Terms

Team

"A group with a specific task or tasks, the accomplishment of which requires the interdependent and collaborative efforts of its members" (Baldwin & Tsukuda, 1984, p. 421).

Interdisciplinary Team

"The interdisciplinary team is comprised of a mix of professionals from diverse backgrounds frequently situated in the same work site and employed by the same agency. However, unlike the multidisciplinary team, it has an identity as a collective which is more important than the individual professional status of each member." Interdisciplinary team members share common goals, collaborate, and work interdependently in planning, problem solving, decision making, evaluating team-related tasks, and assuming leadership roles and functions to assure progress. Great import is given to the interactional processes of the group including methods of communication, role definition, and negotiation (Takamura & Stringfellow, 1985).

Teamwork

"A special form of interactional interdependence between health care providers, who merge different, but complimentary, skills, or viewpoints in the service of a patient and in the solution of his or her health problems" (Baldwin & Tsukuda, 1984, p. 421).

Quality of Life

Although it is widely accepted that the field lacks a consensus definition of quality of life (Farquhar, 1995), for the purposes of this discussion, the definition proposed by Holmes and Dickerson is used. The authors describe quality of life as an "abstract and complex term representing individual responses to the physical, mental and social factors which contribute to normal daily living. It comprises many diverse areas, all of which contribute to the whole" (Holmes & Dickerson, 1987, p. 17). Gurland and Katz (2006) classify quality of life under 19 domains, each of which includes a set of challenges to the adaptive abilities of older persons in order to sustain quality of life.

Systematic Team Evidence-Based Problem Solving

Systematic team evidence-based problem solving is a seven-stage process of identifying problems and corresponding solutions to complex patient management or system-wide challenges that affect quality of life for patients and caregivers. The team problem-solving process includes the following seven steps: defining the problem, brainstorming solutions, choosing solutions, reviewing evidence-based literature, planning ways to implement solutions, carrying out the plan, and evaluating the solutions (see Miller, 1993; Miller & Toner, 1991; Toner, Miller, & Gurland, 1994). The systematic evidence-based problem-solving process has been applied to geriatric mental health (Toner, 1994a, 1994b; Toner, 2002) and disaster preparedness.

INTERDISCIPLINARY TEAM PROCESS: DEVELOPMENT, MANAGEMENT, AND MAINTENANCE

Interdisciplinary teams don't just happen! They require training as a team to empower them to work effectively. Training can be either formal or informal and can be initiated and implemented by the team members themselves and their team leadership (Toner, 1994a) or by facilitators who lead the team to effective team functioning. Interactive learning methods have been described as particularly successful in promoting interdisciplinary teamwork, particularly with learners from different disciplines (Howe & Sherman, 2006; Howe, Hyer, Mellor, Lindeman, & Luptak, 2001; Mellor, Hyer, & Howe, 2002). The interdisciplinary treatment team training described in this chapter is the product of over 25 years of interdisciplinary team facilitation conducted by these authors in health care settings in all parts of the country and abroad. Recent research by these authors suggests that incorporation of the quality of life choice and choosing process (Gurland & Gurland, 2008a, 2008b) within interdisciplinary team training may "provide a vehicle for successful and effective interprofessional team development, team management and team maintenance" (Gurland et al., 2009, p. 111).

Recently, these authors have applied their evidence-based interdisciplinary team process methods to the development of specialized teams in disaster preparedness. Using the methods listed in Table 13.1, the authors have facilitated team development, team management, and team maintenance with the goal of empowering health care professionals to prepare for disasters and function more effectively as a team once a disaster strikes. Table 13.1 lists evidence-based methods that team leaders and interdisciplinary team members can use to effectively develop, manage, and maintain the team. These methods have been successful in helping team members work with one another by collaboratively setting goals for the

Table 13.1

INTERDISCIPLINARY TEAM TRAINING PROCESS ACTIVITIES

GOAL	ACTIVITY	REFERENCE
TEAM DEVELOPMENT	Group member roles	Sampson & Marthas, 1990
	Leadership orientation	Bolman & Deal, 1991
	Establishing group norms	Bion, 1959; Miller, 2004; Rubin, Plovnick, & Fry, 1975; Sampson & Marthas, 1990
	Shared/rotating leadership; CORE mission statement; prioritizing team concerns	Miller & Toner, 1991; Toner, Miller, & Gurland, 1994
TEAM MANAGEMENT	Team working contract	Miller & Toner, 1991
	Systematic team evidence-based problem solving	Haley, 1978; Levenstein, 1972; Miller & Toner, 1991; Toner, Miller, & Gurland, 1994
	Team problem-solving scenarios	Toner & Meyer, 1988
	Orientation to the process of assessment	Nathanson, Moscou, Sheehan, & Toner, 2007; Toner, 1989, 1990
	Treatment decision guide	Toner, Miller, & Gurland, 1994
TEAM MAINTENANCE	Team process/verbal critique	Drinka & Clark, 2000; Miller, 1989, 2004; Takamura & Stringfellow, 1985
	Videotape review	Toner & Meyer, 1988; Toner, Miller, & Gurland, 1994
	Observation of groups at work	Howe, Callahan, & Banc, 2003; Miller, 1989

team and arriving at appropriate treatment/care decisions for the older people they serve. Table 13.1 also provides citations for each of the activities listed so the reader can explore further these interdisciplinary team process methods.

Team Development

Team development begins with a combination of traditional group dynamics approaches and human relations training. Traditional group dynamics approaches include the following: training in establishing goals and a core mission for the team, role definition/negotiation training, shared/rotating leadership exercises, and training in prioritizing team concerns. The team development exercises involved with role definition and role negotiation are continuous and ongoing as the team gains and loses members.

Team Management

The team management activities listed in Table 13.1 can be used as tools to help the team continue to work together more effectively once it has developed cohesion. Two team management exercises that focus on disaster preparedness have been particularly successful with specialized teams: Systematic Team Evidence-Based Problem Solving (STEPS) and Team Problem-Solving Scenarios. STEPS is a seven-stage process that incorporates an evaluative component. The evaluative component is designed to help the team, whenever possible and appropriate, choose evidence-based solutions shown to be successful in the scientific literature.

The Problem-Solving Scenarios, described here, constitute a problem-solving game simulation in which team members work out solutions for typical disaster-related problems faced by the team.

Table 13.2 describes a sample STEPS disaster preparedness problem-solving exercise that was conducted at the annual Geriatric Scholar Certificate Program in Binghamton, New York, in June 2007. The Geriatric Scholar Certificate Program is a component of the curriculum of the CNYGEC, which has been funded by the U.S. Department of Health and Human Services, Bureau of Health Professions, Health Services, and Resource Administration since 1994. The curriculum has trained teams in the methods of STEPS for over 12 years.

Table 13.2

SUMMARY OF INTERDISCIPLINARY TEAM OUTCOMES FOR THE STEPS EXERCISE

STEPS PROCESS	TEAM OUTCOMES/DECISIONS/ACTIONS
Define the problem (brainstorming phase)	Department for the Aging (DFTA) recruitment of volunteers for disaster/emergency work
	DFTA backup in cases of low volume of volunteers
	Hurricane/storm affecting area with large concentration of older persons
	Educating older persons at risk for dehydration/delirium during heat wave
	Snowstorm isolation of older persons. Risks for medical complications with psychiatric comorbidity
	Nursing home evacuation with staff shortage
	Managing fears of patients/caregivers and mental health risks as media feeds fears of terrorism (alerting vs. fueling fears) Bomb threat at government facility
Define the problem (consensus phase)	How do we manage staff, patient, and caregiver (formal and informal) fears in the face of terrorism/terrorist threats?
Brainstorm solutions	Staff pep talk sessions: We've done this before; we can do it again
	Boost the ability of staff and older residents to help older persons/caregivers/staff to understand coping strategies
	Educate all about the inevitability of terrorism and other disasters
	Establish support groups, educational programs, planning activities
	Help develop a disaster action plan with first phase
	Approach focused on the most vulnerable older persons who can't help themselves
	Develop caregivers support/educational group

	Develop support group in collaboration with faith-based group
	Establish buddy system with practice drills and role-playing exercises
	Develop rituals/defensive habits; define and link types of threats with tailored corresponding responses
	Develop resource manual of what people have learned from previous terrorist threats and disasters
	Develop system for assessing individual needs, medications, hydration, mental health, and social supports to determine which older persons are on psychotropics, dialysis, life support, oxygen, etc.
	Develop checklist to rate psychiatric/medical vulnerability
	Contact and involve public service professionals
	Develop survival kit and educate older persons about its function and use
	Help older persons create their individual Go Bag, a component of a disaster survival kit which includes comfort items such as sleeping bag, whistle, hand/foot and body warmers, etc., tailored to their needs
Choose solutions	1. Develop a disaster preparedness geriatric mental health support group.
	2. Develop/identify assessment tools to identify people at risk during disasters.
Review literature to identify available evidence for the efficacy of chosen solutions	Team members volunteer to conduct literature search
	Volunteer team members agree to report back to team by a specific date. Volunteers compile evidence-based information on chosen solutions.
Implement the solutions	1. Develop disaster preparedness geriatric mental health support group.
	■ Main goal: To educate older participants and staff about disaster preparedness and discuss related issues. Older members/residents meet once a week for 8 weeks. Staff meet once a month for 4 months.
	■ Educational program focuses on coping skills in disasters. Older members program

(*Continued*)

Table 13.2

SUMMARY OF INTERDISCIPLINARY TEAM OUTCOMES FOR THE STEPS EXERCISE (*Continued*)

STEPS PROCESS	TEAM OUTCOMES/DECISIONS/ACTIONS
	develops survival strategies and prepares survival kits, Go Bags, etc. Faith-based support involves inviting members to share their spirituality/faith and partner with someone of the same beliefs/faith. "Iron Sharpens Iron" model. Establish buddy system.
	■ Staff program develops team contract and discusses fears and how to cope. Use stress management program by Toner & Meyer, 2008.
	■ Caregivers program: develop plan for members; invite family and caregivers to workshops; prepare survival kits, Go Bags, etc. Seek donations from community. Establish buddy system: Assess older persons and establish partnering of vulnerable with less vulnerable for support in crisis.
	■ Public educational seminars. Develop and deliver disaster seminars and involve community. Reach out to clergy, fire and police departments, community activists, Area Agencies on Aging, emergency response organizations.
	2. Develop/identify assessment tools to identify older people at risk during disasters.
	■ Main goal: To develop an assessment tool to identify older residents and others in the community who are particularly at risk during disasters.
	■ Assessment tool should be brief and to the point. No more than 10 questions. Target recipients: Older people with higher needs (i.e., oxygen, wheelchairs, and others at high risk) are target. Target settings: homebound, senior centers nutrition program attendees, etc. Integrate tool into existing tools.
	■ Assessment tool questions about physical needs and medications

(psychiatric and nonpsychiatric; psychosocial health support); cognitive abilities/
deficits; housing location/challenges
(i.e., elevator, stairs, etc.); available/reli-
able caregivers (i.e., strength of support
system); coping skills of vulnerable older
person and his or her caregivers
- Identify and conduct survey of older
persons and caregivers. Questionnaire to
include older person's name, emergency
contacts (i.e., name, relationship, alternate contact), telephone #s for older
person and their emergency contacts,
diagnosis, current treatments. Specific
questions: What would you do in case of
an emergency (e.g., fire, power failure,
blackout)?; How would you seek help?
Evacuate your residence? Get downstairs?
Get your medications in case you are
evacuated suddenly?
- Develop vulnerability risk factor checklist with comment section. Label the file
(folder) with color-coded stickers based on
identified risk factors.

Carry out the plan	Use Miller and Toner (1991) Priority Grid to systematically carry out plan.
Evaluate the plan	

Team Maintenance

The final 5 to 10 minutes of every team meeting should be devoted to a self-evaluation discussion focused on the effectiveness of the team meeting. The team should ask themselves about the quality of the meeting, how the meeting achieved its goal, how it could be improved, and what could be done differently at the next meeting. This self-evaluation discussion provides a process by which the team can monitor its performance in a structured and mutually supportive setting. This process of team mainte-nance can counteract the natural tendencies of team members to resist change. According to Miller and Toner (1991, p. 215), "Resistances to change, based on a repertoire of maladaptive defenses, are integral to mal-functioning teams and can be mitigated or eliminated by setting aside time for team process discussions."

PROBLEM-SOLVING SIMULATIONS: DISASTER PREP SCENARIOS

Overview

The following section presents a sample problem-solving simulation for disaster preparedness. The section also includes a guide for team leaders or facilitators to illustrate useful methods for implementing the simulations with the team. The Disaster Prep Scenarios are role-playing exercises that are easy to use by the interdisciplinary treatment team and easy to facilitate. Each Disaster Prep Scenario takes approximately 45 minutes to 1 hour and should be followed by a discussion period of at least 30 minutes.

The Disaster Prep Scenarios are problem-solving exercises that represent common clinical management challenges experienced during disasters by health care staff and teams in long-term-care facilities and community-based services. The scenarios are easily adapted for use by the interdisciplinary team during team meetings. Each scenario includes roles for older residents/patients, family members or significant others, and interdisciplinary team members. The format of the Disaster Prep Scenarios is flexible, so one group of interdisciplinary team members can role-play while the remaining team members observe or numerous groups of team members can role-play the Disaster Prep Scenarios simultaneously.

Procedures

Participants are divided into teams of as many members as are indicated in each script. Each team sits in a circle and a bag of role cards is passed around to all members. The team leader/facilitator instructs each team member to pick a role card at random. The cards identify the character each team member will role-play in the exercise and the specific concerns or issues of that character. Participants are instructed not to tell their character's private information to the other people in the group; they will reveal their hidden agendas during the discussion period after the role-play.

The team members are given 5 minutes to read their role cards silently and a few minutes to introduce themselves to each other. Subsequently, the team leader/facilitator hands a script to the participants. The script tells the *disaster story* the participants will enact during the role-play. The team leader/facilitator reads the script out loud while the team members read along. Next, the team leader/facilitator instructs the participants that they will be attempting to solve the problem stated in the script. Through role-playing, the participants suggest solutions to the presenting disaster-related crisis. The participants are instructed at the beginning that by the end of the role-playing exercise they must agree on a solution to the presenting problem.

While the Disaster Prep Scenario participants—the interdisciplinary team members—are role-playing, the team leader/facilitator listens to the interactions of the participants and encourages those who are reticent to become involved. The facilitator may also become involved in the Disaster Prep Scenario by talking in the voice of the character a participant is role-playing. For example, the facilitator uses language such as "I said" instead of "he said" or "she said." After approximately 5 to 10 minutes have elapsed and the participants have become familiar with their characters, the facilitator asks one of the participant team members to pick a contingency card at random. The team member reads the contingency card aloud to the group. Each member considers the contingency within the context of his or her character. The participants use the contingency in their discussion and pay attention to how the contents of the contingency card change the problem-solving approach of the group. Contingency cards are introduced approximately every 5 minutes until all the contingency cards are used or until it is determined the Disaster Prep Scenario has ended.

Sample Disaster Prep Scenarios

Script: The Darlings and the Earthquake

Charley (age 89) and Doris (age 72) Darling live on the top floor of a six-story apartment building in west Los Angeles with their two dogs, Binky and Minky. Married for 20 years, they spent much of their time traveling for fun and visiting Charley's children and grandchildren in New York, Ohio, Portland, and San Diego. Previously they were active participants in their book club, bridge group, gym, and temple. Charley, a retired manufacturer, can no longer drive at night, has trouble walking, has difficulty remembering simple directions, and tends to become angry and belligerent easily. He also is drinking more when he is alone. Doris, depressed at the loss of their happy times and her own macular degeneration, has been thinking of discussing their future with the family but has not yet done so. She has confided some of her fears to her best friends and neighbors, Mac and Sue Back, and has made allusions about her concerns to their young rabbi, Josh Moss.

The current time is 5 AM and there has just been a 7.8 earthquake centered about 4.5 miles away. The catwalk to the Darling apartment has collapsed. Power is out. Elevators are not working. Fires have started across the street. There has been severe damage to the building, and the tenants must be evacuated and relocated.

What to do?

Cast of Characters for "The Darlings" Disaster Prep Scenario

Charley Darling, 89 years old; Doris Darling, 72 years old, his wife; their children: Dan Darling, 52 years old, residing in San Diego; *Mickey Darling, 48 years old, residing in New York City; *Tom Darling, 45 years old, residing in Portland, Oregon; and *Marilyn Darling, 43 years old, residing in Ohio; and Marcella Bella, MSW, 25 years old, social worker; Terry Berry, RN, 35 years old, nurse; Fred Bledd, 30 years old, fireman; *John Good, 28 years old, fireman; Simon Pure, 65 years old, temple volunteer; *Rabbi Josh Moss, 27 years old; *Mack Back, 77 years old, neighbor; *Sue Back, 69 years old, neighbor. (Asterisks indicate optional players.)

Character Role-Play Cards

The following 14 character role-play cards are to be selected by the participants at random. Participants are given approximately 5 minutes to read their character's role-play card silently to themselves and to briefly prepare to introduce themselves to the other participants. All participants introduce themselves *in character* to the other participants. Subsequently, the facilitator distributes the script to all participants and reads the script as the participants follow along.

Character Role-Play Card #1

Charley B. Darling: age 89, has been married to Doris for 20 years and has 4 children and 10 grandchildren from a previous marriage. He is a retired golf ball manufacturer. He was very active socially and in community affairs but lately has experienced some physical and mental problems and is slowing down, but not happily. *Concerns:* "I can't remember. I worry about Doris's eyesight. I wish the grandchildren lived closer and visited more often." *For my eyes only* (not to be shared with the group): "I'm scared. Who will take care of me? Where's my mother?"

Character Role-Play Card #2

Doris Z. Darling: age 72, married to Charley for 20 years, was previously married for 30 years and widow of Chip Zipp, no children, retired administrative assistant. Doris loves being busy, social activities, tennis, bridge, and travel. Recently diagnosed with macular degeneration. *Concerns:* "I worry about Charley's fits of rage and his drinking, which has started to get out of hand. I am worried about my sight." *For my eyes only* (not to be shared with the group): "I don't want to go through taking care of a dying husband again. I don't have the strength. Where are his kids when we need them? I'm not leaving without the dogs."

Character Role-Play Card #3

Dan D. Darling: age 52, Charley's son, is a computer programmer, married and lives with wife, Della, and her widowed mother in San Diego. Dan has two children, Donald (30 years of age) and Diane (29 years of age), who live and work in New York City. Diane is married with three children. Dan is active in sports and is a ham radio operator. Della is an elementary school teacher. Dan was never close to his dad when a young adult and is even less so after Charley married Doris. *Concerns:* "I wish my brothers and sister lived closer so that I wouldn't have to do this alone. I think dad is fading. I can't take them in. I have enough on my plate." *For my eyes only* (not to be shared with the group): "My rotten sister should be doing this, not me. She always gets the praise and the money but never takes the responsibility. And my brothers are no better. They're holier than thou but no better than my sister."

Character Role-Play Card #4

Mickey Darling: age 48, Charley's son, is an unmarried aspiring actor and part-time waiter. He has been a movie grip, video salesman, house painter, and mover. He lives in Brooklyn, New York, in a rental apartment. He is not particularly close to his siblings since he has borrowed money from them often and has had trouble repaying his debts. *Concerns:* "I hope that dad and Doris are okay out there. They really should move into a senior residence." *For my eyes only* (not to be shared with the group): "I hope they don't make me take care of them because I'm the only one without a family. I love my dad, but I can't stand spending time with him now."

Character Role-Play Card #5

Tom Darling: age 45, Charley's son, is an accountant in Portland, Oregon, and has been married to Tina (age 43) for 25 years. Tina is a hospital administrator. They have six children, two of whom are adopted from China. Tom also has a child from an earlier relationship whom he does not see but does support. They live in a gated community and are active in local politics. Tom likes Doris but feels she is a bit of a mental lightweight compared to his dad, whom he adores. He likes his brothers but not his sister. *Concerns:* "I'm worried about dad. He isn't as sharp as he was, and Doris doesn't get it. Something has to be done." *For my eyes only* (not to be shared with the group): "I have just been through a major problem in the office. I think we're going to be sued big time. I don't know how I can handle this now, but I know dad needs me. I feel awful."

Character Role-Play Card #6

Marilyn Darling: age 43, Charley's daughter, lives in Dayton, Ohio, with her new husband, Oscar DeCosta, and helps run their dry cleaning business. She was married twice before but has no children from those marriages. She now is the proud mother of 8-month-old Sophie, who is named after Marilyn's deceased mother. Marilyn has been Charley Darling's darling daughter despite former substance abuse, homelessness, and poor investments. Marilyn has had a mixed relationship with her brothers but admires her stepmother even though she misses her deceased mother now, particularly after the birth of the baby. *Concerns:* "I wish I could help more, but what can I do? The baby is so little and takes all my energy. I hope that Doris and dad are okay." *For my eyes only* (not to be shared with the group): "I'd like to visit Doris and dad with the baby when this is all over. Can Oscar handle the store without me?"

Character Role-Play Card #7

Marcella Bella: social worker, age 25. Although this is only her first job, Marcella is a hard-working, intelligent young woman. Prior to her training, she was an aide in a nursing home and worked with developmentally disabled adults. She lives with two roommates in a shared house. *Concerns:* "I hope we can get this couple to relocate to an assisted-living community. They need a more supportive living environment. Where are the children?" *For my eyes only* (not to be shared with the group): "We have to set up a system and network for these people and fast. I hope there are no gas leaks."

Character Role-Play Card #8

Terry Berry: nurse, age 35. Terry has over 10 years experience in nursing, most of which has been in the ICU. She lives with her husband and four children in Santa Monica, not far from the Darlings's building. She is a serious, efficient, and happy person. She sings in her church choir. *Concerns:* "Oh, I hope we can get all these folks out of here before dark. It will be murder at night. Many of these folks need their meds. What can we do?" *For my eyes only* (not to be shared with the group): "We really need more help here. We're going to lose a lot of them. I'd better start praying. I hope there are no more aftershocks."

Character Role-Play Card #9

Simon Pure: volunteer, age 65. Simon is a partially retired math teacher and has been a temple volunteer for 2 years since his wife, Sadie, died. He has three children who live nearby. He needs to be doing something because, as he says, "time hangs heavy." *Concerns:* "I hope everybody is okay. I don't know exactly what to do." *For my eyes only* (not to be shared with the group): "I really shouldn't be here, but I have to help the Rabbi."

Character Role-Play Card #10

Rabbi Josh Moss: age 27. Rabbi Moss is new to the temple (6 months) but very involved in community action. He has, besides his rabbinical degree, an MSW from Hunter College in New York City. He is newly married and has one-month-old twins. *Concerns:* "This is a dangerous situation. It's absolutely necessary for us to help out here. I know the Darlings personally and many of the other residents in the building, too. This is awful!" *For my eyes only* (not to be shared with the group): "I don't know how much help we can give, but we have to do something. *Pray?*"

Character Role-Play Card #11

Fred Bledd: fireman, age 30. Fred is married with two children. Formerly a marine sergeant, he was a fireman in Los Angeles for 5 years. He is strong, thorough, and soft-spoken. *Concerns:* "My father died 4 months ago. My mother is handicapped and lives in a place like this. Can we get these people out of here safely?" *For my eyes only* (not to be shared with the group): "Why doesn't the building have an exit program for emergencies. These people are helpless."

Character Role-Play Card #12

John Good: fireman, age 28. John is single and lives at home with his parents and autistic sister. He has been a fireman for 3 months. Previously, he was a student at Viceroy Community College. He is quick, quiet, and ambitious. *Concerns:* "This is such a mess. I don't know how we can handle this even if these people cooperate. Our radio communications are not working." *For my eyes only* (not to be shared with the group): "How can I convince this lady to leave without the dogs? Don't they realize that their lives are in danger?"

Character Role-Play Card #13

Mack Back: neighbor, age 77. Mack is a retired shoe store owner. He lives with his wife, Sue, and their cat Chagall. They are good friends of the Darlings. Mack is strong, resourceful, and pleasant but also very hard of hearing and arthritic. *Concerns:* "I hope that Charley and Doris can get out of this okay." *For my eyes only* (not to be shared with the group): "How many times have I told them that they should move to a lower floor?"

Character Role-Play Card #14

Sue Back: neighbor, age 69. Sue is a retired bookkeeper, superb card player, tennis player, and wife of Mack for 45 years. She dotes on their three grandchildren. *Concerns:* "I worry about them. Neither one is in great health, and I know she won't leave without the dogs." *For my eyes only* (not to be shared with the group): "I am so glad we're on the first floor. I hope Mack doesn't try to be a hero here. I'll kill him if he does."

Disaster Prep Scenario Contingency Cards

After approximately 5 to 10 minutes of role-playing have elapsed and the participants have become familiar with their characters, the facilitator asks one participant team member to pick a contingency card at random. The team member reads the contingency card aloud to the group while each member stays *in character*. The participants use the contingency in their discussion. After approximately 5 minutes, another contingency card is introduced into the role-playing in the same manner. The process continues until all the contingency cards are used or until the facilitator instructs the group to conclude the Disaster Prep Scenario.

Contingency Card #1

The Darling children have been frantically trying to reach their parents by phone and e-mail with no luck. They call each other every 2 hours to learn if anyone has gotten through. None of the children know the numbers of any neighbors or friends. Dan Darling, living closest to his parents, decides to drive to Los Angeles to find out what is going on.

Contingency Card #2

Temple Sinai sends a team of volunteers headed by Simon Pure to the building complex to see if they can help in any way. Simon trips over debris and breaks a leg.

Contingency Card #3

The fire department arrives to evacuate the buildings. Charley, confused, frightened, and angry, refuses to leave without the dogs. He then punches Fireman Bledd in the face. Doris is hysterical and seems confused as well. She locks herself in the bedroom with the two dogs. Fireman Good is overcome by smoke in the hallway.

Contingency Card #4

The local hospital sends a team to help. Marcella Bella tries to call the Darlings's children. Terry Berry is hit by a flying shutter but nevertheless tries to get information about the Darlings's health records. Dan Darling is stuck in traffic 1 hour away from Los Angeles.

Contingency Card #5

Sue and Mack Back, who live on the ground floor, are evacuated from the building. They tell Rabbi Moss the names and locations of the Darlings's children so his team from the temple might reach them. Marcella Bella and Terry Berry get stuck on the third floor as a large section of the fourth floor collapses onto their floor.

Team Leader/Facilitator's Guide

This scenario is designed to elicit discussion on a variety of topics related to mental health in older persons during disasters. Following is a list of issues to be addressed during or after the role-playing exercise. The scenario and its role-playing are designed to elicit discussion on the topics in the list. The list is by no means exhaustive, and participants may introduce additional concerns. The team leader/facilitator may, if appropriate, briefly stop the action of the role-play to interject comments and have the group focus on concrete resources available to alleviate a problem being discussed. The team will resume the role-play after the particular issue has been discussed satisfactorily and a plan of action has been developed. Usually, however, the team leader/facilitator will allow the role-play to continue for the full period until all the contingency cards have been used. During the post-play feedback period, the team leader/facilitator reviews the issues addressed by the team and adds any items from the list that have not been covered. Possible solutions to the problems, as well as resources, techniques, and steps in planning actions, should be included by the facilitator and group at this time.

CONCLUSION

Health care professionals and allied health care workers need an effective vehicle for identifying older people at risk for developing a wide range of mental health problems during a disaster or emergency. The interdisciplinary team can be the key vehicle for identifying risk and making informed treatment decisions regarding older patients and clients. The interdisciplinary team also can be a vehicle for managing the normal stress related to caring for chronically ill older persons and especially managing the stress associated with caregiving during disasters and emergencies.

Interdisciplinary health care team members also need practical tools to guide them in preparing for the provision of patient/client care during and after a disaster. This chapter describes strategies that can be used to develop, manage, and maintain effective interdisciplinary teamwork. The chapter also provides a guide regarding the requisite knowledge and skills required for team development, management, and maintenance. As demonstrated in Table 13.1, the requisite knowledge and skills can be learned and can result in increased team effectiveness and efficiency.

The interdisciplinary team training models described in this chapter, particularly STEPS and the Disaster Preparedness Scenarios and Problem-Solving Simulations, offer a unique approach that can be incorporated into the structure of any interdisciplinary team. This can be accomplished regardless of the conditions under which the interdisciplinary team operates or its specific mission. This is true for almost all health care settings that have interdisciplinary teams, with the exception of acute care and other short-term care settings, where time constraints may limit the application of this model.

REFERENCES

American Association for Geriatric Psychiatry Disaster Task Force. (2009). *A consumer guide for preparing and coping with disaster: Mental health issues for older adults.* Bethesda, MD: AAGP/Geriatric Mental Health Foundation.

Baldwin, D., & Tsukuda, R. (1984). Interdisciplinary teams. In C. Cassell & J. Walsh (Eds.), *Geriatric medicine: Medical, psychiatric, and pharmacological topics: Vol. II* (pp. 421–435). New York: Springer-Verlag.

Banerjee, S., Willis, R., Graham, N., & Gurland, B. J. (2009). The Stroud/ADL Dementia Quality Framework: A cross-national population-level framework for assessing the quality of life impacts of services and policies for people with dementia and their family carers. *International Journal of Geriatric Psychiatry, 25,* 26–32.

Barr, H., Koppel, I., Reeves, S., Hammick, M., & Freeth, D. (Eds.). (2005). *Effective interprofessional education: Argument, assumption, and evidence.* Oxford, England: Blackwell Publishing.

Bion, W. (1959). *Experiences in groups.* New York: Basic Books.

Bolman, L., & Deal, T. (1991). *Reframing organizations: Artistry, choice, and leadership.* San Francisco, CA: Jossey-Bass Publishers.

Clark, P. (1995). Quality of life, values, and teamwork in geriatric care: Do we communicate what we mean? *The Gerontologist, 35,* 402–411.

Drinka, T., & Clark, P. G. (2000). *Health care teamwork: Interdisciplinary practice and teaching.* Westport, CT: Auburn House Publishers.

Farquhar, M. (1995). Definitions of quality of life: A taxonomy. *Journal of Advanced Nursing, 22,* 502–508.

Gurland, B. J., & Gurland, R. V. (2008a). The choices, choosing model of quality of life: Description and rationale. *International Journal of Geriatric Psychiatry, 24,* 90–95.

Gurland, B. J., & Gurland, R. V. (2008b). The choices, choosing model of quality of life: Linkages to a science base. *International Journal of Geriatric Psychiatry, 24,* 84–89.

Gurland, B. J., Gurland, R. V., Mitty, E., & Toner, J. A. (2009). The choices, choosing model of quality of life: Clinical evaluation and intervention. *Journal of Interprofessional Care, 23*(2), 110–120.

Gurland, B., & Katz, S. (2006). Quality of life in Alzheimer's and related dementias. In H. Katschnig, H. Freeman, & N. Sartorius (Eds.), *Quality of life in mental disorders* (2nd ed., pp. 179–198). New York: John Wiley & Sons.

Haley, J. (1978). *Problem-solving therapy.* San Francisco: Jossey-Bass Publishers.

Herman, J. L. (1997). *Trauma and recovery: The aftermath of violence.* New York: Basic Books.

Holmes, S., & Dickerson, J. (1987). The quality of life: Design and evaluation of a self-assessment instrument for use with cancer patients. *International Journal of Nursing Studies, 24*(1), 15–24.

Howe, J., Callahan, E., & Banc, T. (2003). *Introduction to the role of interdisciplinary teams in health care: A resource kit.* New York: The Bronx Veterans Affairs Medical Center GRECC/Mount Sinai Interdisciplinary Team Project.

Howe, J. L., Hyer, K., Mellor, J., Lindeman, D., & Luptak, M. (2001). Educational approaches for preparing social work students for interdisciplinary teamwork on geriatric health care teams. *Social Work in Health Care, 32*(4), 19–42.

Howe, J. L., & Sherman, D. W. (2006). Interdisciplinary educational approaches to promote team-based geriatrics and palliative care. *Gerontology and Geriatrics Education, 26*(3), 1–16.

Institute of Medicine. (2001). *Crossing the quality chasm: A new health system for the 21st century.* Washington, DC: National Academy Press.

Institute of Medicine. (2008). *Retooling for an aging America: Building the health care workforce.* Washington, DC: National Academy Press.

Levenstein, A. (1972). Problem-solving through group action. In A. C. Bennett (Ed.), *Improving the effectiveness of hospital management* (pp. 355–372). New York: Metromedia Analearn Publications.

Mellor, M. J., Hyer, K., & Howe, J. L. (2002). The geriatric interdisciplinary team approach: Challenges and opportunities in educating trainees together from a variety of disciplines. *Educational Gerontology, 28*(10), 867–880.

Miller, P. (2004). Interdisciplinary teamwork: The key to quality care for older adults. In L. M. Tepper & T. M. Cassidy (Eds.), *Multidisciplinary perspectives on aging* (pp. 259–276). New York: Springer Publishing.

Miller, P. (1993). Problem-solving in long-term care: A systematic approach to promoting adaptive behavior. In J. Toner, L. Tepper, & B. Greenfield (Eds.), *Long term care: Management, scope, and practical issues.* Philadelphia, PA: Charles Press.

Miller, P. (1989). Teaching process: Its importance in geriatric teamwork. *Physical and Occupational Therapy in Geriatrics, 6*(3/4), 123–133.

Miller, P., & Toner, J. (1991). The making of a geriatric team. In W. Myers (Ed.), *New techniques in the psychotherapy of older patients* (pp. 203–219). Washington, DC: American Psychiatric Press.

Nathanson, M., Moscou, P., Sheehan, C., & Toner, J. (2007). Section 4: Geriatric mental health and disasters: Individual and community mental health outcomes. In J. Howe, A. Sherman, & J. Toner (Eds.), *Geriatric mental health disaster and emergency preparedness curriculum* (Portal of Geriatric Online Education [POGOe] Product No. 18848). Retrieved September 11, 2009, from http://www.pogoe.com

Reeves, S., & Sully, P. (2007). Interprofessional education for practitioners working with the survivors of violence: Exploring early and longer-term outcomes on practice. *Journal of Interprofessional Care, 21*(4), 1–12.

Rothschild, B. (2006). *Help for the helper.* New York: Norton.

Rubin, I., Plovnick, M., & Fry, R. (1975). *Improving the coordination of care: A program for health team development.* Cambridge, MA: Ballinger Press.

Sampson, E., & Marthas, M. (1990). *Group process for the health professions.* Albany, NY: Delmar Publishers.

Sully, P., Wandrag, M., & Riddell, J. (in press). Supervision and facilitated reflective practice as central to disaster preparedness services to the older adult: A national and cross national model. In J. Toner, T. Mierswa, & J. Howe (Eds.), *Geriatric mental health disaster and emergency preparedness: Evidence-based care practices.* New York: Springer Publishing.

Takamura, J., & Stringfellow, L. (1985). Team process. In L. Campbell & S. Vivell (Eds.), *Team training in geriatrics: Project report and leader's manual* (pp. 75–86). Sepulveda, CA: Veterans Administration Medical Center; and Los Angeles, CA: UCLA/USC Long Term Care Gerontology Center.

Toner, J. (2008). Depression in dementia: Assessment and its role on the interdisciplinary team. In E. Capezuti, G. Siegler, & M. Mezey (Eds.), *The encyclopedia of elder care* (2nd ed., pp. 230–231). New York: Springer Publishing.

Toner, J. (2002). Developing and maintaining links between service disciplines: The program for organizing interdisciplinary self-education. In J. R. M. Copeland, M. T. Abou-Saleh, & D. G. Blazer (Eds.), *Principles and practice of geriatric psychiatry* (2nd ed., pp. 795–798). New York: Wiley & Sons.

Toner, J. (1994a). Developing and maintaining links between service disciplines: The program for organizing interdisciplinary self-education (POISE). In J. R. M. Copeland, M. T. Abou-Saleh, & D. G. Blazer (Eds.), *Principles and practice of geriatric psychiatry* (pp. 1022–1028). New York: John Wiley & Sons.

Toner, J. (2006). Effective interprofessional education: What is the evidence? [Review of the article Effective interprofessional education: Argument, assumption, and evidence]. *Journal of Interprofessional Care, 20*(2), 217–218.

Toner, J. (1994b). Interdisciplinary team training in geriatric psychiatry: A model of university-state-public hospital collaboration. *Gerontology & Geriatrics Education, 14*(3), 25–38.

Toner, J., Howe, J., & Nathanson, M. (2007). Section 3: Overview of aging and mental health. In J. Howe, A. Sherman, & J. Toner (Eds.), *Geriatric mental health disaster and emergency preparedness curriculum* (Portal of Geriatric Online Education [POGOe] Product No. 18848). Retrieved September 12, 2009, from http://www.pogoe.com

Toner, J., & Meyer, E. (1988). Multidisciplinary team training in the management of dementia: A stress management program for geriatric staff and family caregivers. In R. Mayeux, B. Gurland, V. Barrett, A. Kutscher, L. Cote, & Z. Putter (Eds.), *Alzheimer's disease and related disorders: Psychosocial issues for the patient, family, staff, and community* (pp. 81–102). Springfield, IL: Charles C. Thomas.

Toner, J., Miller, P., & Gurland, B. (1994). Conceptual, theoretical, and practical approaches to the development of interdisciplinary teams: A transactional model. *Educational Gerontology, 20*(1), 53–69.

14 Geriatric Assessment for Differential Diagnosis

MARK R. NATHANSON

This chapter focuses on the mental health assessment of older persons after a disaster. The goal of this evaluation is to identify signs and symptoms of psychological distress—alterations in behavior, mood, cognition, and thought process—that will aid in the formulation of a differential diagnosis and a treatment plan tailored to the individual. Geriatric mental health assessment after a natural or man-made disaster must proceed in a logical and orderly fashion, avoiding premature diagnosis and allowing time for both comprehensive data collection, including information from families and collateral sources, and tailored biopsychosocial intervention (Albert, 2004). This chapter deals with the risk for psychological distress in older persons, what clinical syndromes and presentations the treatment team should understand and determine during the initial and subsequent evaluations, and the important questions to ask of all older people assessed for the mental health consequences of disasters.

CASE IDENTIFICATION

In order to do an assessment, we must have access to the at-risk or affected population. How do we identify those who are in distress? It is known that older persons underutilize mental health services due to ageism, stigma, inaccessibility of services, a fear of being labeled as *mental patients,* and a cohort effect where mental health treatment is seen as outside the realm of acceptable services to access (Brown & Harris, 1989). Of particular concern are frail older adults who are less likely to have their broad needs met after a disaster (Sanders, Bowie, & Bowie, 2003). Older persons tend to utilize available services less frequently than the general population (Zatzick, 2007). They may not take advantage of counseling or support services, they may be embarrassed to accept handouts, or they may feel others are more deserving of assistance than they are (Oriol, 1999). Case finding becomes a critical issue and calls for creative solutions including the delivery of mental health services in multidisciplinary teams, which have the ability to outreach into the community where stigma can be reduced. Mental health services at a primary care medical clinic or senior citizens' center may be practical solutions to this problem by minimizing the stigma of evaluation at a mental health facility.

RISK FACTORS AND PSYCHOLOGICAL IMPACT OF DISASTERS

The chronological age of the individual is not the critical issue in the development of psychological distress subsequent to a disaster. Relative independence, pre-disaster health and mental health status, social support, economic status, employment status, marital status, and access to services predict mental health stability after a disaster (Brown, 2007). The frail elderly, seniors who function with a limited margin for additional physical and psychological burden and are dependent on a support system for their day-to-day care; the institutionalized elderly in nursing homes; and clients with pre-disaster PTSD or psychopathology are at highest risk for psychological distress after a current disaster (Capezuti, Boltz, Renz, Hoffman, & Norman, 2006). The psychological impact of disasters on older persons has been a matter of debate. Frail older adults with chronic medical and mental disorders are more likely than the healthier or younger population to require assistance to evacuate, survive, and recover from a disaster (Fernandez, Byard, Lin, Bensen, & Barbera, 2002). The type of disaster, its severity and longevity, the efficiency of the advanced warning system, the pre-disaster health and mental health status of the individual, and access to resources and economic constraints are variables implicated in the psychological vulnerability of older persons (Bolin & Klenow, 1982). The proximity to the disaster, the length of exposure, the threat of loss of life to oneself or family, social isolation, lack of independence as measured by scales of ADLs and IADLs, chronic medical and mental illness, current medication use, and prior use of health services determine the risk of pathology.

The physical and psychological distress of being uprooted from one's residence or institutional setting during a disaster has been labeled *transfer trauma,* implying that any disruption from an individual's normal surroundings in the chaos of a disaster leads to worsening anxiety, depression, and cognitive blunting. The amount of time needed for the transfer and the individual's needs on the other end have been underestimated, leading to worsening anxiety and distress on the part of the older client (Mangum, Kosberg, & McDonald, 1989). Nursing home staff who have handled transfers of clients from their facilities have a wealth of experience and information and should continue to share this knowledge with program directors. For example, nametags on all residents, many of whom have dementia and cannot give their name and are thus more likely to become confused, are valuable in reducing further psychological distress in these clients (Aldrich & Benson, 2008).

The process of packing one's possessions quickly in the midst of an impending disaster and being herded onto buses or planes and ending up a day or so later in a new city, a temporary shelter, the unfamiliar home of a stranger, or even the comfort of a family member's home is disquieting, upends equilibrium, and can worsen mental confusion or underlying cognitive impairment or emotional instability. Follow-up studies of older persons relocated from their homes after disasters show that 6 months to several years later there was a higher rate of depression, anxiety, and dread (Burns, et al., 1993).

Older persons, who are prone to multiple sensory impairments, are vulnerable because they do not receive early warnings about disasters, are less likely to respond to information regarding an impending disaster, and have less capacity to plan ahead (Friedsam, 1960). However, older persons may be less impacted by disaster and seem to have a *resourcefulness* and coping ability greater than the younger population. Older adults often have time-limited psychological distress after a disaster that resolves over a period of several months without treatment (Burns, et al., 1993). This may reflect prior learned coping strategies and life experiences, which may aid them in the management of disaster conflicts (Raphael, 2003). Older persons may have fewer current-life stressors and less need for additional conflict resolution subsequent to a disaster. There may be a learned effect from prior trauma for coping and problem solving (Verger, et al., 2004). Frail older persons—those with serious physical, cognitive, economic, and psychosocial problems—are at especially high risk (Fernandez, et al., 2002). The risk factors for developing psychological distress after a disaster relate to the ability of the affected individual or community to assess and respond to the warnings of a disaster; to prepare ahead and organize one's life to prepare for escape routes; to hunker down, establishing and maintaining contact with social supports; and to possess the resources and forethought to have on hand adequate supplies of medication.

During the Gulf Coast hurricanes of 2005, frail older persons in nursing homes, unable to independently manage and negotiate a chaotic system, were the most affected. The highest incidence of death of any segment of the cohort was from nursing home elderly residents who were unable to be relocated during the crisis (Summers, Hyer, Boyd, & Boudewyns, 1996). Before hurricanes Katrina and Rita in 2005, adults aged 60 or older made up only 15% of the population of New Orleans, Louisiana. However, 71% of those who died because of the hurricanes were over age 65 (White House, 2006). For all segments of the population, it is clear that the closer one is to the heart or ground zero of a disaster, the higher the risk for the subsequent development of PTSD, anxiety, substance and tobacco use, alcohol abuse, depression, and impaired functioning in the daily activities of life.

Older persons who lived below Canal Street in New York City, which was designated a *frozen zone* for weeks after the terrorist attacks of September 11, 2001, are a case in point. These frail homebound older persons could not receive any communication from outside support for days on end. This was the group most likely to decompensate in their mental and physical health. Members of this group are often unable to ambulate due to the typical chronic medical illnesses affecting this population, including chronic respiratory illness, debilitating arthritis, cardiovascular disease, and stroke. The home attendants who served this group were unable to reach their clients. It is noted that more intensive efforts were organized to retrieve at-risk homebound pets than older persons.

The greater the impact of a disaster directly on one's life, the greater the risk for the onset of psychological distress, so in the assessment we must understand where the person was at the time of the disaster: were they moved or forced to remain in place? Did they have any support or companionship at the time of the disaster, and was the support consistent or fleeting?

Frail older residents who choose to remain in their homes during a hurricane are not unusual and, in fact, are the norm for the older population. Whether we use the term *set in their ways* or *too old to change*, it is clear that older persons are less likely to respond to requests to vacate their premises and move to safer areas. This is likely also related to the length of time

they have lived in their current residence, their attachment to their surroundings, and the age cohorts that comprise the residents in their home
(Gibson & Hayunga, 2006). If they live alone or with a spouse, it may be
easier to remain in place than respond to an evacuation call.

A strong risk factor for psychological distress from a current disaster
is having had psychological distress from a prior disaster event. Fifty to 75%
of older persons in the community have experienced at least one disaster
in their lifetime, and this data holds up for the population in general. If
we examine those clients who have experienced disasters in the past, we
can ask if the new disaster experience will uncover biological or psychological vulnerability. Prior disaster experience has been hypothesized to
cause an inoculation effect—protection afforded for having experienced
a prior trauma (Eysenck, 1986).

OLDER POPULATIONS STUDIED

Significant interest in the research on trauma psychology in older persons
has focused on combat veterans, prisoners of war, survivors of the Nazi
Holocaust, and aging Vietnam veterans (Beckham, et al., 1998; Danieli,
1981; Yehuda, et al., 1996), and more recently older hurricane survivors in
the Gulf Coast. Findings of psychological distress in acute and longitudinal
studies vary. Older Holocaust survivors have been shown to have considerable strength and coping skills. In contrast, Israeli Holocaust survivors
during the Persian Gulf were found to have a significant incidence of PTSD
symptoms and acute distress (Solomon, Neria, Olny, Waysman, & Ginzburg, 1994).

The assessment of the older client must include an understanding of
cultural issues particular to the client that may impact on the extent and
severity of symptoms, the expression of distress, and reasonable treatment
options. For example, older clients with Asian backgrounds tend to be unable to express their emotions outright and will often somaticize their distress. Anxiety and depression may present with weakness, lethargy, and
fatigue.

The Impact of Loss on Psychopathology

The assessment of psychological distress in the older client must include
a complete review of the impact of the disaster on their lives: the loss of
cherished persons, belongings, and function. The death of a spouse, child,

friend, caregiver, or other close person is a certain risk factor for ensuing emotional instability, bereavement, and grief; it also creates a gaping hole in one's sense of support. An individual's sense of security is demolished in the context of a disaster; the basic fear that one is unprotected will resurrect primitive fears of childhood insecurity, abandonment, and separation anxiety (Zatzick, 2007).

The loss of possessions, familiar households, cherished mementos of the past, and familiar space are key determinants in worsening cognition and a sense of disorientation, dread, and insecurity. The transplanted nursing home residents in New Orleans gave up the basic remnants of their surrounding when they were relocated. They were likely predisposed to confusion and anxiety. Over 50% of nursing home residents have a dementing disorder that adversely affects their ability to manage safely and negotiate their existence outside an institution. Strategies learned from previous disasters include developing crisis intervention teams that can assess older persons in the community and provide basic services such as housing, financial assistance, and securing a sense of safety (Phifer, 1990).

Exposure to some types of traumatic events may also be higher in rural areas. For example, injury-related death rates are 40% higher in rural populations than in urban populations. Many rural older adults experience low levels of social support and high levels of isolation. Rural areas often have fewer resources—such as transportation, community centers, and meal programs—that foster social contact and disaster relief coordination, case finding, and mental health treatment capabilities.

Pre-Disaster Psychopathology: How Does This Impact on Postdisaster Psychopathologic Presentations?

It appears that the best predictor of postdisaster psychological distress and maladaptive functioning is pre-disaster psychological distress and psychiatric symptoms (Kessler, Sonnega, Bromet, Hughes, & Nelson, 1995). Older clients who have a chronic mental illness such as schizophrenia, bipolar disorder, anxiety disorder, dementia, or personality disorder are at increased risk for the reactivation of a previously dormant disorder, the development of new distress, or worsened psychosocial function during and for an extended period of time, perhaps years, after a disaster. The main areas that need to be assessed are in the realms of mood symptoms, cognitive functioning, and thought process and behavioral control. The nature of the disaster may be critical in the production of new symptoms such as paranoid delusions. A 70-year-old male with chronic schizophrenia may have been stable living in the community and functioning at a baseline level of independent self-care with supervision from a case manager, therapist, and psychiatrist. The attacks of September 11, 2001, witnessed repeatedly on a television screen could easily resurrect a delusional belief that terrorists were following this person and poisoning his food or medication. In response to these new delusions, the client might fear taking his medication, going outside, or eating his usual meals. The individual would quickly continue to worsen due to the lack of his usual regimen of antipsychotic medication, adequate nutrition, and reality testing obtained by routine psychosocial contacts. A lack of social support and social isolation also increase the risk of future psychological distress (Norris, Freidman, & Watson, 2002).

ASSESSMENT PROCESS

Given workforce limitations and shortages of mental health personnel with training in geriatric mental health assessment, it is most useful to work in an interdisciplinary team approach.

Assessment is a process that requires the use of all one's senses in an evaluation of the client. For example, the evaluator may note that a 70-year-old female appears confused and has a foul smell of urine. This may be a clue to an untreated urinary tract infection now causing delirium. If the examiner did not follow up on the foul odor, the etiology of the delirium would have been missed. The timing of the assessment is a key factor in informing further process. The nursing home resident who is evaluated in the immediate aftermath of a hurricane may have a mental state revealing shock, fear, and other features that may meet criteria for ASD. The mental confusion, lack of awareness of one's surroundings, and confusion may also be indicative of a delirium (Silverman & Weston, 1995).

The timing of the assessment is important. Are we evaluating someone in a triage setting during a disaster? Is the crisis still ensuing, and are we performing a triage process to determine which clients need immediate mental health treatment and which can wait for some time? In an immediate ongoing disaster, the setting is not as important as a brief evaluation of the mental state of the client. In this case, we are also trying to determine if the presentation of psychiatric or psychological symptoms are a manifestation of a delirium.

Delirium is a medical emergency and has a mortality rate of 15%. Thus, the assessment during a disaster needs to identify those persons who are suffering from delirium, for if we do not identify them in a timely manner, they may succumb to the underlying process causing the delirium. If the client is interviewed and examined 1 month after a traumatic event, there may be less overt signs of ASD. However, older persons, similar to a younger cohort, may have delayed onset of psychological distress. We must include this fact in our assessment of a disaster survivor. The duration since the disaster is important in our understanding of the underlying issues and pathology.

The assessment should take place in a quiet setting free from noise or distraction in a comfortable room that can accommodate the possible handicaps of the client. Doorways should be large enough to access a wheelchair. The presence of other family members or assistants must be carefully considered as we aim to obtain the most information and make our client feel at home. We do not want to frighten him or her any further. In this regard, it is often useful to interview the client with a familiar person in the room. This may include a spouse, adult child, or even a home health aide or home attendant. Asking the client if they prefer to have their family or attendant present is important and lends an air of respect to the interview process. We do not want to unnecessarily alienate the client before we have even begun the interview process. This would only lead to further anxiety and may cut the interview short.

Is the assessment to occur in a comfortable location such as the client's residence—apartment or house, nursing home, or adult home—or are we interviewing our client at the bedside in a hospital after an acute injury subsequent to a disaster? Did the client have an acute injury causing a limitation of function? For example, if we are to perform a mental health assessment in a hospital setting following a hip fracture in an 80-year-old man, we must carefully consider the influence of the surroundings in the mental status evaluation. Do we have privacy or is our client in a multibedded setting?

We are well aware that older clients are reluctant to reveal issues related to emotional content, and even if they are willing, they may lack the language necessary to describe emotional distress. This is referred to as alexithymia. This concept will be important in our understanding of the physical presentation of psychological symptoms of distress in our elderly clients (Klap, Unroe, & Unitzer, 2003). For example, the anxiety and depression associated with postdisaster stress may manifest in older persons as a pain complaint, gastrointestinal disturbance, headache, weakness, or marked lethargy.

The duration of time spent on the assessment of geriatric mental health will often relate to the setting, the availability of staff, and the urgency of others in the vicinity in crisis. A complete assessment may require several hours, but this may be unreasonable given the circumstances and nature of the disaster, setting, and skill of the examiner. Most critical information regarding mental disorders can be obtained in an hour or less if the examiner is trained to assess for those factors of most concern. A brief triage to determine category or extent of pathology can easily be done within 15 minutes. The staff should have had training on the basic features of the mental status examination and its components. They should be able to obtain this information in one session. It also may be useful to extend the assessment process over several sessions. The assessment should always inform the later diagnosis and treatment planning and therefore should be completed so as to initiate treatment based on the severity of the problem. For example, if the client appears to have severe symptoms of anxiety and dread several days after living through a hurricane, the examiner must complete the examination in order to make a referral to rule out any age-related medical causes of anxiety. Commonly, medications may not be available to the client, and the presentation of anxiety may be a sign of withdrawal from a sedative, such as diazepam, that the client has been taking regularly for years but now does not have access to.

We must prepare for and anticipate all difficulties in communicating with our clients. This may include having translators available or making arrangements for telephonic translation services. Many of our older clients will have sensory impairments of one kind or another that will require us to have sign language translators and amplification devices for hearing, which can be obtained from electronic stores. Can the person speak since they had a stroke? Are they able to write? In planning ahead and anticipating services after disasters, these assistive devices are important to have on hand. It is also useful to know prior to a disaster which clients are unable to communicate due to neurological or physical problems, which clients may have had a stroke, which are hearing impaired, or which are aphasic.

The functional status of the client pre- and postdisaster is important in understanding the capacity of the client for self-care, the need for in-home assistance, the need for referral to an institutional setting, or the augmentation of in-home services. The standard scale for ADL assessment should be performed at the onset of the evaluation and afterward at 3-to-6-month intervals. Does the client ambulate alone? Can she bath and dress herself? Does she need any assistance with meal preparation, shopping, cooking, and house cleaning? Can she pay her bills or are they found scattered around the house in boxes with piles of other papers? The assessment of functional status is a critical factor in determining the impact of a disaster on an older client. The assessment of the client's ability to perform

ADLs (Katz, Ford, Moskowitz, Jackson, & Jaffe, 1963) and IADLs (Stuck, et al., 1999) will predict his or her future need for services, need for institutionalization, and level of care for outside support services.

HISTORY AND MENTAL STATUS EXAMINATION

The history of the present illness or the exploration of current signs and symptoms starts from the moment the clinician makes contact with the client or begins to have clinical information presented. For example, the clinician may have advanced word that an 80-year-old man is being transferred to the clinic due to behavioral problems, violence, and aggression. The clinician now runs through a series of possibilities as to the likely cause of this behavior. Is there a prior history of this behavior? Does the man have a violent tendency? Or perhaps this is a man with Alzheimer's disease who has been displaced from his home and since becoming confused believes he is back on the battlefield in Europe. What are the known or suspected patterns of alcohol or substance abuse? All information that relates to the patient is important and should be documented carefully in a medical record.

The examination proceeds when the client arrives. Note his behavior and his attitude toward the examination. Note what he is wearing, the state of his hygiene, and the cleanliness of his clothing and hair and, for a woman, note makeup and the state of her skin, nails, and extremities. Is the person relaxed or anxious, agitated, pacing, restless, or aggressive? Can the client sit still and maintain composure through the examination, or is he restless and fidgeting with items on the desk? The orientation of the client is tested by asking him where he is, where he was earlier in the day, and the components of the date including month, day, date, year, and season. Prompts can be given, but these must be noted in the record. Confabulation can be present at this point in the examination. A memory-impaired client will use this device to avoid the catastrophic reaction of being found out or discovered to have cognitive limitations. The orientation of the client is an important aspect in the diagnosis of dementia, delirium, and mood disorders such as depression. Demented and delirious patients will be unable to answer questions of orientation based on the severity of their underlying illness, whereas depressed clients may give a response indicating they have no interest in the question—"Don't bother me, leave me alone."

The mood and affect are to be considered next. The mood is a report of how the patient is feeling in his or her own words. The affect is the range of emotion evident from the examination. It may be broad, labile, or constricted to a narrow range. One also looks for congruence between the apparent affect and the mood state. If the patient reports feeling fine yet shows marked affective constriction, this is noteworthy and should be subject to further exploration. The client's ability to communicate coherently is noted. Do the sentences and words used make sense? Are words used correctly? This is the point in the examination to look for neurological deficits or disorders such as aphasia or evidence of damage to the language areas of the brain. Often associated with aphasia are significant depressive symptoms since the client is embarrassed and frustrated that he cannot communicate normally.

It is useful at this time to test the client's ability to read, write, and draw and copy simple diagrams such as the pentagon in the Mini Mental State Examination, or MMSE (Folstein, Folstein, & McHugh, 1975). Another task that provides a good deal of information is asking the client to draw the face of a clock—that is, a circle in which they will place the clock numerals and then draw the hands to a certain time. The quality of the drawing, the client's ability to comprehend the task, the positioning of the numbers and hands, and the entire use of the space will give indications of spatial relational disturbances, memory impairment, poor concentration, and attention.

Are there delusions present, false fixed beliefs that are not easily changed? They may take the form of paranoid persecutory thoughts that others are plotting against them or following them, setting traps, or coming into the client's home to harass them. This may also be a manifestation of cognitive impairment or memory disturbance. Perceptual disturbances such as auditory, visual, tactile, or olfactory hallucinations may be present. These may be indicative of underlying neurological impairment, particularly the presence of hallucinations; visual hallucinations should be considered the result of an underlying medical illness or condition such as a withdrawal state from alcohol or a benzodiazepine.

There are many similarities in the presentation of clinical syndromes or disorders in the geriatric population. The three Ds of geriatric mental health—depression, delirium, and dementia—may all appear similar at some point in time. They have considerable differences, however, in their onset, time course, tendency to improve or relapse, prognosis, and treatment implications. As a general rule, the examiner must have a high index of suspicion that a medical illness is masquerading as a psychiatric disorder. For example, pneumonia in older persons may present with the same signs as a depressive disorder—depressed mood, slowed motor behavior, mental dullness, and lethargy. The natural history of depression is that it presents early in life in one's 20s or 30s. Therefore, a careful history of previous psychiatric illness is important in the context of understanding new symptoms in the patient.

The client with mild symptoms of a dementia such as Alzheimer's disease or vascular dementia may also easily be affected by a disaster in a number of deleterious ways. Having cognitive difficulties at baseline, the client then becomes more disoriented and confused in the chaos or relocation to new surroundings and the subsequent loss of familiar persons and cues in the environment and as a result may experience a sense of insecurity and dread. The client may develop a worsening ability to manage ADLs or self-care or be unable to communicate his or her distress to caregivers in the community.

The assessment of prior mental illness in the geriatric client is crucial to understanding the current presentation of any psychiatric symptoms. Are we dealing with a completely new disorder without any roots in the past? Are we observing the recurrence of an underlying disorder that has lain dormant but has become activated by the disaster, or are the present symptoms an extension of an active psychiatric illness that was not adequately treated prior to the disaster and is now worse due to the stress of the current disaster? In this assessment, we will also look at the onset of previous psychiatric illness; the history of prior treatment and its success; and treatment providers, including all member of the treatment team, case managers, the therapist, assertive community treatment teams, and any agencies that have been involved in the care of the client. For example, if adult protective services had a prior relationship with the client and arranged through the courts for a guardian, this information is necessary prior to making decisions to care for the client in the disaster and postdisaster setting.

BEHAVIORAL DISTURBANCES

The assessment of the mental state of older persons must include a complete evaluation of behavior. Often behavioral changes will be early manifestations of another psychopathologic entity such as depression or anxiety. The older person may become increasingly withdrawn and isolative and refuse to leave his or her bed; not attend to personal hygiene, dressing, and changing of clothing; not pay bills; and exhibit other abnormalities in routine. The key element to investigate is change of behavior from the client's baseline. This requires direct interview as well as information from collat-

eral sources as older persons often are not reliable in describing their underlying mood states or distress.

As previously noted, many disorders may manifest with similar clinical
presentation. Social isolation may be a sign of depression or delirium. Agitation is often seen in depression, anxiety states, delirium, and dementia as
well as substance-induced intoxication or withdrawal. Attention-seeking
behavior—the acting out of inner emotional conflicts—may also be the
only way the older client knows to ask for emotional help in response to a
crisis. Alexithymia is common in this cohort and will result in alternate ways
to express emotional distress. Physical symptoms such as fatigue, weari-
ness, chronic pain, and somatic preoccupations may indicate psychological
distress. Therefore, the assessment should include a thorough review of systems from all major medical and organ systems to determine any physical
symptoms related to underlying psychological distress. The older client, for
example, may present with worsening pain complaints masking a progressive depressive disorder. In our society, and particularly with this aging cohort, it is more acceptable to present with physical rather than psychological
distress (Horowitz, 1976).

Such patients are often categorized as difficult or even hateful as they
are persistent in holding onto physical symptoms and are not *good patients*
in the sense that they do not want to get better. This confounds the treatment team, frustrates their efforts, and may lead to unconscious punish-
ment of the client. For example, a repeat visitor to a clinic who has shifting
medical complaints may be labeled a *crock* and deemed not worthy of careful attention. The examiner must understand that such patients are using
meta-requests as please for help and should offer them support, gentle encouragement, and a clear plan for follow-up and treatment. The message
most successfully implied is that the treatment team hears the complaint
and will do what they can to relive distress. Treating clients in a rapid, cur-
sory manner only compounds their fears that they do not matter and are
worthless and insignificant. This may then lead to worsened depression,
withdrawal, social isolation, and even suicidal behavior.

The older cohort uses physical symptoms to manifest underlying psychological conflict. The hypochondriac who focuses on specific symptom
complexes may have a depressive or anxious disorder at the core of his or her
pathology, and it is the work of the examiner to tease this out through careful questioning, reviewing the client's current clinical functioning, and reviewing the meaning of the client's symptoms. Older persons will commonly
express emotional distress through pain complaints, such as headache,

gastrointestinal upset, and vague symptoms that do not respond to standard therapy (Boscarino, 1997).

The help-seeking behavior of the depressed and anxious patient often manifests with a somatic presentation and the client needs to be encouraged to reveal the cause of the distress. Often in the somatic disorders, however, the goal may not be a cure but rather symptom relief. The client may be excessively using sedatives, hypnotics, or opiates. A careful assessment includes all medication's side effects, dosing, and the nature of their use. The education of the client focuses on the dangers of the excessive use of medication—such as falls and mental confusion or the risk of addiction. We may see the overuse of emergency rooms, office visits, or clinic appointments to seek relief from the psychological distress of the untreated effects of a disaster.

Delirium

The current assessment must focus on the acute presentation of psychological symptoms and signs of illness. The most pressing and urgent to detect is delirium. Delirium—also referred to as acute confusional states, encephalopathy, or acute brain failure—is an acute mental status change presenting with confusion, disorientation, global cognitive impairment, the inability to attend to a situation, reversal of the sleep-wake cycle, and agitation or marked inactivity and social withdrawal (American Psychiatric Association, 2000). The etiology may be multifactorial, and the outcome in 15% of cases of delirium will be death. The frail elderly in a disaster are vulnerable to the onset of delirium. Medication may be a significant issue if taken in excess, if not taken at the right time, or if not taken at all. A patient with cardiac disease who is prescribed a daily dosage of digoxin may be stable on her usual medication regiment. During a disaster, her medication may be misplaced, or she may be overwhelmed and forget to take her usual dose. This may lead to worsened cardiac function, decreased blood flow to the brain, congestive heart failure, and subsequent mental confusion. Any disruption of blood flow, oxygen, or glucose to the brain will result in some degree of mental confusion. A patient with mild cognitive impairment who is taking such heart medication may forget they have taken their daily dose and take one or two extra for the day. Digoxin has a narrow therapeutic index, and accidental overdose can cause mental confusion. The list of medications that can result in mental confusion or delirium in excess or when not taken at the appropriate time is extensive. Common offenders that should be carefully considered included steroids, beta agonists, antihypertensive medications, caffeine, stimulants, sedatives, hypnotics, tranquilizers, analgesics, and anti-inflammatories. Any medication, even an over-the-counter medication, can cause mental confusion. The examiner needs to make a thorough list of the client's medication and dosing schedule and also obtain a sense of the client's medication adherence.

Another area of assessment for delirium relates to a careful mental status examination of the client's ability to maintain a lucid, cogent train of thought or logical thought process as manifested by his or her ability to pay attention despite outside stimuli. Hallucinations may accompany a delirium. These are typically visual or tactile hallucinations—perceptual disturbances that are immediate, appear real, and are usually terrifying to the client. Auditory hallucinations are not as common but may manifest as one or several voices inside or outside the head giving a running dialogue of critical or derogatory statements. This type of hallucination is more commonly seen in the patient with schizophrenia.

Delirium is most worrisome in the older client as it is easily mistaken for depression. Delirium tends to present in two ways. The first, most dramatic is the psychomotorically agitated person ranting, screaming, and pulling out intravenous lines in the hospital. He is disoriented, paranoid, and terrified. Any prior experience of captivity, imprisonment, or battle may emerge during this state, so real and immediate that the person truly is on the field fighting off the enemy. The second type of delirious presentation, more likely to be confused with depression, is the motorically slowed person who is lethargic, curled in a fetal position, and barely responsive. Such a person likely would be confused and disoriented with clouding of consciousness. He would appear depressed and sullen; if the underlying cause of the delirium were not quickly ascertained, he would further lapse into more profound mental clouding, coma, or death.

Dementia

It cannot be overstated that a client with a dementing disorder prior to a disaster is at significant risk for functional decline in the context of a disaster setting. Estimates in the population are that 10%–30% suffer some form of cognitive impairment (Albert, 2004). The distress associated with a disaster; the disruption in the basic safeguards of one's existence; and the loss of power, food, supervision, and safety pose significant concerns for this vulnerable cohort. The assessment of the patient with dementia requires compassion, skill, and basic human concern for a vulnerable person unaware of the gravity of the circumstances. The patient's historic information is critical and raises the issues of early case identification, preparation, and planning. When did the person start showing signs of dementia? What is their baseline functioning in terms of ADLs and IADLs? Dementia patients with prior exposure to disasters often present an uncovering of symptoms as the cognitive impairment progresses. A baseline assessment of cognitive status using the MMSE is valuable.

Affective Disorder

The assessment of affective disorder includes alterations of mood states, fear, terror, helplessness, rage, guilt, despair, depression, and hopelessness. These may arise amidst the disaster or days or months after the event. Such factors depend on the client's premorbid functioning, previous psychiatric illness, and proximity to the disaster. Nursing home residents moved from their original locations into temporary or sheltering nursing homes in the Gulf Coast reported increased prevalence of depression and anxiety (Laditka, et al., 2008).

The assessment of older persons for mental distress must include a careful understanding of their suicide risk, intent, and plan. The examiner should not fear that inquiry into suicidal intent would put the idea in the client's head. Rather, suicidal intent and ideation is fraught with ambivalence and uncertainty. Asking about suicide relieves the person, enables them to share their frightening thoughts, and brings to their attention that there is a compassionate listener. The risk of suicide is complex and multifactorial. We must understand such variables as advanced age, gender, history of prior suicide attempts, depression, and family history of suicide. The client who appears depressed, refuses to speak, or shrugs off the examiner is worrisome. Successful suicide generally takes planning and is not an impulsive act. The clinician should look for recent behavioral changes, isolation, decline in function, and reluctance to contact close friends or family. The suicidal client may prepare by making a will, drafting letters to his or her loved ones, and getting his or her affairs in order. One recent patient was noted to have systematically sent all her photographs back to the persons in the pictures and removed her possessions, packing them neatly in bags along the corridor. A suicide note was found on a cabinet shelf.

Acute and Posttraumatic Stress

ASD and PTSD are categorized as anxiety disorders and have considerable overlap and similarity with other anxiety disorders, such as generalized anxiety, panic, and obsessive-compulsive disorders. The examiner should be familiar with the diagnostic categories as outlined in the *DSM-IV*. The features of persistent anxiety and dread, re-experiencing of the traumatic event, avoidance, and increased arousal may be seen in acute and post-traumatic stress disorder, generalized anxiety disorder, and panic states. The anxiety disorders are the most commonly diagnosed disorders in the general population, and older persons are frequently diagnosed with generalized anxiety disorder, panic disorder, and isolated panic attacks. The goal of the assessment process is to differentiate the premorbid diagnosis of anxiety disorder from the effects of a disaster, to understand the baseline functioning of the person, and to develop a comprehensive treatment plan that incorporates all the patient's symptoms and signs of the disorders in a coherent and workable plan; the ultimate goal is to alleviate suffering and allow the person to go on with their usual activities as much as possible.

There are no unique issues for ASD pertinent to the older population. We must assess the exposure to a traumatic event and the threat of death, serious injury, or threat to the physical integrity of the patient or his or her loved ones. Responses may involve intense fear, helplessness, horror, and dissociative symptoms such as numbing, detachment, absence of emotional response, reduced awareness of one's surroundings, derealization, and depersonalization and dissociative amnesia (Yehuda, et al., 1996). Re-experiencing the event also occurs as vivid dreams, flashbacks, or daydreams associated with the intense mood states of anxiety, fear, and dread. This may recur after a trigger or reminder of the event as in the case of images of the twin towers. Avoiding places or reminders of the event may occur. Associated with these symptoms are sleep disturbance, excessive startle responses, anxiety, poor concentration, and cognitive dulling (Averill & Beck, 2000). These can easily impair functioning in the usual setting, and the assessment should include a measure of the patient's current ability to perform ADLs and IADLs. The timing of these symptoms according to the *DSM-IV* (American Psychiatric Association, 2000) is for onset within 4 weeks of the disaster event, lasting for at least 2 days up to 4 weeks.

Anxiety disorders—such as ASD, PTSD, generalized anxiety disorder, panic disorder, or obsessive compulsive disorders—invoke intense fear and threat to self of death, self-harm, or fear of harm or death of a loved one. Symptoms may be acute, time limited, chronic, or intermittent. PTSD has many similar features to ASD but the chronicity and timing of onset are different. PTSD is diagnosed when the symptoms exceed 1 month in duration. A further categorization into acute PTSD, lasting for less than 3 months, and chronic PTSD, for symptoms persisting for more than 3 months, is useful. PTSD is diagnosed when the constellation of symptoms has been met. As in ASD, these include the three hallmark categories of avoidance, re-experiencing, and arousal. The risk of PTSD appears to be greater for those previously exposed to a severe disaster setting; the impact of total disaster involvement may be cumulative over a lifetime (Engdahl, Eberly, & Blake, 1996; Fields, 1996). Therefore, the combat veteran of WWII evacuated from a nursing home who has early dementia and physical limitations may have a resurgence of PTSD symptoms previously held in check. There does not appear to be an increased risk for the geriatric client to develop PTSD. As noted earlier, there may be some degree of inoculation effect from experiences in a previous disaster, learned strategies, life skills, coping methods, and the ability to organize oneself amidst a new crisis.

WWII veterans admitted to a psychiatric unit for other mental health issues were found to have a 54% prevalence of prior PTSD; 27% had current criteria for PTSD (Fontana & Rosenheck, 1991).

Alcohol, Prescription Drug, and Substance Use

There is a strong comorbid relationship in the general population between PTSD and alcohol and substance abuse disorders (Chilcoat & Menard, 2003). One third of patients with PTSD have a substance abuse disorder, and 6% of those with a substance abuse disorder have comorbid PTSD (Kessler, et al., 1995). The older client may turn to alcohol, prescription drugs, or illicit drugs during and after a disaster. The pattern of alcohol use in older persons tends to be in two major groupings: the chronic alcohol abuser and the moderate drinker. The first is the client who has engaged in habitual use of alcohol and may have increased the use recently to excessive levels. The person who has used alcohol for many years will show consequences of its use such as signs of alcohol-related dementia, hepatitis, poor self-care, comorbid tobacco use, and a history of multiple falls and fractures. This group is known to be inattentive to their health concerns and may have multiple chronic medical problems such as cardiovascular disease, diabetes, chronic respiratory illness, and hypertension. They may have a pattern of excessive use of alcohol since adolescence with or without efforts to curtail their drinking.

As disaster may lead to anxiety, fear, and dread, the older client who reports minimal alcohol use also may turn to alcohol for self-medication of symptoms. Since alcohol is a depressant, this use over time only makes mood symptoms worse, and the client may sink deeper into despair. The examiner should always inquire into the patterns of the client's current use of alcohol.

Prescription drug use may escalate after a disaster. The older client is likely to have been prescribed some type of sedative or hypnotic prior to a disaster. Older persons are often overmedicated by their primary care physicians and mental health specialists with an array of psychotropic medication, each of which increases the risk of falls, confusion, and cognitive slowing. After a disaster, it is a knee jerk reaction by physicians to prescribe sedatives to ease anxiety and distress, yet there is a substantial risk of worsening the overall functioning of the client.

Over-the-counter medications are not benign. The examiner must inquire into all medication taken by the client and urge them to carry an updated medication list on their person at all times. The client may have multiple health care providers, each prescribing their own medication but unaware of what the others have prescribed. Following Hurricane Katrina, a survey of 680 evacuees living in Houston shelters during September 2005 showed that 41% reported having chronic health conditions such as heart disease, hypertension, diabetes, and asthma; 43% indicated they were supposed to be taking a prescription medication and 29% of those said they had problems getting prescriptions filled. Most of those surveyed did not give their age, but many of the people in shelters were older persons (Washington Post, Kaiser Family Foundation, & Harvard University, 2005).

The assessment should include a thorough review of all medication the client is prescribed including dosages, timing, side effects, and recent changes. If making a home visit, the clinician should look through the medicine cabinet and encourage a thorough cleaning. If possible, staff should discard unused medication from the home as older persons tend to stockpile these for no reason. This is very important if the patient has any suicidal or depressive symptoms. The examiner should urge the patient to document and carry on his or her person an up-to-date, complete list of medications from all physicians and health care providers. The clinician should also ask clients if they know what their medical problems are and if they understand what each medication is for, including over-the-counter medications, vitamins, natural remedies, and the like as these are rarely benign and may be taken in excess.

Schizophrenia and Chronic Mental Illness

Schizophrenia is a chronic psychiatric illness that manifest in late adolescence or early 20s. In regard to disasters, we must understand that patients with any chronic mental illness may be severely impacted by the distress, fear, and dread common to the general population. The chronic mentally ill tend to have limited support systems and coping skills. Late-life schizophrenia, paraphrenia or late-onset psychosis, or delusional disorder may also occur in the older client. Particularly noteworthy are well-organized paranoid delusions, often of a persecutory nature. The client may not have had prior psychiatric treatment. Often the precursor to this late-onset psychosis is a premorbid schizoid personality or paranoid personality disorder. For instance, the extensive media coverage of September 11, 2001, may have induced some patients to have active delusions that terrorists were personally persecuting them. For some older persons, this may have led to acute decompensation of their clinical status. Many times, the decompensation starts with a paranoid delusion that food is tainted or poisoned. The next step may be nonadherence with medication, typically an antipsychotic, followed by further decline in functioning and increased positive symptoms of psychosis, paranoia, and fear. At this point, the patient might discontinue treatment with the therapist and psychiatrist, isolate himself in his room, and refuse to participate in usual activities. Television coverage of the disaster would continue to reinforce the paranoid thoughts and fears of retribution for imagined crimes.

We should consider that any person with a chronic mental illness is more vulnerable to the impact of a disaster than the general population. The mentally ill are stigmatized, feel shunned and disregarded, and have flaws in self-esteem and sense of self-worth. The disruptive effects of a disaster on their sense of security and safety, further breakdown in their support systems, and disequilibrium all add to a more fragmented sense of self and increased feelings of distress in the chronic mentally ill.

One significant myth in the study of personality disorders in the older client is that personality disorders tend to become less clinically important. To the contrary, personality disorders in older persons tend to be more debilitating regarding individual functioning, self-esteem, and sense of independence. The relationship between personality disorders and disasters is complex. The presence of a highly anxious, passive, dependent personality disorder is a risk factor for escalating anxiety, dread, and disequilibrium after a disaster. The person who has difficulty with independent planning, self-care, and organization of surrounding supportive networks is left after a disaster with increased distress, bewilderment, and panic.

A CASE

A disaster will have a noticeable impact on a person with a prior history of traumatic abusive assault, long-standing physical or sexual abuse, rape, or domestic violence and is likely to unleash and uncover emotions perhaps buried for years under a defensive cover. The person may have learned to block out uncomfortable feelings related to their former assault by using denial or other defensive mechanisms, thus allowing the individual to continue on in life with some semblance of normality. However, a disaster may be the swift, startling event that throws all this to the wind and leaves the person feeling raw, empty and alone, exposed, terrified, and uncertain how to continue in his or her daily existence. It is the disruption of equilibrium, the sheer terror and profound sense of being out of control, that may hearken back to an event such as a sexual assault. In our example, a 65-year-old female working in the World Trade Center saw the jet crash into her building and uncertainly made her way out of the tower to the ground level. There she witnessed the bodies of her fellow workers plunging to the ground around her. She does not recall how she made her way home to Astoria, Queens. She believes she was pushed along by the terrified crowds. She continued to have nightmares and flashbacks of the event and also developed symptoms of paranoia. She was convinced her neighbors were stealing from her, coming into her yard, and rearranging the garbage cans. She called the police several times to report their illegal acts only to be told it was all in her head. She then began having vivid memories of a sexual assault that had taken place 30 years prior. This earlier trauma had occurred on her way home from work one evening. She did not know the assailant and never reported the event to anyone, including her family. However, after surviving the World Trade Center attacks and finally regaining some sense of normality in her life, she continued to have these recurrent vivid dreams of the sexual assault. She sought counseling and was able to make a connection between the common mood states of the September 11, 2001, disaster and the previous assault. She identified a sense of being completely out of control, unsafe, and at the mercy of another power. She continued to be terrified but was relieved to have counseling to get her fears out in the open after all these years. It is not unusual for victims of assault to have such an uncovering of previous events after a disaster as the crisis recreates the environment of insecurity, dread, and feeling out of control.

CONCLUSION

The goal of this chapter is to heighten the awareness of participants in the psychological assessment of older persons following a disaster. An assessment carried out in a multidisciplinary team approach with a longitudinal sense of ongoing assessment and treatment planning is the most effective approach. Risk factors for psychological distress, including the nature and severity of the disaster, the vulnerability of the client before and during the disaster, threat to life, previous history of psychological disturbances, past treatment efficacy, and current access to mental health services are all considerations. The elements of the treatment plan that are developed from the assessment are discussed in the next chapter.

REFERENCES

Albert, S. (2004). *Public health and aging: An introduction to maximizing function and well-being.* New York: Springer Publishing.

Aldrich, N., & Benson, W. F. (2008). Disaster preparedness and the chronic disease needs of vulnerable older adults. *Preventing Chronic Disease, 5,* 1–7.

American Psychiatric Association. (2000). *Diagnostic and statistical manual of mental disorders* (4th ed., text revision). Washington, DC: Author.

Averill, P., & Beck, G. (2000). Posttraumatic stress disorder in older adults: A conceptual review. *Journal of Anxiety Disorders, 14,* 133–156.

Beckham, J. C., Moore, S. D., Feldman, M. E., Hertzberg, M. A., Kirby, A. C., & Fairbank, J. A. (1998). Health status, somatization, and severity of posttraumatic stress disorder in Vietnam combat veterans with posttraumatic stress disorder. *American Journal of Psychiatry, 155,* 1565–1569.

Bolin, R., & Klenow, D. J. (1982). Response of the elderly to disaster: An age-stratified analysis. *International Journal of Aging and Human Development, 16,* 283–296.

Boscarino, J. (1997). Diseases among men 20 years after exposure to severe stress: Implications for clinical research and medical care. *Psychosomatic Medicine, 59,* 605–614.

Brown, L. (2007). Issues in mental health care for older adults after a disaster. *Generations, 31*(4), 21–26.

Brown, G., & Harris, T. (1989). *Life events and illness.* New York: Guilford.

Burns, B., Wagner, H., Taube, J., Magaziner, J., Permutt, T., & Landerman, L. (1993). Mental health services use by the elderly in nursing homes. *American Journal of Public Health, 83,* 331–337.

Capezuti, E., Boltz, M., Renz, S., Hoffman, D., & Norman, R. (2006). Nursing home involuntary relocation: Clinical outcomes and perceptions of residents and families. *Journal of the American Medical Directors Association, 7,* 486–492.

Chilcoat, H., & Menard, C. (2003). Epidemiological investigations: Comorbidity of posttraumatic stress disorder and substance use disorder. In P. C. Ouimette & P. J. Brown (Eds.), *Trauma and substance abuse: Causes, consequences, and treatment of comorbid disorders* (pp. 9–28). Washington, DC: American Psychological Association.

Danieli, Y. (1981). The aging survivor of the Holocaust: Discussion on the achievement of integration in aging survivors of the Nazi Holocaust. *Journal of Geriatric Psychiatry, 15,* 191–215.

Engdahl, B., Eberly, R., & Blake, J. D. (1996). Assessment of posttraumatic stress disorder in World War II veterans. *Psychological Assessment, 8,* 445–449.

Eysenck, H. (1986). Stress, disease, and personality: The "inoculation" effect. In C. Cooper (Ed.), *Stress research* (pp. 121–146). New York: Academic Press.

Fernandez, L., Byard, D., Lin, C., Benson, S., & Barbera, J. (2002). Frail elderly as disaster victims: Emergency management strategies. *Prehospital Disaster Medicine, 17*(2), 67–74.

Fields, R. (1996). Severe stress in the elderly: Are older adults at increased risk for posttraumatic stress disorder? In P. E. Ruskin, & J. A. Talbott (Eds.), *Aging and posttraumatic stress disorder* (pp. 79–100). Washington, DC: American Psychiatric Press.

Folstein, M., Folstein, S., & McHugh, P. (1975). Mini-mental state: A practical guide for grading the cognitive state of patients for the clinician. *Journal of Psychiatric Research, 12,* 189–198.

Fontana, A., & Rosenheck, R. (1991). Traumatic war stressors and psychiatric symptoms among World War II, Korean, and Vietnam War veterans. *Psychology of Aging, 9,* 27–33.

Friedsam, H. (1960). Older persons as disaster casualties. *Journal of Health and Human Behavior, 1*(4), 269–273.

Gibson, M., & Hayunga, M. (2006). *We can do better: Lessons learned for protecting older persons in disasters.* Retrieved June 1, 2009, from http://www.aarp.org/research/health/disabilities/better.html

Horowitz, M. (1976). *Stress response syndromes.* New York: Jason Aronson.

Katz, S., Ford, A., Moskowitz, R., Jackson, B., & Jaffe, M. (1963). Studies of illness in the aged: The index of ADL: A standardized measure of biological and psychosocial function. *Journal of the American Medical Association, 185,* 914–919.

Kessler, R. C., Sonnega, R., Bromet, E., Hughes, M., & Nelson, C. B. (1995). Posttraumatic stress disorder in the National Comorbidity Survey. *Archives of General Psychiatry, 52*(12), 1048–1060.

Klap, R., Unroe, K. T., & Unutzer, J. (2003). Caring for mental illness in the United States: A focus on older adults. *American Journal of Geriatric Psychiatry, 11*(5), 517–524.

Laditka, S. B., Ladtika, J. N., Xirasagar, S., Cornman, C. B., Davis, C. B., & Richter, J. V. E. (2008). Providing shelter to nursing home evacuees in disasters: Lessons from Hurricane Katrina. *American Journal of Public Health, 98*(7), 1288–1292.

Mangum, W., Kosberg, J., & McDonald, P. (1989). Hurricane Elena and Pinellas County, Florida: Some lessons learned from the largest evacuation of nursing home patients in history. *Gerontologist, 29,* 388–392.

Norris, F., Friedman, M., & Watson, P. (2002). 60,000 disaster victims speak: Part II. Summary and implications of the disaster mental health research. *Psychiatry, 65,* 240–260.

Oriol, W. (1999). *Psychosocial issues for older adults in disasters.* Washington, DC: U.S. Department of Health and Human Services, Substance Abuse and Mental Health Services Administration, Center for Mental Health Services. Retrieved January 17, 2009, from http://download.ncadi.samhsa.gov/ken/pdf/SMA99-3323/99-821.pdf

Phifer, J. (1990). Psychological distress and somatic symptoms after natural disaster: Differential vulnerability among older adults. *Psychology and Aging, 5*(3), 412–420.

Raphael, B. (2003). Early intervention and the debriefing debate. In R. J. Ursano, C. S. Fullerton, & A. E. Norwood (Eds.), *Terrorism and disaster: Individual and community mental health interventions* (pp. 123–130). Cambridge, UK: Cambridge University Press.

Sanders, S., Bowie, S., & Bowie, Y. (2003). Lessons learned on forced relocation of older adults: The impact of Hurricane Andrew on health, mental health, and social support of public housing residents. *Journal of Gerontological Social Work, 40*(4), 23–35.

Silverman, M., & Weston, M. (1995). Lessons learned from Hurricane Andrew: Recommendations for care of the elderly in long-term care facilities. *Southern Medical Journal, 88*(6), 603–608.

Solomon, Z., Neria, Y., Ohry, A., Waysman, M., & Ginzburg, K. (1994). PTSD among Israeli former prisoners of war and soldiers with combat stress reaction: A longitudinal study. *American Journal of Psychiatry, 151,* 554–559.

Stuck, A. E., Walthert, J. M., Nikolaus, T., Bula, C. J., Hohmann, C., & Beck, J. C. (1999). Risk factors for functional status decline in community living elderly people: A systematic literature review. *Social Science and Medicine, 48*(4), 445–469.

Summers, M., Hyer, L., Boyd, S., & Boudewyns, P. (1996). Diagnosis of later life PTSD among elderly combat veterans. *Journal of Clinical Geropsychology, 2,* 103–115.

Verger, P., Dab, W., Lamping, D. L., Lozes, J., Deschaseaux-Voinet, C., Abenhaim, L., et al. (2004). The psychological impact of terrorism: An epidemiologic study of posttraumatic stress disorder and associated factors in victims of the 1995–1996 bombings in France. *American Journal of Psychiatry, 161*(8), 1384–1389.

The Washington Post, Kaiser Family Foundation, & Harvard University. (2005, September). *Survey of Hurricane Katrina evacuees.* Menlo Park, CA: The Henry J. Kaiser Family Foundation.

The White House. (2006). *The federal response to Hurricane Katrina: Lessons learned.* Retrieved July 19, 2009, from http://library.stmarytx.edu/acadlib/edocs/katrinawh.pdf

Yehuda, R., Elkin, A., Binder-Brynes, K., Kahana, B., Southwick, S. M., Schmeidler, J., et al. (1996). Dissociation in aging Holocaust survivors. *The American Journal of Psychiatry, 153*(7), 935–941.

Zatzick, D. (2007). Interventions for acutely injured survivors of individual and mass trauma. In R. J. Ursano, C. S. Fullerton, L. Weisaeth, & B. Raphael (Eds.), *Textbook of disaster psychiatry* (pp. 206–227). New York: Cambridge University Press.

15

Bereavement and Grief: What Is Normal in Disasters and Emergencies?

D. PETER BIRKETT

Disasters kill the young and bereave the old. To some extent, this is a matter of definition. Deaths of the young are regarded as more disastrous than those of the old. The deaths of 116 children from a landslide at Aberfan, Wales, in 1966 that engulfed a school and of 186 children from a terrorist massacre at Beslan, Russia, in 1994 horrified the world. An influenza epidemic that increases deaths among the aged by several thousand barely registers on public consciousness.

PTSD VERSUS GRIEF

In many cases, the most common psychiatric disorder caused by a disaster is PTSD, but it also may be grief in one of its forms. The distinction is not always complete. Those who were not in danger themselves may suffer grievous loss. Sometimes both physical danger and bereavement occur at the same time so that ASD and PTSD are combined with grief.

On September 11, 2001, those killed ranged in age from 3 to 85 but were mainly young adults. We still see people affected by the aftermath of the 2001 event. In some cases, survivors were in terrifying danger. Many young adults escaped with resulting acute stress or PTSD but were not bereaved of close family members. Typical older victims, on the other hand, were frequently the parents of those killed. Their major continuing emotional suffering is caused by grief.

THE ROLE OF MENTAL HEALTH WORKERS

What do mental health workers do for the bereft in the wake of such disasters? Can they really be of measurable help? What can we do to prepare them to be helpful? Some of the help given is not measurable and can never be truly evidence based to Cochrane standards (Cochrane, 1999). Nevertheless, coping with grief amongst survivors is a task that demands expertise.

At least one member of every disaster preparedness team should be familiar with the principles of grief counseling or at least have read through such texts as Worden's 4th edition of *Grief Counseling and Grief Therapy* (2009) and Colin Murray Parkes's 3rd edition of *Bereavement: Studies of Grief in Adult Life* (1998), if not Stroebe, Hansson, Schut and Stroebe's massive *Handbook of Bereavement Research and Practice* (2002).

One of the major tasks of the mental health professional in a disaster is that of counseling the helpers, and this counseling often takes the form of advice about what to expect in grief-stricken people. The most urgent question posed by helpers will be whether the extreme disturbances they see are *normal*. The bereaved themselves will sometimes ask if they are going mad. In such circumstances, the concept of normal becomes tenuous.

Is grief an illness? Many manifestations of extreme grief resemble those of mental illness, and it seems to be a semantic issue as to whether they constitute psychosis. The standard nomenclatures are ambiguous. The International Classification of Disease, or ICD-10 (World Health Organization, 1992), says almost nothing about grief, although it recognizes an enduring personality change after bereavement to be coded as F62.8. The *DSM IV-TR* (American Psychiatric Association, 2000) puts bereavement in its V category of conditions that are not quite mental illness.

Definitions of illness and disease can be a matter of dispute. One of the hallmarks of a disease is that it runs a predictable course. As Darwin pointed out in *The Expression of the Emotions in Man and Animals* (1872), the course of grief runs through certain predictable stages and shows many predictable symptoms. Among the phenomena that can be objectively observed and are described herewith are the following: agitation and weeping; religion, disbelief, or forgetting; hallucinations that can be formed and vivid; panic attacks and phobias; anger to the point of violence; and a prolonged stage similar to clinical depression with weight loss, insomnia, and self-neglect.

In spite of the persuasive evidence of a disease model, the idea persists that grief is not a medical matter. Failure to experience grief is sometimes regarded as a moral failure rather than a sign of good mental health. Existentialist philosophers from Kierkegaard to Sartre have regarded our ability to suffer grief as a sign of our humanity and would have looked askance at attempts to devise an effective antigrief medicine.

Freud, in *Mourning and Melancholia* (1917/1982, p. 197), pointed out that grief could produce severe mental abnormality but felt that any attempt at medical treatment was inadvisable or even harmful (Freud, 1917/1957, p. 125).

MANAGEMENT OF SYMPTOMS

Agitation and Weeping

Tears and wailing are the most familiar reactions to acute bereavement. They are described by Darwin (1872, p. 45) as follows, "When a mother loses her child sometimes she is frantic with grief. . . . She walks wildly about, tears her clothes or hair and wrings her hands."

Darwin regards these reactions as the earliest response, but they are often delayed. Their familiarity does not mean they are easier to deal with. Shouting, wailing, moaning, and keening occur. The bereaved may run wildly, disregarding all social restraints. They may throw themselves on the corpse and refuse to be parted from it. Such extremes are difficult to witness, and caregivers themselves can become distraught and tearful.

In spite of these extremes of behavior, such reactions can be expected and regarded as normal. Many caregivers, often from their own experience, have learned their own ways of responding. These emotional expressions of grief are socially sanctioned to such an extent that failure to manifest them can arouse concern. If numbness is not followed by this type of reaction, caregivers may believe that emotion is being repressed and that this is a bad thing. The public, and some professionals, fear that repressed emotions will eventually surface in harmful ways. Caregivers may turn to mental health professionals to express their anxiety at this supposed suppression.

Many culturally determined rituals have evolved around mourning. Such rituals may even mandate loud shouting and tearing of clothing. It is important for helpers to try to learn about these.

Religion

Spirituality can be helpful in resolving grief (Walsh, King, Jones, & Blizard, 2002), and the elderly are more likely than the young to be involved in organized religion and attend a place of worship. Training helpers should include instruction by clergy. Many of the theological issues related to grief are complex and demand knowledge of matters such as liturgy and interdenominational differences as well as pastoral counseling. Questions arise regarding theodicy, that is, the belief in God's goodness in spite of the existence of evil in the world, especially in disaster situations. Theodicy is dealt with in popular works such as Kushner's *When Bad Things Happen to Good People* (2001) but can be best understood and expounded upon by a qualified priest, minister, or rabbi.

Disbelief or Forgetting

Disbelief, or forgetting that a loved one has gone, also occurs in non-disaster situations. In everyday life, we sometimes experience memory lapses or cognitive dissonance when something familiar changes. Such disbelief provides transient anesthesia but gives rise to renewed paroxysms of grief when remembrance of reality returns. A complication in disaster situations is that there may be actual uncertainty due to compromised communication systems.

Another complication is that older bereaved persons may already have memory problems. Outside of disaster situations, demented older persons may continue to believe long-departed spouses are still alive. A frequent problem in geriatric practice is that of informing a demented patient about the loss of a close relative. The family will often come to the health professional and ask him or her to perform this task. It is recommended that this should only be done once. After the initial information has been understood, there is no need for reminding, and we can presume that disbelief is comforting to the demented patient.

Hallucinations

Hallucinations are very common in bereavement and occur in about half of those widowed (Rees, 1971). They may be a sense of the presence of the dead person as more well formed and vivid. When hallucinations are auditory, they assume the voice of the lost and are felt to be genuine. The hearer insists the dead person is talking to them.

Such voices may be thought of as evidence of mental illness by an observer, but they differ from the auditory hallucinations of schizophrenia in their phenomenology. Multiple voices are not heard, and the hearer, although he or she insists on the validity of the experience, does not expect others to be able to share it. Thus, it is necessary sometimes to reassure both hearers and caregivers that this manifestation is part of the grieving process. It may be suggested that such hallucinations can be comforting. In some cases, of course, such hallucinations readily fit in with cultural or religious beliefs about an afterlife.

Panic Attacks and Phobias

Panic attacks and severe anxiety are especially common when the grieved death was sudden and unexpected as occurs in disasters. In cases where the bereaved person shared in the disaster, other features of PTSD can be present. Questions of whether to start benzodiazepines—a type of medication typically prescribed for anxiety and phobia—and how and when to stop such treatment often arise. Several recent reviews, such as the American Psychiatric Association's "Practice Guidelines" (2004), cover the topic of the management of PTSD.

In many cases, the circumstances of a disaster will give rise to a phobia of things connected with it, which can be treated by the usual methods for treating phobias. In some cases, this may require instruction by a mental health professional using behavior therapy or hypnosis, but return to everyday living may be sufficient. For example, following an automobile accident in which there were deaths, the survivors, at least in rural and suburban America, often remain phobic for about 6 months. The daily necessity of driving produces a deconditioning by the end of that time.

Anger

Anger is often the most difficult emotion for helpers to deal with, especially because caregivers may find themselves as the objects of anger. Caregivers from an outside agency may be regarded as agents of those responsible for the disaster. The bereaved may convince themselves the disaster was avoidable. Their anger builds up like a liquid under pressure. Once it flows in a particular direction, the stream becomes unstoppable and efforts to divert it fail. Attempts to assuage the anger can be perceived as arguments supporting authority. Under the influence of anger, the subject confuses attempts at explanation with justification. The caregiver who tries to give a reason for the disaster is readily thought to be giving an excuse. If the disaster was the result of a human attack, then any discussion of the motives of the attackers can be seen as defending their actions.

In some cases, anger can give rise to litigation, as will be discussed later.

Depression

This prolonged stage of grief is similar to the melancholic type of clinical depression and manifests as weight loss, insomnia, and self-neglect. Recurrent thoughts of the loss pervade each day. There is a risk of suicide. The similarities and differences are well described by Freud in his 1917 paper cited earlier. More recent studies, using sophisticated modern statistical techniques, have mostly confirmed what Freud said. The only clear distinction between the symptoms of clinical depression and those of grief is the fact of bereavement (Kendler, Myers, & Zisook, 2008).

Delusional guilt feelings distinguish depression from normal grief, but in disaster situations this diagnostic point may be obscured by survivor's guilt. Yet a further complication is that the survivor's guilt may not be entirely irrational.

These subtle phenomenological differences may test the skills of even experienced mental health professionals. The differentiation between grief and clinical depression is often made intuitively on the basis of what has been lost. Severe symptoms following the loss of a pet or photographs are more readily assigned to mental illness than those following the loss of a child. As we shall discuss, however, this can be deceptive.

Antidepressant Medication

Given the similarities of grief to a type of depression that often responds well to organic treatments, the question arises of whether antidepressant medications can help. Three open-label and one randomized controlled trials of such treatment have been reported (National Cancer Institute, 2009). Medications found helpful are desipramine, nortriptyline, and bupropion.

The Length of Mourning

The length of mourning is another point of differentiation often invoked. Some religious customs have specified periods of mourning. *DSM IV-TR* (American Psychiatric Association, 2000, p. 299) allows only 2 months before the symptoms qualify as a "major depressive episode."

To what extent does grief counseling resemble the psychotherapy of depression? As we have seen, the classical psychodynamic methods are considered inapplicable by some authorities. The cognitive therapy of Beck, Rush, Shaw, and Emery (1979) and the rational-emotive therapy of Ellis (Ellis & Dryden, 2007) also have intrinsic limitations in the face of grief. These therapies involve trying to convince the patient that things are not really as bad as they think. Advocates of Klerman's *Interpersonal Therapy* (Klerman, Weissman, Rounsaville, & Chevron, 1984, p. 5) recommend concentrating on the "here and now" for treating depression regardless of the possible influence of such factors as childhood bereavement.

Grief Counseling

The principles of grief counseling are well described in works such as that of Worden (2009). Severe grief may have a negative effect on family, friends, and therapists such that there may be a tendency to avoid the grieving person. Family, friends, and caregivers, including therapists, should be encouraged to *avoid such avoiding*.

Experts differ about the need to work through the stages of grief. There is no consensus that this is necessary or helpful, although reminiscence and ventilation must at least be allowed. In talking about the deceased, we encourage survivors to remember them during life. Talk directed toward memories of the loved one during life often brings a smile and slight relief. Talk about the exact circumstances of death tends to increase distress. Much of the counseling is intuitive; sensitive helpers will assess what helps, what is to be avoided, and when advice and commiseration are needed.

The bereaved often say the most effective comforters are those who have been though a similar loss. Support groups of several kinds exist to facilitate this and are included in the resources section of this book.

As in the stage of acute agitation, there are demands for sleeping medication. The philosophical objection to these is, for some reason, less than the objection to antidepressants. Again, the medications most frequently used are benzodiazepines and benzodiazepine-receptor targeted drugs marketed as sleeping aids, such as zolpidem (Ambien). Knowledge of the patient's previous drug and alcohol use is important. There are always a million reasons to drink, and bereavement is one of them. A relapse into alcohol abuse by one mourners can add to the distress of the others

As time goes on, caregivers have to focus more on functional impairment. Functional impairment is distinguished from the sheer pain and poignancy of grief. The impaired mourner may require help with grocery shopping and housework. Money may be needed if there is no steady income due to the inability of the impaired griever to return to work. Dealing with impairment involves social service work and practical advice. As time goes on, there is a return to preloss activities and functioning.

Is Treatment Evidence Based?

The efficacy of all forms of psychotherapy has been questioned. The possibility even exists that it may be harmful. In controlled trial described by Beem and colleagues (1999), widows who received grief counseling experienced more sleep difficulty and other symptoms than did a control group.

Many trials have shown that when psychotherapy alone is compared with organic treatments in severe psychotic illnesses, the organic treatments have been superior. Strictly controlled trials of psychotherapy in other conditions are difficult to carry out. A major obstacle is that anecdotal evidence indicates that much depends on the individual psychotherapist.

The training of psychotherapists is more a matter of apprenticeship than acquisition of formal academic credentials. In order to regularize this situation and establish exactly what is being learned, some practitioners have produced manuals with step-by-step instructions. By following the manual exactly, a uniform kind of therapy can be produced and reproduced. *Manual-based psychotherapy* can then be tested by controlled trials. Several such manual-based therapies have been shown to be successful, although meta-analysis has cast doubt on many of the claims (Speilman, 2009). The difficulties facing research trials of psychotherapy in general are magnified in bereavement studies. As we have seen, there are ethical quandaries about even attempting to treat grief as a medical condition.

Neimeyer (2008) concluded from a literature review that the evidence for the general effectiveness of grief therapy relative to no treatment is weak. Eberl (2008) found that no rigorous evidence-based recommendations could be made regarding the treatment of bereaved persons.

Two trials of manual-based therapies for grief have been reported (National Cancer Institute, 2009). Shear, Frank, Houch, and Reynolds (2005) carried out a trial in which they compared their complicated grief treatment (CGT) with manual-based interpersonal therapy (Klerman, et al., 1984). CGT was found to produce superior results on several measures. Boelen, de Keijser, van den Hout, and van den Bout (2007) found that a version of cognitive-behavioral therapy was superior to supportive counseling.

ASSESSMENT OF THE RELATIONSHIP BETWEEN SEVERITY AND POIGNANCY OF GRIEF

Several scales have been devised to measure the severity of grief, such as the Texas Revised Inventory of Grief (Neimeyer, Hogan, & Laurie, 2008). Such scales attempt to establish prognostic criteria and separate the component factors. A distinction that can be made both intuitively and from studies of resulting data is between the poignancy of grief and its effect on functioning. Consider the following two vignettes:

A prosperous professional couple in the United States has one child. She is intelligent, happy, healthy, and pretty. When she is 6 years old, she is killed in a school bus crash.

A 70-year-old woman, living in a country without social security or state pensions, has suffered years of abuse from a violent, domineering husband. She cannot read or write or drive a car. Her husband is killed when her village is bombed.

In the first case, the parents suffer severe pain, but they return to a kind of functioning that externally appears normal. In the second case, the pain from the loss of companionship is minimal, but the widow faces destitution.

Scales such as the Social Readjustment Scale measure the impact of life events on function (Holmes & Rahe, 1967). On such scales, the effect of a loss may not have a direct relationship to its poignancy. Widowhood is considered by Holmes and Rahe to be the most severe of life-changing events, in spite of the fact that not all husbands are loved. It is the knowledge that widowhood is often accompanied by a series of other life-changing events that increases its stressfulness.

Some human relationships give rise to such strong bonds that breaking them is especially painful. This may be stating the obvious, but it is necessary to state the obvious so as to quantify and examine it. In this case, we must examine which relationships cause specific levels of grief.

Sanctioned and Unsanctioned Grief

However scant the consolation, society endorses, recognizes, and finds ways to support the distress caused by some kinds of bereavement. The language of bereavement contains separate words for those who have lost spouses or parents. Governments and charities often provide for widows and orphans. In many parts of the world, however, the person who has lost a lifelong gay partner has no special legal status.

When older persons lose their possessions in disasters it may be thought they are mourning a merely material loss. Rescuers accustomed to e-mailing digital pictures can find it hard to appreciate the significance of old and faded photographs. A common part of grieving is to preserve, or to be unable to destroy, the clothing or possessions of a dead child, spouse, or partner. In this way, these objects have more than material meaning for their owners.

Grieving for pets is a complex matter. In some cases, the pet may be a transitional object connected with a deceased person, or it may be the sole companion of someone otherwise solitary.

Are the Old Less Grieved For?

Some lives are considered, overtly or covertly, more valuable than others. Rescuers in disaster situations may find themselves making distinctions. A triage rescue system that apparently leaves the old to fend for themselves may not be entirely the result of discrimination.

World War II bombings killed 50,000 British civilians. To try to reduce the danger, civilians were evacuated from their homes in the targeted cities. Initially the plan was to move children and older persons. So many of the older persons refused to leave their homes that efforts were eventually limited to the evacuation of children.

The lesser value of the life of an older person can be rationalized in several ways. Actuarially, their lives have less value because they are closer to natural death. If they are slow and infirm they may impede rescuers. They are liable to have multiple physical illnesses reducing their quality of life. They are also more liable to have mental illnesses, especially dementia, that alter their status as persons worthy of saving. People with these illnesses are often segregated into institutions such as nursing homes (Birkett, 2001). Such considerations suggest that all life is not equally valuable, which may not be openly expressed when officially preparing for disasters. In the actual situation when a choice has to be made between saving those trapped in a nursing home and those trapped in a school, ageism may become a factor.

LITIGATION

Does DNR Mean Do Not Rescue?

DNR, meaning *do not resuscitate,* was originally an informal coded message left on the charts of some terminal hospital patients at the discretion of doctors. Such informal reliance on medical authority has now given way, in most jurisdictions, to a proliferation of living wills, health care proxies, and so forth. Many controversies surround this area. Questions have been raised about whether euthanasia and assisted suicide should be legalized and whether those who suffer from severe depression or dementia are capable of deciding their own fates. It was hoped that the wisdom of governments would resolve these issues, but doubts remain, especially in emergency situations (Hoffman, 2006).

The resuscitation referred to in DNR is narrowly defined in most American states. It refers only to procedures such as cardiopulmonary resuscitation or advanced cardiac life support and does not prohibit a life being saved in other circumstances. The existence of a DNR order could possibly affect the zeal of aid workers under stress. It could also give rise to suspicions and misunderstandings.

In 2005, when New Orleans was flooded by Hurricane Katrina, the following message were sent:

> This is quick; don't know how much longer we have use of the computer. Things are really bad. Please take a minute to call for someone to ask for more assistance for us. We are at Memorial Medical Center. One of the nurse's husband is here—he is a lawyer, made some calls so help may be coming. I will be in touch—the plan is to evacuate the sickest first then

families, then us. They will pick us up in helicopter, fly to where there's no water and drop us off.

—Rafay, 2005

The seventh floor of Memorial Hospital in New Orleans was run as a separate entity called Lifecare Hospital. It contained long-term patients who needed special machinery to survive. These patients could not be evacuated easily in the aftermath of Hurricane Katrina. No help arrived for 4 days. When help arrived, four patients were dead. The families concluded that the patients must have been killed and brought legal action against the caregivers.

The motives of those who brought suit in the New Orleans Memorial Hospital case are, at first sight, baffling. One might suppose the natural targets of litigation would be those allegedly responsible for the disaster. The concepts of retributions and justice are understandable, and we can see how these might bring a kind of solace to the grief stricken. In cases such as the Beslan massacre and the September 11, 2001, terrorist attack, the actual perpetrators are dead and the search for vengeance is more complicated. The desire for justice and retribution can lead to civil litigation. The motives for such litigation may be suspect as the concept that cash can assuage grief is often hard to empathize with.

One possibility is that those who have lost an older institutionalized relative feel the need to demonstrate that they care. It is a way of demonstrating their concern. We must also accept the possibility, cynical though it may seem, that health care workers and hospitals are natural targets of litigation because they have supposedly deep pockets and probably carry malpractice insurance.

After a certain point in time, the problems for the helping professionals change from managing grief to managing chronic problems of money, housing, and physical and/or mental illness.

HOLOCAUST SURVIVORS

The Nazi concentration camps were liberated in 1944, and their victims are now a concern of geriatrics. Most survivors of Nazi concentration camps are now dead, while those who are left are in their 80s. Those who survived may be people of unusual toughness and resilience (Collins, Burazeri, Gofin, & Kark, 2004), but they continue to have psychiatric symptoms attributable to their experiences. Their utilization of psychiatric medications, for example, exceeds that of a control group (Stessman, et al., 2008), and they have a higher number of suicide attempts (Barak, 2007).

When approaching an older patient of European immigrant background, it is useful first to ask a caregiver where the patient was during the war. If the reply indicates a Holocaust experience, the question then becomes how the patient feels about talking about it. Responses typically range from acceptance to more dramatic reactions, such as weeping that continues until the patient breaks down.

Some Holocaust survivors' children are now moving into the geriatric age group. Anecdotal accounts and clinical experience suggest that these offspring may be psychologically affected by what their parents went through, although objective studies have not been able to confirm any lasting damage (Sagi-Schwartz, et al., 2003).

Diagnostic Issues

All Holocaust survivors I have known were bereaved as well as victims. Those seeking treatment now have lost siblings or parents. It is possible they experienced some of the symptoms of the deprivation of maternal care described by Bowlby (Bretherton, 1992). Those who lose parents between the ages of 5 and 18 continue to have less well-being than those who do not (Lis-Turlejka, Luszczynski, Plichta, & Benight, 2008).

Several distinct syndromes among survivors were noted after World War II and are now tracking into geriatric psychiatry. Some investigators (Yehuda, et al., 2008) classify Holocaust survivors as suffering from PTSD. As with other forms of bereavement, there is a concern from an existential point of view that these syndromes do not belong to psychiatry because "the process of diagnosis is dehumanizing and the evil nature of the perpetrator is neglected" (Kellerman, 1999, p. 55). Such considerations could lead to the denial of needed treatment. Over the last 50 years, I have treated several survivors who became clinically depressed and responded well to organic treatments, such as electroconvulsive therapy (ECT).

Holocaust survivors with dementia and agitation may exhibit geriatric delusional patterns, such as "phantom boarder delusions" (Birkett, 2001, p. 115). These may be interpreted as due to the revival of memories.

A demented 90-year-old woman was distressed because she believed starving children were coming into her apartment looking for food and she had none to give them. Her family felt this was a recrudescence of her wartime sufferings in the Warsaw Ghetto.

ABERFAN

Aberfan exemplifies a disaster in which the geriatric survivors were not themselves placed in physical danger. The children killed in 1966 were between 5 and 11 years old. Their parents are now in their 70s and 80s. They are reluctant to be interviewed, and studying them systematically has presented ethical problems (Morgan, Scourfield, Williams, Jasper, & Lewis, 2003). Anger remains a salient emotion among the parents of these disaster victims, and there is guilt—entirely misplaced but real enough—on the part of those who tried to save their children but failed. They did everything that could possibly have been done but they will not forgive themselves for failing (Humphreys, 2006).

Clifford Minett lost two children at Aberfan. He estimates that he and his wife are 2 of around just 30 surviving parents left in the village:

> We have buried quite a few of them in recent times. I estimate that we lose a higher number every year because of what happened here.
>
> I know for a fact that it puts a lot of them in their graves with broken hearts. They just can't forget what happened, and it can take years off their life. A lot of them—friends of mine—should have lived a lot longer than they did. But I think quite a few of them couldn't put up with it any longer. You see it's not like the outside world. We will mark what happened this year as we always do with the annual memorial service. But there is no 40th anniversary, or 30, or any special anniversary, because for us it's here all the time. It never goes away and it happens every day. (Humphreys, 2006)

SUMMARY

In disaster situations, grief and PTSD often occur together. Grief particularly affects older survivors who may not have been in physical danger. Disaster workers should be familiar with the manifestations of grief. The features are similar to those of clinical depression and can include severe agitation, sleep disturbance, and hallucinations. Several writers have descried methods of grief counseling, but their effectiveness has not been proven by controlled trials. Some feel it is inappropriate to treat grief as a mental illness. Many forms of mourning are ritualized and even socially sanctioned or obligated.

Few controlled trials on drug use in the treatment of grief have been undertaken. Benzodiazepines are often used in large doses to deal with agitation and promote sleep. Any dosage reduction of these medications must be gradual. Antidepressants were found helpful in one controlled trial.

The formation of bonds of affection is a complex and variable process. In general, the loss of children is felt with the greatest pain, but the loss of a spouse produces the greatest loss of function. Social services and financial assistance may be needed to cope with the loss of a spouse. The life of the old is often considered less valuable, which can affect the priority of rescue attempts. The role of DNR orders in triage situation has not been codified.

Grief can take the form of anger, which may be directed at helpers and lead to litigation. Increased mortality, mental disturbance, and suicide rates can be tracked for many years after bereavement in disasters.

REFERENCES

American Psychiatric Association. (2000). *Diagnostic criteria from DSM-IV-TR*. Washington, DC: Author.

American Psychiatric Association. (2004). Practice guidelines for the treatment of acute stress disorder and posttraumatic stress disorder: Part A. Treatment recommendations. *American Journal of Psychiatry, 161*(11, Suppl. 1–31).

Barak, Y. (2007). The aging of holocaust survivors: Myth and reality concerning suicide. *Israeli Medical Association Journal, 9,* 196–198.

Beck, A. T., Rush, A. J., Shaw, B. F., & Emery, G. (1979). *Cognitive therapy of depression.* New York: Guilford Press.

Beem, E. E., Hooijkaas, H., Cleiren, M. H., Schut, H. A., Garssen, B., Croon, M. A., et al. (1999). The immunological and psychological effects of bereavement: Does grief counseling make a difference? A pilot study. *Psychiatry Research, 85,* 81–93.

Birkett, D. P. (2001). *Psychiatry in the nursing home.* Binghamton, NY: Haworth Press.

Boelen, P. A., de Keijser, J., van den Hout, M. A., & van den Bout, J. (2007). Treatment of complicated grief: A comparison between cognitive-behavioral therapy and supportive counseling. *Journal of Consulting and Clinical Psychology, 75,* 277–284.

Bretherton, I. (1992). The origins of attachment theory: John Bowlby and Mary Ainsworth. *Developmental Psychology, 28*(5), 759–775.

Collins, C., Burazeri, G., Gofin, J., & Kark, J. D. (2004). Health status and mortality in Holocaust survivors living in Jerusalem 40–50 years later. *Journal of Traumatic Stress, 17,* 403–411.

Cochrane, A. L. (1999). *Effectiveness and efficiency: Random reflections on health services.* London: Nuffield Provincial Hospitals Trust.

Darwin, C. (1872). *The expression of the emotions in man and animals* (Rep. ed.). New York: Barnes and Noble Publishing.

Eberl, M. M. (2008). *Bereavement interventions: Evidence and ethics.* Retrieved June 9, 2009, from http://www.bioethics.buffalo.edu/bereavement

Ellis, A., & Dryden, W. (2007). *The practice of rational emotive behavior therapy* (2nd ed.). New York: Springer Publishing.

Freud, S. (1957). Mourning and melancholia [trauer und melancholia]. In J. Rickman (Ed.), *A general selection from the works of Sigmund Freud* (p. 124–140). New York: Doubleday Anchor. (Original work published 1917).

Freud, S. (1982). *Studienausgabe band III, psychologie des unbewussten*. Frankfurt am Main, Germany: Fischer Wissenschaft, Fischer Taschenbuch Verlag. (Original work published 1917).

Hoffman, J. (2006, October 10). The last word on the last breath. *New York Times*. Retrieved June 10, 2009, from http://www.nytimes.com

Holmes, T., & Rahe, R. (1967). The social readjustment scale. *Journal of Psychosomatic Research, 11*, 213–218.

Humphreys, J. (2006). *John Humphreys returns*. Retrieved June 15, 2009, from http://www.dailymail.co.uk/news/article-406691/John-Humphreys-returns-Aberfan.html

Kellerman, N. P. (1999). Diagnosis of Holocaust survivors and their children. *Israel Journal of Psychiatry and Related Sciences, 36*, 55–64.

Kendler, K. S., Myers, J., & Zisook, S. (2008). Does bereavement related major depression differ from depression associated with other stressful life events? *American Journal of Psychiatry, 165*, 1449–1455.

Klerman, G., Weissman, M., Rounsaville, B. J., & Chevron, E. S. (1984). *Interpersonal psychotherapy of depression*. New York: Basic Books.

Kushner, H. S. (2001). *When bad things happen to good people* (20th Anniversary ed.). New York: Random House.

Lis-Turiejska, M., Luszczynski, A., Plichta, A., & Benight, C. C. (2008). Jewish and non-Jewish World War II child and adolescent survivors at 60 years after war: Effects of parental loss and age at exposure on well-being. *American Journal of Orthopsychiatry, 78*, 369–377.

Morgan, L., Scourfield, J., Williams, D., Jasper, A., & Lewis, G. (2003). The Aberfan disaster: A 33-year follow-up of survivors. *British Journal of Psychiatry, 182*, 532–536.

National Cancer Institute. (2009). *Bereavement, mourning, and grief* (Health professional version). Retrieved October 18, 2009, from www.cancer.gov/cancertopics/pdq/supportivecare/bereavement/HealthProfessional

Neimeyer, R. A. (2008). Grief and bereavement counseling. In C. Bryant & D. Peck (Eds.), *Encyclopedia of death and human experience*. Thousand Oaks, CA: Sage.

Neimeyer, R. A., Hogan, N. S., & Laurie, A. (2008). The measurement of grief: Psychometric considerations in the assessment of reactions to bereavement. In M. S. Stroebe, R. O. Hansson, H. Schut, & W. Stroebe (Eds.), *Handbook of bereavement research and practice* (pp. 133–161). Washington, DC: American Psychological Association.

Parkes, C. M. (1998). *Bereavement: studies of grief in adult life* (3rd ed.). Madison, CT: International Universities Press.

Rafay. (2005, August 31). Untitled message posted to http://neworleans.metblogs.com

Rees, W. D. (1971). The hallucinations of widowhood. *British Medical Journal, 4*, 37–38.

Sagi-Schwart, A., Van IJzedoorn, M. H., Grossmann, K. E., Joels, T., Grossmann, K., Scharf, M., et al. (2003). Attachment and traumatic stress in female Holocaust survivors and their children. *American Journal of Psychiatry, 160*, 1086–1092.

Shear, K., Frank, E., Houch, P. R., & Reynolds, C. F. (2005). Treatment of complicated grief: A randomized controlled trial. *Journal of the American Medical Association, 293*, 2601–2608.

Speilman, G. (2009). Does cognitive behavioral therapy work or not. *The Carlat Psychiatry Report, 7,* 9.

Stessman, J., Cohen, A., Hammerman-Rozenberg, R., Bursztyn, M., Azoulay, D., Maaravi, Y., et al. (2008). Holocaust survivors in old age: The Jerusalem longitudinal study. *Journal of the American Geriatrics Society, 56,* 470–477.

Stroebe, M. S., Hansson, R. O., Schut, H., & Stroebe, W. (2002). *Handbook of bereavement research and practice: Advances in theory and intervention.* Washington, DC: American Psychological Association.

Walsh, K., King, M., Jones, L., & Blizard, R. (2002) Spiritual beliefs may affect outcome of bereavement. *British Medical Journal, 324,* 1551–1553.

Worden, J. W. (2009). *Grief counseling and grief therapy* (4th ed.). New York: Springer Publishing.

World Health Organization. (1992). *ICD-10 classification of mental and behavioral disorders.* Geneva, Switzerland: Author.

Yehuda, R., Schmeidler, J., Labinsky, E., Bell, A., Morris, A., Zemelman, S., et al. (2009). Ten-year follow-up study of PTSD diagnosis symptom severity and psychosocial indices in aging holocaust survivors. *Acta Psychiatrica Scandinavica, 119*(1), 25–34.

Zisook, S., Schucter, S. R., Pedrelli, P., Sable, J., & Deauciuc, S. C. (2001). Bupropion sustained release for bereavement. *Journal of Clinical Psychiatry, 62,* 227–230.

Special Populations

16

The Experience of Vulnerability in Geriatric Combat Veterans With Posttraumatic Stress Disorder During Times of Disaster

JOANNE IZZO

On the morning of September 11, 2001, veterans and staff of the Post Traumatic Stress Disorder (PTSD) and Mental Hygiene Clinic at the Brooklyn VA Medical Center stood shoulder to shoulder, aghast, as they watched the attack on the World Trade Center towers unfolding. Looking out the north-side windows of the clinic, they saw Tower 1 on fire. In the clinic that morning were Vietnam, Korean, and World War II veterans. The work of that day took on a different dimension; clinicians roamed the clinic and checked on each veteran and on one another. It was an *open-door-policy* day. Some veterans were able to sit with a mental health provider and process how they were feeling. Other veterans simply walked up to an open door and met with an available counselor. Over the next 48 hours, there was an atmosphere of mutual support as veterans expressed their concern for the staff with statements such as: "I see the work that you are doing. Are you all right? Is there anything I can do for you?" The terrorist act of violence brought out feelings among the veterans ranging from outrage to anxiety, concern for others, and a desire to be of service.

Thematic statements expressed to staff over the next week among the cohorts of veterans from World War II, Korea, and Vietnam included: "Now you have a sense of what the experience of combat is like. Sadly, now America knows in a way what it means to be vulnerable." The attack on the twin towers, while not leveling the playing field between

317

citizen-solider/veteran and citizen provider, created an opportunity for the veterans to apply Shakespeare's words from King Henry V, Act 4, Scene 1—"teach others how to prepare."

Just as New York City and the United States have adapted to the realities of a post–September 11 world, so too geriatric veterans have adapted. While they often re-experience feelings of vulnerability as a result of September 11, veterans are utilizing what they learned on the field of battle and in therapy. Many veterans who are in therapy for PTSD at our Brooklyn VA Hospital PTSD program have chosen a path of healing. This path requires them to accept rather than deny their actions or inactions during war. Combat veterans on this path progressively learn to recognize their maladaptive avoidance behavior and to examine their beliefs about their actions. This process teaches veterans to challenge faulty thinking about the past that supports irrational core beliefs about themselves. The end result of this process is a more realistic self-image. Combat veterans are able to access valuable life lessons to live by and to pass on to others, lessons previously inaccessible as a result of their avoidance of the traumatic material.

The events of September 11 functioned as the touchstone in reshaping the framework of therapy with geriatric combat veterans diagnosed with PTSD. In our work, we speak of healing rather than cure, symptom reduction rather than remission. A person may heal from the most painful and debilitating aspects of trauma, but inasmuch as the memory lingers after the level of distress has been reduced significantly or neutralized, the person lives with the trauma. The memory of a lived event cannot be excised from the mind, and so cure is not a fitting concept to apply. Similarly, PTSD symptoms as subjectively experienced and objectively measured may be reduced with therapy to a subthreshold level for combat trauma.

INTRODUCTION

This chapter introduces the reader to three generational cohorts of older American veterans. The similarities and differences among these three cohorts, as well as the hopes and values characteristic of each, are discussed. The purpose of this chapter is to offer the reader a basic impression of this population as seen through the lenses of clinical observation and experience rather than of research. There is a small but excellent body of research on these three age cohorts conducted by the National Center for

PTSD in West Haven and authored by some of the leaders in this field: Robert Rosenheck, Al Fontana, Paula Schnurr, Matthew Friedman, Allan Spiro, Paula Resick, and others whose efforts and work have contributed to a better understanding of geriatric veterans with PTSD. There is also a growing body of literature written by the mental health community outside the VA that discusses the needs and problems of an aging veteran population with PTSD. Research on this aging veteran population is consistent with our experience at the Brooklyn Campus of the New York Harbor Healthcare (NYHHC), VA Medical Center, and also confirms the observations and experience of other mental health professionals who treat these populations. It is important for the reader to keep in mind that the discussion in this chapter is limited to those veterans with chronic and often severe PTSD who are in active treatment. This chapter aims to enhance the reader's understanding of how this population continues to be affected by their beliefs about their combat experiences. Some veterans diagnosed with PTSD may become disabled as a result of the severity of their symptoms. Their disability manifests as an impairment of social, industrial, or familial function or a combination.

This chapter also focuses on the impact of terrorism and war upon the beliefs and behaviors of the cohorts in this population, particularly in relation to the expression of PTSD symptomatology. The effects of aging and memory and the psychological dynamics of powerlessness, vulnerability, and hopefulness as manifested by this population are examined. The spiritual and existential implications of veterans who are thought to have lived far beyond their days of greatness are explored. The chapter concludes with a brief summary and suggestions for practice working with a geriatric veteran population.

DEFINITION OF TERMS

Veteran

A veteran is a person who has been employed and/or had years of experience in a service or occupation (especially military).

Combat Veteran

For the purposes of this chapter, a combat veteran is a soldier who served in a war zone either in direct combat or in a support unit located in the theater of activity.

Posttraumatic Stress Disorder

Over the centuries, this disorder was recognized by physicians and psychiatrists and described in a variety of ways. In the Civil War, what we now call PTSD was known as *soldiers heart* (Tick, 2005) and *war nostalgia* (Hyams & Wignall, 1996). The term *shell shock* (Figley, 1985) came into use in WWI and the terms *war neurosis* or *traumatic war neurosis* during WWII (Friedman, Keane, & Resick, 2007) continuing through the Vietnam War. In 1985, the Committee of Anxiety Disorders for *DSM-III* defined the term *posttraumatic stress disorder* (Friedman, et al.).

PTSD usually manifests as a mixture of anxiety and depression and varies in degree and severity from individual to individual. The range of possible symptoms is as follows: repeated, disturbing memories, thoughts, and images of the traumatic event(s); repeated, disturbing dreams of the traumatic event(s); suddenly acting or feeling as if the event were happening again; feeling very upset when something is reminiscent of the stressful or traumatic event; physical reactivity such as palpitations, difficulty breathing, and sweating when reminded of the traumatic event; avoidance of thinking or talking about the event; avoidance of activities that remind the person of the event; difficulty remembering aspects of the event; loss of interest in things one used to enjoy; feeling distant or cut off from others; emotional numbness and difficulty having and expressing loving feelings toward those close to the person; negativistic thinking; a sense of a foreshortened future; difficulty falling asleep and remaining asleep; irritability and angry outbursts; difficulty with concentration; hypervigilance; and hyper-reactivity (American Psychiatric Association, 2000).

PTSD as a condition can be classified as *subthreshold* (i.e., the disorder's impact on the functioning of the individual is minimal, with little to no impairment reported) to *moderate or severe* (indicating a substantial impairment in each sphere of a person's life). PTSD also may be classified as *chronic* when the individual has lived with the disorder for an extended period of time prior to entering treatment (Engdahl & Eberly, 1994). As with any medical or psychiatric condition, the longer treatment is delayed the more entrenched the symptoms become in the person's lifestyle.

Geriatrics

Geriatrics is a concentration in health sciences that focuses on the process of aging and diseases typically found in older adults.

For the purposes of this chapter, Vietnam veterans are considered to be geriatric for two reasons: (1) because some are already within this category, and (2) because they are the fastest growing geriatric cohort in relation to the rates of decline among the WWII and Korean War veterans (U.S. Department of Veterans Affairs, 2008). To be more specific, the youngest Vietnam veteran is 55 years old today, and the oldest Vietnam veteran could be into his late 70s. Within the next several years, geriatric combat veterans of the baby boomer generation may become the largest consumer group of medical and mental health services and products.

INTERVENTIONS

The instrument commonly used to assess for combat trauma is the PCL-M (Weathers, Husk, & Keane, 1991). This instrument is a 17-item list that translates the *DSM-IV-TR* criteria for PTSD into questions, asking the subject to indicate *how much they have been bothered by each item in the past month* (Weathers, Husk, et al.). A score below 50 is considered subthreshold for combat trauma (Weathers, Litz, Herman, Huska, & Keane, 1993). In addition to this widely used instrument, which is an integral part of the monitoring process in the treatment of PTSD, often within the first few sessions a structured interview for PTSD known as Clinical Aided, PTSD, or CAPS (Blake, et al., 1998), is conducted. The CAPS is an extensive evaluation that allows for greater objective assessment of the expression of subjective symptoms experienced by the veteran.

A veteran may experience a period of symptom reduction after completing a course of therapy in which one or two target symptoms were addressed in the context of examining the veteran's most traumatic experience. Veterans who experience a reduction in symptoms endorse improved familial, social, or industrial function. However, improvement does not preclude the possibility of symptom exacerbation triggered by an external event (Schnurr, 1994). These exacerbations may require a return to therapy for stabilization. In some cases, further exploration of the cognitive distortions and beliefs that may have surfaced is warranted.

Since the events of September 11, 2001, two subjects have taken center stage in the therapeutic dialogue: the potential for another attack and, after 2003, the wars in Iraq and Afghanistan. Veterans have utilized their own capacities for resilience by drawing upon their experiences as survivors of war and stepping into renewed roles as contributors, providers, and protectors of their family and friends. For those who have yet to claim this role, clinicians have focused on the enhancement of coping skills. At the same time, veterans have been encouraged to address their underlying feelings of anxiety and dread connected to unresolved, unconscious beliefs about the present as related to the past.

As part of their therapy regime at Brooklyn VA Medical Center, clinicians have taken advantage of *disaster drill days* that often are staged at the medical center without prior notice. The purpose of the drill is to simulate what would happen if a disaster occurred during normal hours of operation when the facility is at maximum activity. A disaster drill involves an announcement over the public address system—"Disaster in effect"—followed by an alarm. Prior to the drill, every service personnel and most noncommissioned staff are assigned specific task assignments to be activated in a disaster situation. This interruption of the normal flow provides an opportunity to revisit the protocol that went into effect after September 11 and to explore the veterans' response to a biochemical or nuclear attack. These drills are often anxiety provoking for the veterans until they are notified that it is a drill. Yet the drills have helped heighten their awareness of the implications of being away from home in the event of a disaster.

These drill days have provided another benefit—they have identified the most optimal means for the facility to meet the needs of the veterans. The disruptions have been recast into a therapeutic forum for discussion in which the veterans have been better able to identify (1) what they would need to do and have in a disaster and (2) what the facility would need to do and have on hand to assist this population in the event of a disaster. As a result of these ad hoc sessions, the following therapeutic interventions have been added: (1) periodic and deliberate psychoeducation in disaster preparedness; (2) discussions about disaster plans that involve the family; (3) group therapeutic activities such as trips to restaurants, the theater, or other activities that include spouses; and (4) facilitating veterans' voluntary initiatives such as fund-raising and direct assistance to soldiers returning from Iraq or Afghanistan.

Traditionally, the inclusion of discussion regarding political and social issues in individual or group therapy has been discouraged. This is grounded in the belief that to focus on these more global issues in a process group enables the veterans to avoid identifying and working through their own personal feelings (i.e., helplessness, abandonment, and betrayal) and thereby misses the opportunity to use therapy for insight into how their beliefs and behaviors contribute to maintaining their symptoms. However, the events of September 11, 2001, precipitated an awakening within many combat veterans and a movement toward confronting their past in an unprecedented way. Many veterans at the Brooklyn VA Medical Center have begun to challenge long-held, irrational core beliefs about their behavior in war in a more realistic way. As a result, some have come to recognize a previously held irrational belief (i.e., I am evil) as connected to a behavior that they want to change (i.e., social isolation). New cognitions such as "I am okay as I am" or "I can make mistakes and still be a good person" have replaced the old dysfunctional beliefs. As the belief about self changes, the behaviors of social isolation begin to yield to increased social activity.

Responsiveness is a thought process integral to the neocortex. Reaction belongs to the limbic system. In boot camp, training in quick, decisive reactions is the central component to survival. This training is aimed at the limbic system. Many veterans have become more aware of *a global perspective* related to our interdependence and connectedness as human beings. The veteran population has come to greater acceptance that (1) there is little in life that is predictable and (2) that we have little control over anything beyond our choice to respond rather than react to a situation.

Some WWII veterans often demonstrate a positive view supported by their belief that good will triumph over evil in the end. Some Korean War veterans are not as optimistic and endorse a more aggressive stance as inevitable and the only solution to the present chaos.

The Expression of PTSD Symptoms in the Geriatric Veteran Population

> Wretched I was, wretched I am: Battered by sorrows. From now on I must live alone with none—no companion in the days to come, and in misery I shall die—sad sad sad! Doomed to the sufferings I have had and for as many Horrible days.
>
> —Sophocles

Philocetetes, a play written by Sophocles at age 87, is about a Greek citizen-soldier gone off to fight in the war against the Trojans. Philocetetes sustains a festering wound from a snakebite and is dropped off on an isolated island by his comrades in arms. Isolated and alone, he mourns two losses: the life he knew as a citizen and the life he knew as soldier. Heracles makes a gift of a magic bow to this mournful and isolated citizen-soldier. In the end, the military leader learns from the god Heracles that the war against Troy cannot be won without the wounded Philocetetes. This imposes upon the military the responsibility to heal his wound and to reintegrate him into the society of soldiers so he may return home as a citizen-soldier.

So, too, has been the mission of the VA and in some respects the military: to seek healing for those soldiers physically or psychologically wounded by exposure to traumatic events in the course of combat. PTSD, currently classified as an anxiety disorder, shares an overlapping symptom spectrum with depression (American Psychiatric Association, 2000). Different symptoms of PTSD may manifest at different stages in the lives of many veterans. Agitated depression in younger, more virile years may manifest as vegetative depression in later years. The young, angry, and isolated veteran often does not lose his anger but either learns to channel it into constructive activities or becomes more deeply entrenched in depression.

While intrusive memories and nightmares continue to a lesser degree, the geriatric combat veteran may express a deeper feeling of nostalgia. These reminisces sometimes are accompanied by a clarification of an internal emotional conflict around guilt and shame—guilt about things done or left undone or shame about oneself as inadequate, defective, or weak. Alongside these feelings is an alternative self-image of strength as a survivor under horrible conditions. The *PCL-M* (Weathers, et al., 1991), which was completed by a sample of all three cohorts at the Brooklyn VA campus, suggests that symptoms continue over time to meet the criteria for severe PTSD even though some symptoms are not as distressing as in the past.

Reestablishing a civilian life—including providing for a family, seeing one's children launched, and watching one's children's children grow—on some level removes the feelings of fear, failure, and survivor's guilt. Ironically, these successes, including perhaps the shock of having lived so long, challenge the fundamental belief of a foreshortened future rather than a happy life entrenched in a depressive symptom of negative thinking. The ever-present question, "Was I good enough?" was aptly expressed by Private Ryan at the conclusion of his silent journey in the movie *Saving Private Ryan* (Bryce & Spielberg, 1989). Acknowledging how much time one has left in this world lessens the mechanism of avoidance and propels the geriatric combat veteran into a purposeful use of therapy. While such questions are normal for the general population, most do not seek out therapy or become increasingly anxious. For those with untreated PTSD, the shock of retirement, the unstructured time available for reflection, and enforced limits on daily activity due to health are a few factors that may lead combat veterans into treatment at this stage in their life's journey.

The impact of war, terrorism, and threats of continued terrorist activity brings anxiety to the fore in the general population and particularly in the geriatric veteran population. As older veterans see images of young soldiers on the news, they feel a strong identification with their old unit and their personal experiences. They may re-experience the anxiety and dread of combat, and they also may grieve for those now in combat. Feelings of helplessness, frustration, and vulnerability return. The impact of these memories and their associated feelings is evident particularly in those veterans hospitalized for medical illnesses. A veteran in this circumstance may experience an exacerbation of PTSD symptoms concurrently with a depressive episode or adjustment due to a medical condition.

Reports of enemy war atrocities provoke feelings and expressions of anger and outrage that carry deep within them personal memories and experience. The news may serve as a distraction from thoughts about their illness and may displace feelings of fear and vulnerability that have arisen as they have adjusted to the loss of health and autonomy and the experience of confronting death. Expressions of anger and frustration may either be the manifestation of repressed feelings of helplessness and vulnerability to illness or a reprise of earlier problematic patterns of belief and behavior. It is often the case that combat veterans use anger to mask or avoid feelings of helplessness, weakness, and vulnerability in order to feel strong and safe. However, it may also be that global events bring to the surface unresolved feelings and beliefs about their actions during war in a new way and from a different perspective, thus allowing them to embark on a deeper inner journey toward healing. Their inability to be of service, to offer sacrifice now as they are isolated in sickness, echoes a painful truth concisely expressed in meter by Sophocles, "Wretched I was, wretched I am; Battered by sorrows." How each older veteran makes meaning in this crucial life transition from Erickson's (1980) life stages of generativity versus stagnation to integrity versus despair determines the value each will place upon the sorrows experienced in his life.

Fowler's expanded life cycle stages of human development, which includes the spiritual dimension (Fowler, 1981), and Erickson's works help us understand from a spiritual perspective the dynamics operating in each life stage and in the transitional space between them.

VALUES AND CHARACTER TRAITS IN THE GERIATRIC COMBAT VETERAN

Several years ago, in preparation for a lecture titled "Values and Character Traits in the Geriatric Combat Veteran Population," 82 veterans from all three wars were surveyed. Fifty-one veterans identified their primary concern at present as *acting according to ethical and moral values,* 18 veterans identified their primary concern at present as *becoming who I was meant to be,* 9 veterans identified *the physical dimension of life* as most important, and 4 veterans were undecided (Izzo, n.d.).

The values most frequently identified were family, faith, defense of country, and justice. The character traits most frequently identified were respectfulness, responsibility, fairness, and reverence for life. Overall, there was a congruence of hopes and values among the three generations of combat veterans demonstrating more similarities than differences. Perhaps one impact of a combat experience is a narrowing of the generation gap. Perhaps the agreement and, to a degree, harmony among these cohorts teaches us about the impact of adversity and trauma upon the human character and personality.

Within the environment of war are other aspects of the personality that may have lain dormant and undeveloped and that, for better or worse, may now present themselves. The environment of war brings out subtle and latent aspects of the fundamental character of the person. Often, veterans will speak of themselves as having two personalities, as in Jekyll and Hyde: the *me* I was before combat and the *me* I became in combat. Many long for who they were before the war.

Yet all are unwilling to give up the good they identified doing while enduring much evil. Most veterans cannot recognize a balanced responsibility and readily take blame for negative outcomes over which they may have had little or no control. The challenge of therapy is to give veterans the confidence to acknowledge their own hopes, dreams, and desires to be better than who they were before, during, and after the war—in other words, to be who they are now. Just as the organic and psychological growth and development of a child are shaped by the environment from the womb through the child's early years, it is important for us to consider that we are not finished products. Rather, we are organic living beings continually in a process of change, growth, and development as we adapt to the environment and its changes. Acceptance of the past, of change, and of the present makes the future possible. When the veteran reconnects with the personal integrity that always existed within him in a new and meaningful way, he is free to accept himself and his lived experience and to offer wisdom born of a whole life lived.

SOME GENERAL IDENTIFYING CHARACTERISTICS OF EACH OF THE THREE COHORTS OF GERIATRIC VETERANS

If everybody is thinking alike then somebody isn't thinking.

—G. S. Patton, 1947

There are technically four cohorts of geriatric combat veterans: veterans of WWI, WWII, Korea, and Vietnam. This chapter does not include a discussion of WWI veterans since there are so few surviving. Of the three remaining cohorts there is a steady decline in the WWII population, relative stability within the Korean veteran population, and growth within the Vietnam veteran's cohort. The following section provides a brief overview of each generation within its historical and sociological context.

Some Characteristics of the Generation of WWII

The Greatest Generation is the appellation given to the veterans of the WWII era, whose battle statistics are noted in Table 16.1. The average age of a WWII draftee in the United States was 25 years old. What were some characteristics of the world in which these citizen-soldiers lived? All were affected to one degree or another by the Great Depression, which began with the stock market crash of 1929. The world then was smaller and more fragmented than the world today since the technology for widespread communication was still in its infancy. Economic hardship was known to most in varying degrees, and for many it formed a common bond that created strong community bonds and neighborhood ties in the inner city. The common struggle fostered an already-present sense of social responsibility and nationalism. The individuals of this generation carried forward from the previous generation a sense of right and wrong, just and unjust. These

Table 16.1

SUMMARY OF WORLD WAR II CASUALTIES
World War II (1941–1945)
Total U.S. Service Members (Worldwide) 16,112,566
Battle Deaths 291,557
Other Deaths in Service (Non-Theater) 113,842
Non-Mortal Woundings 671,846
Living Veterans 2,306,000
From "America's Wars," U.S. Department of Veterans Affairs, Office of Public Affairs, 2008.

values and beliefs were American, yet they also reflected the desire of immigrant populations to alter their traditions to be in conformance with and in support of the American ideal. From an historical time line, they are the younger brothers of WWI veterans, the older brothers of the Korean War generation, the fathers of Vietnam veterans, and possibly grandfathers of Iraq and Afghanistan veterans.

These men, for the most part, returned to marriage and families and took up the lives they had laid down during their service. Yet returning home to live the traditional values of work, family, and community that they had fought and saw friends die for brought with it numerous challenges. The world they once knew was now changed. Many of these men returned home to find that women filled their previous jobs. Some returned home to discover that work was not always readily available. When it was available, the camaraderie of the trenches was nowhere to be found in the competitive world of business and industry.

Today, this cohort is very community oriented. They demonstrate the characteristics of resilience and endurance. However, this generation, who thought they were participating in the war to end all wars, has never experienced a world at peace. They found themselves confronted by survival and in many ways became isolated. There is an excellent illustration of these internal conflicts, from intrusive memory through existential angst and beyond to marital conflict, in the film *The Man in the Grey Flannel Suit* (Zanuck & Johnson, 1956).

Our experience at the Brooklyn VA has demonstrated that the fathers and grandfathers of Iraq and Afghanistan war veterans are very active in supporting troops abroad and the wounded at home. They are strong voices for peace along with Korean and Vietnam War veterans. A good percentage of this cohort may be primary caretakers for their spouses or provide care for younger grandchildren. Most have some medical illness; many are active and involved in various activities within the VA and veterans organizations to the extent they are able, which brings them into contact with the larger community.

Some Characteristics of the Generation of the Korean Conflict

The generation of the Korean conflict listened to the radio as President Roosevelt announced the bombing of Pearl Harbor and the declaration of war on Japan. They saw their older brothers or their friends' fathers deployed to either Europe or the Pacific. They saved tinfoil and metal and lis-

Table 16.2

SUMMARY OF KOREAN WAR CASUALTIES
Korean War (1950–1953)
Total U.S. Service Members (Worldwide) 5,720,000
Battle Deaths 33,739
Other Deaths (in Theater) 2,835
Other Deaths in Service (Non-Theater) 17,672
Non-Mortal Woundings 103,284
Living Veterans 2,307,000
From "America's Wars," U.S. Department of Veterans Affairs, Office of Public Affairs, 2008.

tened to the news on the radio or saw newsreels at the movies. They saw their brothers and friends' fathers return home from war and saw gold stars in the windows of mothers whose sons did not return as illustrated in Table 16.2. By 1947, some had joined the Reserves or the National Guard or had gone into active duty. Those activated to serve in the Korean conflict, as it was known at the time, were men who had served in WWII and who were still under the 7-year obligation to serve as Inactive Ready Reserves (IRR). Reserve units and National Guard units, as well as draftees, were enlisted into service during this conflict.

This generation went to war with their peers from other countries. Quietly, they were drafted; slowly, and with less fanfare, they went missing from their neighborhoods, jobs, and families. Just as quietly, they returned a year or two later and went about the business of picking up their lives just as their older brothers and friends' fathers had before them. This cohort of American veterans ate WWII rations and for the first 18 months or so of the war had the wrong clothing for the season. They experienced what no other soldier had experienced before—a tactic thoroughly counter to any training, in which thousands of soldiers charged simultaneously and fired their weapons. This was referred to as *human wave attacks*. As they moved from point to point, many soldiers encountered children half naked, starving, orphaned, or separated from their families. Where and when they were able, they would feed, clothe, and care for the children. How many of these soldiers—once younger brothers themselves, now older brothers and fathers—saw with broken hearts these unspoken victims of war?

These men returned to face similar problems as the veterans of prior wars: little or no gainful employment. As the Cold War developed over the next few years, theirs was the generation that built the fallout shelters and taught their children what to do when the air raid siren sounded.

But the picture has not been totally bleak for the soldiers of the Korean War. Theirs is the only generation of soldiers that continues to be held in esteem by the nation they fought to preserve and protect. The government and people of South Korea have broken the silence of this forgotten war by bringing soldiers from all the nations who served back to Korea as honored guests. No longer anonymous victors, this generation has lived to return and see peace and prosperity. They rejoice in a bittersweet way as they discover the battlefield they knew is now merely a memory. Their memory is the only marker of where an American soldier was wounded or where a buddy was killed. Trees, towns, homes, and businesses have now replaced the former killing grounds. These veterans have found recognition and continue to come forward and identify themselves to family, friends, and neighbors.

Some Characteristics of the Generation of the Vietnam War

American involvement in Vietnam began in 1959 and ended in 1975. As Table 16.3 indicates, it produced more American deaths and lasted longer than the prior wars of the century. With each passing year, more and more Baby Boomers who formed the cohort of Vietnam veterans become part of the geriatric population. This cohort has helped a nation reconsider the effects of war upon the personality, soul, and psyche of individuals and a nation. The average age of a draftee for this war was 18 years of age. During WWII, soldiers could serve with a unit for years. During the Korean War, a point system was instituted before rotation out of the war zone. During the Vietnam War, each branch of service developed its own policy with regard to the duration of a tour of duty in a combat zone—a tour did not exceed 13 months in the Marine Corps and could be as short as 6 months for naval personnel.

This generation grew up in the shadow of missile silos and fall-out shelters. They faced the Cuban missile crisis at a moment in American his-

Table 16.3

SUMMARY OF VIETNAM WAR CASUALTIES
Vietnam War (1964–1975)
Total U.S. Service Members (Worldwide) 8,744,000
Deployed to Southeast Asia 3,403,000
Battle Deaths 47,434
Other Deaths (in Theater) 10,786
Other Deaths in Service (Non-Theater) 32,000
Non-Mortal Woundings 153,303
Living Veterans 7,125,000

From "America's Wars," U.S. Department of Veterans Affairs, Office of Public Affairs, 2008.

tory that perhaps opened the door to larger questions about government policy. This generation grew up in a time of changing values and turmoil as the rules of society, old values, ideals, and standards were slowly challenged. They lived in that uncomfortable liminal place between the old and the yet undefined new. This generation returned and opted in or out of society. Many sought to do as their fathers, uncles, and grandfathers had done—pick up where they had left off and attempt to live the life they had expected to have before going off to war. This generation experienced entire neighborhoods and zip codes targeted for the draft and found those neighborhoods dramatically changed upon their return. This generation returned home to find a different kind of war at home: the awakening of a country to civil rights for all. The effects of war were experienced more deeply and dramatically than in previous cohorts partially due to exposure to war at a younger age, increased exposure to the widespread use of chemical hazards such as dioxin (Agent Orange), increasing resistance to the war at home, and a lack of world stability.

Many in all three generations have complex medical profiles. Of these generations, the Vietnam veterans often are in poorer health compared with Korean War and WWII veterans during similar ages. The effects of

Agent Orange appear to be the main culprit. Currently, Agent Orange has been implicated in the diagnosis of certain cancers, heart disease, and diabetes, as well as having been a precipitator of psychological stress upon the human body.

The connection between psychological stress, trauma, and the body is better understood than in previous generations. The Vietnam veteran has lived between institutional resistance to acknowledge that exposure to dioxin could be harmful and a lack of understanding of the impact of psychological stress upon the body. The persistence of Vietnam veterans in advocating for government accountability for the soldiers it sends to war has opened the doors of advocacy to veterans of WWII and Korea. Further, the veterans of more recent wars have benefited from the results of the Vietnam veterans' call for accountability and have adopted similar strategies.

In the chapel on Fort Hamilton Army Base there is a small wooden plaque on the north wall with the following words carved into it: *The soldier is the first to pray for peace.* The truth of this is seen in the eyes, heard in the voice, and witnessed in the actions of geriatric combat veterans who, having seen war, desire peace. It is their hope and prayer; it is the source of internal psychological conflict in the light of terrorist attacks; and it is central to their feelings of despair.

ENTERING THE WORLD OF THE COMBAT VETERAN

In basic training, the military recruit undergoes, among other things, a narrowing of perspective. The individual is subordinated first to the country, then to their particular branch of service, then to the division in which he or she serves, and finally to their particular company or barracks. The focus on division and company creates a corporate identity and pride that filter down to the platoon or squad of which the soldier is a member. Within this squad, the world grows smaller still—first to my buddy, then to the one who watches my back, and finally to the one whose back I watch. While the archetypes of nation, soldier, and warrior are at play in the conscious mind of the soldier, there is another process occurring: that of attachment. Most soldiers form a fraternal attachment to one or more men in their unit. Under the conditions of war, these new attachments are formed because one's life depends upon others. Attachment theorists recognize that adversity and trauma create an environment that shapes and promotes attachment choices. Theorists also are examining more deeply the adult formation of attachments. It is critical to understand how and why attachments are formed during combat in order to fully comprehend and effectively treat survivors' guilt and their impairments to interpersonal relating and social and familial functioning.

When the ego is encouraged to identify with larger archetypal categories, it is a short step to living out the self in an archetypal drama of war—identifying the self as hero. When this happens, the boundaries of real and perceived power blur, moral judgment is impaired, and personal feelings become marginally or completely inaccessible.

Martha Nussbaum (2007) suggests, in her work *Upheavals of Thought*, that the affective component is so critical to informed thinking and decision making that its absence impairs the individual capacity for moral/ethical right judgment and decision making.

When the combat veteran returns home, he or she does not easily or frequently shed the thought distortions acquired in the combative experience. Similarly, the combat veteran is unconscious of changes in his or her personality; these changes are not self-apparent, although they might be apparent to others. Many are disinclined to express emotion and demonstrate a tendency to repress tender and sensitive feelings as well as feelings associated with vulnerability and anxiety. Combat veterans identify their postwar life as one of survival but not living. Countless veterans with chronic and severe PTSD shun the feelings that accompany many nonthreatening and pleasant activities of living. For many, their families become the new squad; the veterans' role is to keep everyone safe. Even their health and mental health providers may be viewed as members of a squad from whom they expect safety and protection and for whom they will provide safety and protection if needed.

There are four typical behaviors of combat veterans with severe PTSD: avoidance, withdrawal, protection, and reaction. All these behaviors are designed to ward off anxious feelings and thoughts. These behaviors correlate to the five basic problematic areas identified in cognitive processing therapy, or CPT (Resick, Monson, Price, & Chard, 2007), as beliefs that are evident in many areas of life. These cognitive distortions manifest in relation to safety, trust, power and control, self-esteem, and intimacy.

The Avoidance of as Many Stressors in Daily Life as Possible

The avoidance of remembering events from war, as well as the avoidance of as many stressors in daily life as possible, consumes a large portion of veterans' psychic attention and energy. Avoidant behaviors may range from avoiding anxiety-provoking situations—such as not answering the telephone because there is a strong belief that it will be bad news—to avoiding abandonment by not telling or showing a spouse or partner your love because if you do you will be hurt when they die or leave. These behaviors also encompass not taking an active role in raising children—because it is your fault if something bad happens because you failed to protect them—to seeking anonymity in the workplace.

Withdrawal From Relationships and Intimacy

To a large degree, the veteran does not develop the usual network of interpersonal relationships. The veteran keeps social and family contacts to a superficial minimum. Perceptions of being an outsider or being different than others because of one's combat experience play a significant role. Particular core beliefs about veteran versus civilian and beliefs about self as unworthy and others as unsafe or untrustworthy underlie this behavior.

Protection

Veterans feel a need for power and control based on a belief that the more control they exercise the safer their world will be. Veterans with PTSD often invest time and energy into creating a secure home environment to ensure their spouses and children are protected. The more the veteran can demonstrate to his own satisfaction that he has created a safe environment the more in control and therefore less anxious the veteran feels in this regard.

Reaction

The veteran maintains a posture of hypervigilance in order to feel safe and in control. The veteran fears losing control over his environment by becoming complacent. The reactive mode, particularly in crisis, allows the veteran to feel superior and in control of a potentially threatening or dangerous situation. This behavior operates at a more primitive or pre-rational functioning level within the brain that is connected to the basic instinct of survival. It is associated with the fight, flight, or freeze reaction characteristic of the limbic system and the amygdala. This is the area of the brain stimulated during boot camp and matches perfectly to the primitive circumstances of combat. A combat veteran's belief about losing one's edge by letting down one's guard is believed by many in the field to be the one symptom most resistant to nearly all clinical interventions.

LIFE AFTER SEPTEMBER 11, 2001, FOR COMBAT VETERANS

Since 2002, each cohort of geriatric combat veterans at the Brooklyn VA has participated in discussions and psychoeducation sessions on the topic of safety planning in the event of attack. They have participated in various surveys about the impact of September 11 upon their behavior, beliefs about safety, and beliefs about the future. These veterans have been invited to reflect upon changes they may have observed with regard to their subjective experience of PTSD. Thirty veterans per cohort currently participating in treatment at the Brooklyn Campus of NYIIIIC were asked to respond to the following questions:

- Since 2001, has your concern about the threat of attack (weapons or biochemical) increased, decreased, or remained the same?
- Since 2001, has your behavior changed significantly with regard to travel, particularly into New York City, for reasons other than medical or financial?
- Since 2001, have you developed safety and emergency plans with your families and/or friends?
- Since 2001, have you experienced an increase, decrease, or no change in your experience of PTSD symptoms?

The results of this discussion revealed the following:

Increased concerns about safety: 60% of WWII, 50% of Korean War, and 40% of Vietnam veterans indicated a greater concern for safety (U.S. Department of Veterans Affairs [Veterans Affairs], n.d.).

Changes in behavior: 75% of WWII, 75% of Korean War, and 67% of Vietnam veterans reported changes in behavior resulting in a decrease in social activities and travel (Veterans Affairs, n.d.).

Development of a safety plan: 75% of WWII, 75% of Korean War, and 80% of Vietnam veterans reported not developing a safety plan as a precaution in case of attack (Veterans Affairs, n.d.).

Subjective experience of PTSD: 90% of WWII, 80% of Korean War, and 80% of Vietnam veterans reported exacerbation of PTSD symptoms since 2001 (Veterans Affairs, n.d.).

We have continued to provide an annual psychoeducational session and open discussion with each of the cohorts around the issues of safety planning. The beliefs and fears about future acts of war or terrorism are often the content of the group process. The results of a survey conducted in 2009 indicate that a significant number of veterans continue to meet the criteria for chronic and severe PTSD. These results suggest that for the population of geriatric combat veterans diagnosed with chronic and severe PTSD, most of whom were in treatment prior to September 11, there is marginal qualitative change in their beliefs and behaviors. As was stated previously, incremental gains are understood as improvement in this population.

The combat veteran in general may subjectively experience an increase in symptoms of PTSD even after 50 years and participation in therapy (Schnurr, 1994). The veteran, as well as his or her family members and health care provider, may note increased anxiety in the face of the current global situation. This particular population may be more profoundly affected by such changes, which may manifest as an exacerbation of a preexistent condition that may or may not have been diagnosed and treated.

For some within this population, a belief that was either left unspoken or said in hushed tones in the sanctuary of the clinical office has come to haunt them. That belief, born of fear or guilt or shame, is that somehow war has followed them home—it is here now. The inner battle they have lived through personally on a daily basis is matched externally in world events. The enemy within exists externally, and both are beyond their control.

Suppressed feelings of helplessness and powerlessness surface and require attention. These veterans also express specific hopes that civilians will better understand at least some parts of their wartime experiences and treat them with more compassion and less criticism. This desire to be understood and received applies to their own families, many of whom have reacted to the veteran's behavior without fully comprehending its origins or meaning. The desire to be understood and accepted is indisputably fundamental to all human beings, and it is no less true of combat veterans. Finally, many see the present situation as an opportunity to confirm the values they acquired in combat: there are some things worth fighting for and worth the cost of peace of mind. But many, although they endorse this belief, do not rest any easier at night or in their quiet solitary moments. Perhaps they reach backward to the archetype of the warrior in search of the self lost in the depth of this conflict: the self that had to survive and react rather than respond, or the self that found choices limited— each one uglier and more distasteful than the last—but that chose within the limits and lives now in fear of those limits.

As was indicated in the first section, psychosocial rehabilitation offers a context in which to develop strategies to reduce feelings of helplessness, powerlessness, and frustration. Veterans' expressed need to be of service to and involved with military personnel serving in Iraq and Afghanistan has resulted in some providers in mental health clinics encouraging, supporting, or starting such initiatives. These therapeutic activities include packing boxes of needed items for shipment to units or individuals, visiting the wounded in the hospital, and participating in social activities with the wounded through the Wounded Warrior Program.

Another area in which some older veterans participate is mentoring younger veterans as they attempt to confront their trauma, encouraging them to make use of the opportunity for therapy. Other older veterans also help young veterans find their way around the hospital. It doesn't matter whether or not the geriatric veteran has received a warm welcome, a cold reception, or no acknowledgment at all. By and large, they are moving out of their once-insular world and treating this newly returning cohort with sensitivity, dignity, and respect. Ironically, the activities focused on the newest cohort have served to bridge a gap among the differing cohorts of geriatric combat veterans. They have created some unity, which has overcome the competitive and bitter feelings of the past about who were the victors and who were the vanquished.

A number of the existential and spiritual questions raised by these veterans emerge out of the growth and reflections normal to this and the previous stage of the life cycle. For some, these questions are not new but were ever present on the horizon of their consciousness. Often one or more of these questions is related to the early presentation for treatment. These questions, for some, may become submerged in the initial phase of treatment as the worst trauma is confronted and its impact is understood. Over time, as the traumatic material is processed and integrated, these existential or spiritual questions resurface and become the focus of therapy:

- Am I capable of doing good?
- What legacy do I leave?
- What is left for me to do?

- What do I need to repair?
- Will I forgive?
- Was I good enough? Am I good enough?

All these questions are challenging and sometimes anxiety provoking for anyone at any given time. Some of these questions are grounded in false beliefs, irrational cognitions, and misperceptions about the self and are best dealt with using a cognitive behavioral approach. Other questions can be the focus of therapy, pastoral counseling, or spiritual direction relative to the veteran's stated preference. By clarifying which existential/spiritual questions are most significant to the veteran, the provider is better equipped to understand the impact of trauma upon the whole person. Such understanding typically illuminates problematic patterns of behavior and the persistence of irrational thinking confirming unhealthy guilt. These elements often support avoidance and ambivalence in the treatment process. How these questions relate to the veteran's perceptions of the current global crisis and threats of future acts of war or terrorism is crucial to understanding where the veteran is on his or her own journey toward healing and the integration of past combat trauma.

THE USE OF EVIDENCE-BASED PRACTICE (EBP) WITH GERIATRIC COMBAT VETERANS

There are a variety of EBPs that have gained the attention and endorsement of the VA and/or Department of Defense (DOD) for the treatment of PTSD. Among these are cognitive processing therapy (Resick, et al., 2007), prolonged exposure (Foa, Hembree, & Rothauma, 2007), and psychosocial rehabilitation (Foa, Keane, & Friedman, 2000). These CBTs primarily have been used successfully with the younger cohorts of veterans and to date have not been adequately used and studied with WWII and Korean combat veterans. CBT methods, however, whether applied to younger or older combat veterans, require extensive therapist training. Untrained professionals or paraprofessionals should not utilize them.

Psychosocial Rehabilitation Model (PRM)

One of the most successful EBPs that has been used with older veterans is PRM. The model seeks to improve and enhance interpersonal relationships in the context of the veteran's social and familial functioning and incorporates psychodynamic group process. Films are used as catalysts for discussion. This has met with a good degree of success with Korean and WWII populations. Movie therapy involves viewing videos followed by discussion during two to three counseling sessions. The movies are selected to challenge the limitations and prejudices of the defense mechanism of avoidance of beliefs about self, others, and the world. The discussions allow the veteran to use the objective narrative of the video to project an aspect of his or her own questions and unresolved material. Such discussions have resulted in increased insight, reduced avoidance, and a reduction in anxiety. There has been a noticeable enhancement of feelings of self-confidence and cognitions/beliefs about safety and trust with regard to the past that are more adaptive, constructive, and realistic. Other psychosocial rehabilitation activities include (1) education about various resources and concrete services available to this population within the VA and the larger community, (2) enhanced social interaction through the use of social activities outside the VA, (3) the support and assistance of veteran-led initiatives related to care for troops and the wounded, and (4) monthly multifamily support groups.

SUMMARY

Presently, there is a very sparse body of literature that discusses the use of EBP, specifically CBT, with the geriatric veteran population. With the trend in the VA to make CBT available to all veterans who either request it or are assessed as potential candidates for this therapy, it is likely that the body of research literature on this population will expand. As discussed earlier, asking basic questions of older combat veterans with chronic and severe PTSD suggests that while some of our therapeutic efforts have been helpful, the overall outcome has not produced an appreciable reduction in symptom expression for this population. Given the therapeutic success with younger veterans, it is expected that CBT would result in a reduction in symptoms in the older veteran population with chronic and severe PTSD. The philosophy and protocols of this type of intervention may help the older veteran understand his or her reactions to the threat of global and local terrorism, war, and biochemical attacks. In this process, perhaps the older veteran will discover his or her inner strength and resources hidden by fear. It is worth repeating that CBT requires extensive therapist training. Untrained professionals or paraprofessionals should not utilize CBT.

REFERENCES

American Psychiatric Association. (2000). *Diagnostic and statistical manual of mental disorders* (text revision). Washington, DC: Author.

Blake, D., Weathers, F., Nagy, L. M., Kaloupek, D. G., Charney, D. S., Gusman, F. D., et al. (1998, July). *Clinician administered PTSD scale for DSM-IV* (Rev.). Boston: National Center for PTSD, Behavioral Science Division.

Bryce, I. (Producer), & Spielberg, S. (Director). (1989). *Saving Private Ryan* [Motion picture]. United States: DreamWorks.

Engdahl, B., & Eberly, R. (1994). Assessing PTSD among veterans exposed to war trauma 40–50 years ago. *NCP Clinical Quarterly, 4,* 13–14.

Erickson, E. (1980). *Identity and the life cycle.* New York: Norton.

Figley, C. (1985). *Trauma and its wake: Stress disorders among Vietnam Veterans: Vol.1.* New York: Brunner/Mazel.

Foa, E. B., Keane, T. M., & Friedman, M. J. (2000). *Effective treatments for PTSD.* New York: Guilford Press.

Foa, E. B., Hembree, E. A., & Rothauma, B. O. (2007). *Prolonged exposure therapy for PTSD.* New York: Oxford University Press.

Fowler, J. (1981). *Stages of faith: The psychology of human development and the quest for the meaning of life.* New York: Harper.

Friedman, M. J., Keane, T. M., & Resick, P. A. (Eds.). (2007). *Handbook of PTSD science and practice.* New York: Guilford Press.

Hyams, K. C., & Wignall, R. (1996). War syndromes and their evaluation: From the U.S. Civil War to the Persian Gulf War. *Annals of Internal Medicine, 125,* 398–405.

Izzo, J. (n.d.). *Values and character traits in the geriatric combat veteran population.* Grand rounds presented at the Brooklyn Campus of the NYHHC, VA Medical Center, Brooklyn, New York.

Nussbaum, M. C. (2007). *Upheavals of thought, the intelligence of emotions.* New York: Cambridge University Press.

Resick, P. A., Monson, C. M., Price, J. L., & Chard, K. M. (2007) *Cognitive processing therapy, veteran/military version trainer's manual.* Washington, DC: Department of Veterans Affairs.

Schnurr, P. P. (1994, Winter). The long-term course of PTSD. *NCP Clinical Quarterly,* 15–16.

Tick, E. (2005). *War and the soul: Healing our nations veterans.* Wheaton, IL: Quest Books.

U.S. Department of Veterans Affairs, Office of Public Affairs. (2008). *America's wars.* Retrieved November 9, 2008, from http://www.va.gov

U.S. Department of Veterans Affairs. (n.d.). [Survey of veterans in treatment at the Brooklyn Campus of the NYHHC, VA Medical Center, Brooklyn, New York, regarding impact of September 11, 2001 events.] Unpublished raw data.

Weathers, F. W., Husk, A. J. A., & Keane, T. M. (1991). *PCL-M.* Boston: National Center for PTSD, Behavioral Sciences Division.

Weathers, F. W., Litz, B. T., Herman, D. S., Huska, J. A., & Keane, T. M. (1993, October). *The PTDS Checklist (PCL): Reliability, validity, and diagnostic utility.* Paper presented at the 9th Annual Meeting of International Society for Traumatic Stress Studies, San Antonio, Texas.

Zanuck, D. (Producer), & Johnson, N. (Director). (1956). *The man in the grey flannel suit* [Motion picture]. United States: 20th Century Fox.

17 Alzheimer's Disease and Related Disorders

JED A. LEVINE AND BETH A. KALLMYER

After a harrowing 8 hours in the car leaving Galveston prior to Hurricane Rita, Brenda Hernandez was at a loss. Her 85-year-old father with Alzheimer's disease was extremely agitated and kept repeating, "Take me home, I want to go home." They arrived at an emergency shelter. It was loud and crowded. Brenda knew that the shelter environment was likely to further upset her father. She only had 2 days worth of her father's medication and was running low on his incontinence products. She kept thinking to herself, *I wasn't prepared for this.*

OVERVIEW OF ALZHEIMER'S DISEASE AND DEMENTIA

Dementia is the leading cause of cognitive impairment in older Americans today.

It is a clinical syndrome of loss or decline in memory . . . and (decline) in at least one of the following cognitive abilities:

1. Ability to generate coherent speech and understand spoken or written language;
2. Ability to recognize or identify objects, assuming intact sensory function;

3. Ability to execute motor activities, assuming intact motor abilities, sensory function and comprehension of the required task; and
4. Ability to think abstractly, make sound judgments and plan and carry out complex tasks.

The decline in cognitive abilities must be severe enough to interfere with daily life. (Alzheimer's Association, 2008)

There are a number of common causes of dementia, including Alzheimer's disease (AD), vascular dementia, Lewy-Body disease, frontotemporal lobe dementia, Parkinson's disease, mixed dementia, and others. Each has its own unique pattern of symptoms and distinguishing biological markers.

Alzheimer's disease is the most common cause of dementia and can last anywhere from 3 to more than 20 years; the average length of illness from onset of symptoms to death is 8 to 10 years. Although people with Alzheimer's and related disorders experience the disease idiosyncratically, there are predictable patterns of loss, beginning with mild forgetfulness and confusion leading to increasing difficulty managing usual activities of personal care, financial management, verbal and written communication, and social and occupational functions and ending in total dependence on someone else for all activities of daily living. The disease is usually described in four stages: early, middle, late, and terminal.

The statistics and projections regarding the prevalence and incidence of Alzheimer's disease in the United States and the world are alarming. According to the 2009 *Alzheimer's Disease Facts and Figures* (Alzheimer's Association, 2009), every 70 seconds someone in the United States will develop Alzheimer's disease. There are an estimated 5.3 million Americans who have the disease, and that number is projected to increase to approximately 16 million by mid-century. Age is the greatest risk factor; 50% of those aged 85 years and over have Alzheimer's or a related dementia. Ten million Baby Boomers are expected to develop AD, with an additional 4 million developing other dementias, if the progression of the disease is not stopped.

Internationally, the numbers are significant and growing. According to Alzheimer's Disease International (2009), there are an estimated 30 million people in the world affected by the disease; that number is expected to grow to 100 million by 2050. India and China, with their large populations, are facing a sizable increase in the numbers of persons with AD.

There is no medical cure for AD at this time. There are four drugs approved by the Federal Drug Administration (FDA) for the treatment of

Alzheimer's disease: donepezil, rivastigmine, galantamine, and memantine. However, the treatments are modestly effective at best. Researchers hope to develop a disease-modifying drug or a method of effectively preventing or delaying the onset of the disease. If the onset of the disease can be delayed by 5 years, its incidence can be cut in half.

NUMBERS AFFECTED IN RECENT U.S. DISASTERS

It is difficult to determine an exact number of persons diagnosed with Alzheimer's or a related dementia who were affected by the September 11, 2001, terrorist attacks, Hurricane Katrina, or other major storms, floods, or disasters in the United States. "It is generally believed that in September 2001 there were 6,300 people living in the immediate area and nearly 19,000 living within a three-block radius of the World Trade Center. However, [the] impact [of the event] was not confined to lower Manhattan" (Jellinek & Willig, 2007–2008, p. 42). Death statistics following Hurricane Katrina illustrate how older persons are disproportionately impacted by disasters. Of confirmed fatalities resulting from Hurricane Katrina, over 70% were aged 60 or older (Rothman & Brown, 2007–2008, p.16).

The decline in cognitive function puts the person with dementia at greater risk in an emergency or disaster. It is imperative that as we discuss the needs of the person with dementia in an emergency situation, we factor in the stage of illness, the individual's residual strengths, and his or her need for support or assistance. Someone in the very early stage of the disease has very different abilities than someone in the middle or late stage. Regardless of the stage of the disease, preserving or enhancing good quality of life and promoting the choice and choosing process in dementia should be the goal of care even during a disaster, when the crisis limits choices. In fact, it has been demonstrated that people with dementia can be encouraged to make choices in all activities of daily living (Banerjee, Willis, Graham, & Gurland, 2009).

THE ALZHEIMER'S ASSOCIATION'S RESPONSE TO THE SEPTEMBER 11, 2001, TERRORIST ATTACKS

The New York City chapter of the Alzheimer's Association helped families who were both directly and indirectly affected by the events of September 11, 2001. Assistance was provided to survivors who lost primary and/ or secondary caregivers and helped relocate older couples who lived near the towers. The association also provided counseling, emotional support, and coordination with community resources. Several of the association staff volunteered to work with Project Liberty[1] or help out in area nursing homes in the immediate days following the terrorist attacks since other staff were unable to come to work when nursing home staff needed a break.

There was increased fear, worry, grief, anger, and generalized anxiety expressed in telephone calls to a 24-hour help line, in support groups, and in education meetings. Families reported that their relatives with dementia exhibited increased confusion and agitation, especially if they were watching the constant television coverage of the disaster. AD patients in the middle stage often have difficulty distinguishing reality from TV. With each viewing, family members reported that their AD relatives experienced the planes hitting the towers as if for the first time. Families were encouraged to limit exposure to TV or radio coverage and to reassure their relatives with dementia that they were safe.

Families were urged to use their natural support systems and the association's support groups to talk about their feelings and to maintain daily routines as much as possible. Others were encouraged to get counseling if needed. Many already-stressed caregivers in New York City expressed that with the added shock of September 11, they were even more overwhelmed than when they had first received their relative's diagnosis of AD or had begun dealing with their relative with AD. They were unsure where they would find the stamina and reserve to continue in their roles as caregivers and cope with their own fears, grief, and profound sadness brought on by the disaster.

DISASTER PREPAREDNESS FOR PERSONS WITH DEMENTIA (PWDS) AND FAMILY CAREGIVERS

Preparing for a disaster is one of the most important things a caregiver can do. A few simple steps may help the person with dementia endure the disaster and may mitigate unnecessary anxiety and distress. Assembling an emergency bag or kit including extra medications, clothes, water, favorite food or snacks, and small items that are comforting to the person with dementia is easy to do, and the kit can be stored in a closet ready for any emergency. If an evacuation is necessary, being aware of the person's risk for agitation and wandering will help the caregiver provide needed support. Finally, asking others for help and informing them about the

Table 17.1

DISASTER PREPAREDNESS RECOMMENDATIONS FOR OLDER PERSONS WITH DEMENTIA AND THEIR CAREGIVERS

DISASTER PREPAREDNESS GOAL	RECOMMENDATION
Advance Preparations	■ If your loved one lives in a residential facility, find out about its disaster and evacuation plans. Ask if you will be responsible for evacuating your loved one. ■ Whether your loved one lives with you, or you are a long-distance caregiver, make sure evacuation plans include his or her specific needs. Check your local Alzheimer's Association and other organizations that provide services for the elderly to see if help is available. ■ Prepare an *Emergency Kit* (See the following for suggestions). ■ Enroll in MedicAlert® + Alzheimer's Association Safe Return®, a 24-hour nationwide emergency response service for individuals with Alzheimer's or related dementia who wander or who have a medical emergency.
If You Know a Disaster Is About to Occur	■ Get yourself and the person with Alzheimer's to a safe place. ■ If the need to evacuate is likely, do not delay. Try to leave as early as possible to minimize long delays in heavy traffic. ■ Alert others (family, friends, medical personnel) that you are changing locations, and give them your contact information. Contact them regularly as you move. ■ Be sure there are people other than the primary caregiver who have copies of the demented person's medical history, medications, physician information, and family contacts. ■ Purchase extra medications. ■ If your loved one uses oxygen, be sure to obtain portable tanks. ■ Get more information on disaster preparedness from the National Hurricane Center.

(*Continued*)

Table 17.1

DISASTER PREPAREDNESS RECOMMENDATIONS FOR OLDER PERSONS WITH DEMENTIA AND THEIR CAREGIVERS (*Continued*)

DISASTER PREPAREDNESS GOAL	RECOMMENDATION
Emergency Kit	Consider preparing an emergency kit in advance. Keep it in a watertight container and store it in an easily accessible location.
	■ Easy on/off clothes (a couple of sets)
	■ Supplies of medication (or minimally, a list of medications with dosages)
	■ Velcro shoes/sneakers
	■ A spare pair of eyeglasses
	■ If the need to evacuate is likely, do not delay. Try to leave as early as possible to minimize long delays in heavy traffic.
	■ Incontinence products
	■ Extra identification items for the person, such as an ID bracelet and clothing tags
	■ Copies of legal documents, such as a power of attorney
	■ Copies of medical documents that indicate the individual's condition and current medications
	■ Copies of insurance and Social Security cards
	■ Use waterproof bags to hold medications and documents
During an Evacuation	People with dementia are especially vulnerable to chaos and emotional trauma. They have a limited ability to understand what is happening, and they may forget what they have been told about the disaster. Be alert to potential reactions that may result from changes in routine, traveling, or new environments.
	■ When appropriate, inform others (hotel or shelter staff, family members, airline attendants) that your loved one has dementia and may not understand what is happening.
	■ Do not leave the person alone. It only takes a few minutes to wander away and get lost.
	■ Changes in routine, traveling, and new environments can cause: 　• Agitation 　• Wandering 　• Increase in behavioral symptoms, including hallucinations, delusions and sleep disturbance

	■ Do your best to remain calm. The person with dementia will respond to the emotional tone you set.
Tips for Preventing Agitation	Reassure the person. Hold hands or put your arm on his or her shoulder. Say things are going to be fine.

■ Find outlets for anxious energy. Take a walk together or engage the person in simple tasks.
■ Redirect the person's attention if he or she becomes upset.
■ Move the person to a safer or quieter place, if possible. Limit stimulation.
■ Make sure the person takes medications as scheduled.
■ Try to schedule regular meals and maintain a regular sleep schedule.
■ Avoid elaborate or detailed explanations. Provide information using concrete terms. Follow brief explanations with reassurance.
■ Be prepared to provide additional assistance with all activities of daily living.
■ Pay attention to cues that the person may be overwhelmed (fidgeting, pacing).
■ Remind the person that he or she is in the right place.

Helpful Hints During an Episode of Agitation

■ Approach the person from the front and use his or her name.
■ Use calm, positive statements and a patient, low-pitched voice. Reassure.
■ Respond to the emotions being expressed rather than the content of the words. For example, say, "You're frightened and want to go home. It's okay. I'm right here with you."
■ Don't argue with the person or try to correct. Instead, affirm his or her experience, reassure, and try to divert attention. For example, "The noise in this shelter is frightening. Let's see if we can find a quieter spot. Let's look at your photo book together."

(Continued)

Table 17.1

DISASTER PREPAREDNESS RECOMMENDATIONS FOR OLDER PERSONS WITH DEMENTIA AND THEIR CAREGIVERS (*Continued*)	
DISASTER PREPAREDNESS GOAL	**RECOMMENDATION**
Take Care of Yourself	■ Take care of yourself by finding a good listener to hear your thoughts and feelings about the event. ■ Find moments to breathe, meditate, and reflect.

Disaster Preparedness. Updated November 2007. Printed with permission. Copyright © 2007 Alzheimer's Association. All rights reserved. This is an official publication of the Alzheimer's Association but may be distributed by unaffiliated organizations and individuals. Such distribution does not constitute an endorsement of these parties or their activities by the Alzheimer's Association. 1-800-272-3900/www.alz.org

situation is very important. Table 17.1 outlines some suggestions for preparedness from the Alzheimer's Association.

Disaster Preparedness From the Caregiver's Perspective

Most discussions related to dementia usually mention the caregiving dyad or family system providing care. Usually there is one primary caregiver, often a spouse or adult child and most often a daughter. Because age is the greatest risk factor for AD, the spousal caregiver is often an older person as well and may be coping with the medical, sensory, and psychological challenges of aging. However, it is important to keep in mind that 10% of all persons with Alzheimer's or related disorders are under the age of 65, usually in their 40s, 50s, or early 60s (Alzheimer's Association, 2005). This form of the disease is referred to as *younger-onset Alzheimer's.*

Under the best circumstances, caregivers experience increased rates of stress and depression and require more doctors' visits. The duration of the caregiving, combined with the excruciating complexity of the tasks required to manage the care of a relative with AD, create high levels of caregiver burden. Frequently, this caregiver burden manifests as an emotional response and may involve a host of feelings including grief, rage, and profound sadness associated with witnessing the decline of the loved one. All of these factors contribute to the stress of caregiving, which results in a caregiver at greater risk for not being as resilient when facing a disaster situation.

Tips and suggestions for preparing for a disaster are helpful for planning. However, the majority of Alzheimer's caregivers are limited in their ability to develop disaster plans by a shortage of time and energy. Many caregivers find it difficult to plan for usual care in a rational and thoughtful way. They are burdened by the demands of caregiving, which compete with career and other family responsibilities. It is important for caregivers to get the support and assistance that can help normalize the range of their emotional responses. Programs that allow caregivers to share their feelings in an accepting environment lessen the likelihood that those feelings will get acted out in ways that are not constructive or result in poor care.

For families caring for those with dementia who live in areas at high risk for natural disasters, it is especially important to plan ahead, to be familiar with evacuation routes, to have a go-bag/emergency kit, and to take other steps as outlined earlier. The consequences of not planning for a disaster if you live in an earthquake-, flood-, hurricane-, or tornado-prone area can be extremely serious. The result may be injury or loss of life, or at very minimum significant disruption for the person with dementia and his or her caregiver. Information in Table 17.1 may provide some guidance for planning ahead.

Understanding the Reactions of Persons With Dementia During Disasters

Disasters and emergency situations are difficult for anyone. The sheer unpredictability of a disaster requires problem-solving skills, flexibility, and an understanding that many things are out of one's control. Because Alzheimer's disease affects all levels of cognition, including memory, judgment, orientation, and abstract thinking, the ability of the person with dementia to understand and cope with a disaster situation is greatly challenged. Complicating matters further, older people with Alzheimer's disease are at greater risk for restriction, abuse, neglect, and mistreatment, especially at times of crisis (Fulmer & Gurland, 1996).

Imagine being faced with an evacuation due to an impending hurricane. There are many things to consider, including gathering your necessary belongings, deciding where to go, determining how to get there, and planning for safety. Now imagine that you have dementia. You might forget from moment to moment what is happening, but everyone around you is busy making preparations. Other people are likely to be anxious, worried, and even panicked, but you don't understand why. Obviously this would be extremely confusing. While any type of disaster causes unavoidable disruption, careful preparation and preparedness along with a well-thought-out response to this vulnerable population can mitigate the devastating effects.

Reactions from a person with dementia are often unpredictable; in the case of a disaster, these reactions are even harder to foresee. Understanding the types of reactions that may occur will help families and caregivers be prepared and respond appropriately. The person with dementia most likely has a limited ability to understand what is happening or what has been communicated and may have difficulty negotiating new surroundings or a change in schedule. Not understanding what is going on can lead to adverse reactions or behaviors.

Wandering

Case Study

Jane Glavin is staying at a shelter after being evacuated from her nursing home in Biloxi, Mississippi. She and the other residents of the Alzheimer's unit have been assigned to cots in a high school gymnasium approximately 150 miles from their home. The shelter is staffed with Red Cross volunteers who are making sure that the 500 people staying at the shelter are checked in, have their meals, and are assigned cots. The nursing home has two staff members at the shelter making sure that the 12 residents are well taken care of. While the staff is busy assisting other residents, Jane decides to use the restroom. Unsure of where the restroom is or who to ask for directions, Jane eventually wanders out the front door of the high school. Two Red Cross volunteers see her exit the building but are unaware of her dementia and therefore have no reason to stop her. About 30 minutes later, the nursing home staff approach the volunteer station to ask if they have seen one of their residents, Jane, as they cannot find her. After learning that Jane was seen leaving the building, they alert the heavily burdened police to the fact that there is a missing person. After 2 hours, Jane is spotted walking down the exit ramp of a busy highway. She is subsequently safely returned to the shelter.

Wandering is one of the most dangerous behaviors for the person with dementia. It often arises as the result of confusion. The aimless and purposeful motor activity that results from wandering causes social problems such as getting lost, leaving a safe environment, or intruding in inappropriate places. Approximately 46% of people who wander will face serious injury or death if not found within 24 hours (Koester & Stooks-bury, 1995). In normal circumstances, up to 60% of people with dementia will wander at some point during the course of the disease. In disaster situations, the risk for wandering may be even greater due to the change in environment and the person's inability to negotiate new surroundings.

In the midst of a disaster, wandering can be even more problematic as the community resources commonly employed to find wanderers are already strained. Additionally, families and caregivers may be unfamiliar with the area, or it may be unsafe for them to conduct a thorough search. The best way to prevent wandering is to avoid leaving the person with dementia alone. Assigning someone to stay with the person at all times can be difficult, but the consequences of not doing so can be tragic. For example, during the evacuation and relocation of a family to a shelter, it is important to make sure the person with dementia is always accompanied to the restroom or other areas to prevent the individual from wandering or getting lost. Alerting shelter staff to the situation and asking for assistance when needed is helpful. Even if the person with dementia evacuates to the home of a familiar family member or friend, it is important to be aware of the risk of wandering and to persistently and cautiously monitor the person. Furthermore, caregivers can be on the lookout for pre-wandering signals including pacing, talking about going home, and other agitated behaviors.

Families or caregivers may want to consider enrolling the person with dementia into the MedicAlert®+ Alzheimer's Association Safe Return Program®, a 24-hour emergency response service for persons with dementia.[2] One component of the program involves inscribing on a bracelet or necklace a personal identification number along with a toll-free number where help can be accessed 24 hours a day. If the person wanders and becomes lost, pertinent contact and relevant medical information is available immediately from the emergency response center of the MedicAlert + Safe Return Program. Calling the emergency response center also activates coordination with local law enforcement and provides support and resources for the family. This type of program provides the peace of mind that reassures caregivers help will be available should the person with dementia get lost.

Catastrophic Reactions

Another type of response from a person with dementia is referred to as a catastrophic reaction. This can occur when a situation overloads the cognitive ability of the person with dementia and results in an exaggerated response such as yelling, making unreasonable accusations, or becoming overly agitated and emotional. While catastrophic reactions can also occur during the course of everyday life, the added stress of a disaster or emergency situation can further impair the ability of the person with dementia to handle frustration. Caregivers can anticipate and possibly reduce the frequency and intensity of these catastrophic reactions by becoming aware of the potential triggers that might precede these reactions, such as overstimulation, pain, hunger, thirst, fear, or an inability to express thoughts or feelings. If a person with dementia experiences a catastrophic reaction, it is essential for the caregiver to remain as calm as possible. The person with dementia will pick up on emotional cues. Speak slowly using short, simple sentences. Validate the person's feelings or emotional state by saying something such as, "I know it is loud in here and you are scared, but I am going to stay with you and keep you safe." Provide continued reassurance that the person is safe and that you will stay with him or her. Try to move the person to a quieter environment. Attempt to redirect the person's attention and, if possible, get the person involved in something they enjoy.

Lingering Effects

Another aspect to be aware of is that the effects of the disaster may linger for the person with dementia. The implications of trauma reactions on people with dementia are not completely understood and vary from person to person, but cases have been documented where PTSD symptoms have been seen during and following a traumatic event. Experiencing the trauma of a disaster can also trigger reactions from past traumatic experiences. Dementia may preclude the person's ability to access coping skills, which can lead to ongoing, adverse emotional and physiological reactions similar to posttraumatic stress symptoms (Van Achterberg, Rohrbaugh, & Southwich, 2001). These types of reactions can be effectively managed using a variety of strategies that include orienting individuals to the present, reassuring them they are safe, and engaging them in distracting and relaxing activities (Flannery, 2002).

CONSIDERATIONS FOR PERSONS WITH EARLY-STAGE DEMENTIA

Another special concern during disasters involves people in the early stages of Alzheimer's disease or dementia. Family and nonfamily caregivers may not expect a person in the early stages of dementia to exhibit adverse reactions because the person's functioning in everyday life has not yet become significantly impaired. However, the impact of a disaster can bring about unexpected challenges for a person with early-stage AD. In order to avoid being caught unaware, families and caregivers need to be sensitive to possible reactions and institute safeguards, including checking in frequently to ensure the person understands the situation, keeping close watch, orienting the person to new surroundings, and staying alert to possible indicators the person is becoming upset or agitated.

Supportive Responses

Overall, caregivers can help the person with dementia manage reactions through close attention and awareness of the person, utilizing knowledge about what calms the person, understanding the potential causes of adverse reactions, and knowing how to respond. Another helpful technique is to establish a consistent schedule as soon as possible. Knowing what to expect helps people with dementia feel safe. During the course of an emergency or disaster this may be difficult to achieve, but it is important to institute a schedule with structured activities as soon as possible. If it isn't possible to establish a consistent schedule, try to involve the person in activities suitable to his or her abilities. Even after things seemingly return to normal, continue looking for episodes of confusion or agitation. Caregivers may feel relief that the disaster has passed, but the person with dementia may experience difficulty readjusting even to what was previously normal.

CONSIDERATIONS FOR RESIDENTIAL FACILITIES

Disaster planning and response in residential facilities poses additional challenges for residential care administrators and staff. While licensed skilled-care facilities are required to have disaster plans in place, the lessons of hurricanes Katrina and Rita highlighted the importance of ensuring the disaster plans are practical, up-to-date, and not merely documents gathering dust on a shelf. Coordinating the plan with local and state disaster management agencies and other nearby facilities is essential. If all the facilities in one area are planning on using a particular bus service for evacuation, administrators need to know there are enough buses. Additionally, ensuring all the facility's staff are trained and know their roles in a disaster or emergency is imperative.

Sixty-nine percent of residents in long-term-care facilities have Alzheimer's or some other form of dementia. Further, only 5.2% of all nursing home beds are part of special dementia care units (Alzheimer's Association, 2008). This means that even if a facility does not specifically cater to persons with dementia, it is essential that they consider this population in their disaster plans.

Because administrators and staff are responsible for the safety and well-being of large groups of people during a disaster, it is even more important that all staff, including nonclinical care staff, have some knowledge and awareness of how to work with people with dementia. It may be that the facility needs to call on office, housekeeping, or janitorial staff for help during an emergency. Providing basic training on Alzheimer's disease and other dementias to all staff can help prepare the facility for a disaster and can lessen the impact of the disaster for residents with dementia. Basic training consists of recognizing dementia, the stages of dementia, appropriate communication and interventions, and managing inappropriate responses. Table 17.1 provides some advance-planning recommendations that can be helpful in advance of a disaster.

Person-Centered Care

An important aspect of quality of life as well as quality care for the person with dementia is called *person-centered care*. This means getting to know the residents' personalities along with their preferences and ways of interacting. It also means fostering the choice and choosing process in the caregiving setting to promote quality of life. Findings suggest that person-centered care enhances quality of life particularly when the choice and choosing process is incorporated in care (Gurland & Gurland, 2008a, 2008b; Gurland, Gurland, Mitty, & Toner, 2009). Furthermore, quality of life may be facilitated particularly well for those with Alzheimer's disease through the use of reliable and valid quality of life assessment tools (Barrett & Gurland, 2001; Barrett, Gurland, Chin, & Rattau, 2000; Gurland & Katz, 2006).

During a disaster, nonclinical care staff may not know personally the residents who are assigned to their care; the development of a personal information form for each resident can be helpful. This form can be placed in an easily accessible place inside a closet door or attached to a folder in the resident's room. A nonclinical care staff member can quickly read the form and gain insight into how best to work with the particular resident. Information on the form could include: what the resident likes to be called, cultural background, names of family members and friends, what upsets them, what calms them, and typical patterns of behavior, in addition to regular drinking and eating habits. This type of knowledge can be pivotal in preventing or managing agitated behaviors.

Nutrition Concerns

During a disaster, it can be very difficult to maintain a regular drinking and eating schedule. However, it is important to be aware that residents with dementia may not be able to ask for food or drink and may need cueing or reminders. Being hungry or thirsty can add stress to a situation for anyone, but for a person with dementia, the added stress can precipitate an adverse or catastrophic reaction.

Challenging Behaviors

Specific training in the management of challenging behaviors that may arise in reaction to a disaster should be included as part of the overall training of all residential care staff. For instance, regular cueing to the environment can help residents feel safer. Making sure they know how to find the restroom, dining room, or who to ask for help is important. Reminders about what has happened, such as, "We had to move because there was a fire and we are going to stay here for awhile," may be necessary. Establishing a consistent routine as soon as possible is also helpful. If the facility is being evacuated, try to have each resident bring a small personal or comforting item with him or her. Finally, engaging the residents in structured activities, including exercise when appropriate, can lesson their anxiety.

Identifying Residents

During the chaos of a disaster, residents with dementia may wander off, get lost, or become otherwise separated from the group. Therefore, it is essential that facilities establish a method to identify residents who may be unable to provide relevant personal information, including their name, names of family members, and critical medical conditions.

There are several ways to identify residents. Some facilities utilize plastic pouches that hold information sheets about the resident. These pouches can be pinned directly to the resident's clothing in the event of an emergency. The Alzheimer's Association MedicAlert + Safe Return program, mentioned earlier, is a jewelry identification that the resident always wears and that will be with the older person during an emergency. If communication is available, one call to a 24-hour response center can provide all necessary information about the resident. There are also electronic tools, such as USB drives that can be plugged into a computer once a resident arrives at a new location, that can assist a facility in identifying residents and accessing medical information.

Communicating With Residents' Families

The family members and caregivers of residents should be educated about the facility's disaster plans. For example, if families know how the facility will handle an emergency or disaster, as well as the conditions under which evacuations will occur and where the facility plans to evacuate, they will be able to respond accordingly. This can help avoid unnecessary confusion and panic for family members and caregivers during and immediately after a disaster.

CONSIDERATIONS FOR FIRST RESPONDERS

The term *first responder* refers to a variety of groups including law-enforcement agencies, fire departments, emergency medical technicians, and disaster response agencies. Each of these groups play different roles during a disaster, and all are trained to work with individuals who are emotionally fragile, scared, and even panicked. They are trained to work quickly, often with lives at stake. However, persons with dementia may pose additional challenges for first responders because cognitively impaired persons may not understand what is happening or realize that the first responders are there to help. Catastrophic reactions or other agitated behaviors may impede the work of the first responders. A basic understanding of dementia and some simple communication tips can help first responders react quickly and effectively move the person with dementia to safety.

Tips for Law Enforcement, Fire Departments, and Emergency Medical Technicians

In disaster situations, the top priority is saving lives and preventing injuries by mobilizing people and resources. A person with dementia may be unable to understand directions or process information. Furthermore, they are especially sensitive to trauma; can be easily agitated, frustrated, or overwhelmed; and can be prone to wander or hide. These types of behaviors will affect the ability of first responders to do their job.

A normal response to someone not following directions during a disaster is to use logic to explain the situation. If the person with dementia does not appear to understand the situation, this type of communication may lead to further frustration and agitation. Instead, the first responder should explain that he or she is there to help. Speak slowly, calmly, and directly to the person while maintaining eye contact. Keep communication simple, and be aware that information may need to be repeated or that the person may need more time to process the information. During a disaster situation, it may not seem wise to slow things down. However, when possible, taking extra time to communicate with a demented person may help avoid having to use physical force or restraints and in the end will likely save time.

Evacuations are generally chaotic. First responders are often responsible for determining where people will go and how they get there. It is essential for first responders to do whatever is necessary and possible to avoid separating persons with dementia from their family members or caregivers. Even in the earlier stages of the disease, persons with dementia may become disoriented and unable to cope on their own. If it becomes necessary to separate a person with dementia from his or her caregiver due to emergency or medical situations, the responders should make sure that the person with dementia has on his or her person identifying and contact information and that family members are told where the person with dementia is being taken.

Tips for Staff of Disaster Response Agencies

One of the roles of disaster response agencies during an emergency or disaster is to provide assistance to those affected by the disaster. Often this assistance is in the form of providing and maintaining emergency shelters where evacuated or relocated individuals live until they can return home. While there are shelters designed for people with special needs and disabilities, it is not always possible for evacuees to get to those shelters. Shelters can often appear chaotic, loud, and overwhelming, even for a person without cognitive challenges. For a person with dementia, a shelter environment is likely to be frightening, which can lead to episodes of challenging behaviors.

Understanding that persons with dementia may not have the cognitive skills to understand what is being communicated or what is happening around them is crucial. It is important for disaster response staff and volunteers to understand effective ways to communicate with persons with dementia in order to avoid unnecessary disruption. Use simple language when communicating instructions. Allow extra time for the person with dementia to process the information, and be ready to repeat information slowly. People with dementia may not understand instructions given to a group, so it may be necessary to provide one-on-one instruction. Agitated persons with dementia should be moved to a quiet space as soon as possible. Staff should be aware that television broadcasts, in particular repeated coverage of the disaster, can overload the coping skills of the person with dementia. Limiting access to that type of television viewing is highly recommended.

Being in a new or chaotic environment creates a high risk for a person with dementia to wander or get lost. It is extremely important that a person with dementia is not left alone even to go to the restroom or dining area. It may be that the person's family member or caregiver needs to attend to urgent personal business or meet with FEMA representatives. Even in these situations, leaving a person unattended can lead to agitation and wandering. When possible, help the caregiver make arrangements so that the person with dementia is not left alone.

NOTES

1. Project Liberty was created in 2001 to provide supportive crisis counseling to individuals and groups affected by the World Trade Center disaster in New York City and 10 surrounding counties.

2. Information about how to enroll is available at http://www.alz.org.

REFERENCES

Alzheimer's Association. (2005). *Early-onset Alzheimer's: I'm too young to have Alzheimer's disease* [Brochure]. Chicago: Author.

Alzheimer's Association. (2008). *2008 Alzheimer's disease facts and figures*. Chicago: Author.

Alzheimer's Association. (2009). *2009 Alzheimer's disease facts and figures*. Chicago: Author.

Alzheimer's Disease International. (2009, September 18). *Statistics*. Retrieved June 19, 2009, from http://www.alz.co.uk/research/statistics.html

Banerjee, S., Willis, R., Graham, N., & Gurland, B. J. (2009). The Stroud/ADL Dementia Quality Framework: A cross-national population-level framework for assessing the quality of life impacts of services and policies for people with dementia and their family carers. *International Journal of Geriatric Psychiatry, 25,* 26–32.

Barrett, V. W., & Gurland, B. J. (2001). A method for advancing quality of life in home care. *Home Health Care Management and Practice, 13*(4), 312–321.

Barrett, V. W., Gurland, B. J., Chin, J., & Ratau, A. (2000). The QoL-100: A new instrument for measuring quality of life. Preliminary utilities. *Journal of Nursing Measurement, 20,* 111–121.

Flannery, R. B. (2002). Addressing psychological trauma in dementia sufferers. *American Journal of Alzheimer's Disease and Other Dementias, 17*(5), 281–285.

Fulmer, T., & Gurland, B. (1996). Restriction as elder mistreatment: Differences between caregiver and elder perceptions. *Journal of Mental Health and Aging, 2*(2), 89–99.

Gurland, B. J., & Gurland, R. V. (2008a). The choices, choosing model of quality of life: Description and rationale. *International Journal of Geriatric Psychiatry, 24,* 90–95.

Gurland, B. J., & Gurland, R. V. (2008b). The choices, choosing model of quality of life: Linkages to a science base. *International Journal of Geriatric Psychiatry, 24,* 84–89.

Gurland, B. J., Gurland, R. V., Mitty, E., & Toner, J. A. (2009). The choices, choosing model of quality of life: Clinical evaluation and intervention. *Journal of Interprofessional Care, 23*(2), 110–120.

Gurland, B., & Katz, S. (2006). Quality of life in Alzheimer's and related dementias. In H. Katschnig, H. Freeman, & N. Sartorius (Eds.), *Quality of life in mental disorders* (2nd ed., pp. 179–198). New York: John Wiley & Sons.

Jellinek, I., & Willig, J. (2007–2008). When a terrorist attacks: September 11 and the impact on older adults in New York City. *Generations, 31*(4), 42–46.

Koester, R. J., & Stooksbury, D. E. (1995). Behavioral profile of possible Alzheimer's disease patients in Virginia search and rescue incidents. *Wilderness and Environmental Medicine, 6*(1), 34–43.

Rothman, M., & Brown, L. (2007–2008). The vulnerable geriatric casualty: Medical needs of frail older adults during disasters. *Generations, 31*(4), 16–20.

Van Achterberg, M. E., Rohrbaugh, R. M., & Southwich, S. M. (2001). Emergence of PTSD in trauma survivors with dementia. *Journal of Clinical Psychiatry, 62*(3), 206–207.

18 Disaster Related Elder Mistreatment (DREM)

IAN PORTELLI AND TERRY FULMER

DEFINITION AND TYPOLOGY OF DREM

Disasters, both natural and man-made, are tumultuous by their very nature and affect all people regardless of race, age, or class. However, the older population is particularly vulnerable during these times. During Hurricane Katrina in Louisiana, 64% of all fatalities were people over the age of 65, with 49% over age 75 (Brunkard, Namulanda, & Ratard, 2008). These numbers are particularly striking in that only 11.7% of New Orleans's population (Baylor College of Medicine [BCM] & American Medical Association [AMA], 2006) were affected by the disaster. Of the older victims, 68% died in nursing homes, with some allegedly abandoned by their caretakers (AARP, 2006). Abandonment is one form of elder mistreatment, a practice potentially more damaging and most frequent in disaster situations (Castle, 2008).

Disaster related elder mistreatment (DREM) as a term is still being adapted and explored to fit the disaster public health realm. The literature does not showcase a single definition to this ontology. For the purposes of this discussion, DREM is defined in the following ways:

1. An intentional action that causes harm or creates a serious risk of harm (whether or not harm is intended) to a vulnerable elder

361

by a caregiver or other person who stands in a trust relationship with the elder

2. Failure by a caregiver to satisfy an elder's basic needs or to protect the older person from harm during a time of disaster

During a disaster actions such as the following can lead to trauma responses that can endanger the life of the older person (Islam, Muntner, Webber, Morisky, & Krousel-Wood, 2008):

1. Physical, sexual, or emotional abuse (Graziano, 1997, 2003)
2. Neglect
3. Financial or material exploitation
4. Abandonment

This chapter will examine the traits of older persons that put them at risk for DREM, along with the steps that aid public health response to recognize and prevent this type of mistreatment.

VULNERABILITY OF THE OLDER POPULATION

Old age is a time of transition in terms of both physical and psychosocial changes. These changes, along with existing cultural and underpinning sociodemographic characteristics, make the older population particularly vulnerable to mistreatment (Geroff & Olshaker, 2006). During times of disaster, these vulnerabilities are exacerbated and stretched to their limits (Kohn, Levav, Garcia, Machuca, & Tamashiro, 2005), increasing the importance of recognizing such traits and ensuring the older population is cared for (Castro, Persson, Bergstrom, & Cron, 2008).

Altered Physical Functioning

The most vulnerable older persons are those with a physical disability. According to Rothman and Brown (2007, p. 16), "people with any disability are the ones most likely to suffer a decline in their functional status during or after a disaster." Physical disability can take many forms, such as general frailty (Cefalu, 2007), a lack of mobility, or even impaired hearing or vision. Such functional impairments hinder the frail older person from performing basic ADLs such as preparing meals, using the restroom, or managing their medications and, in effect, make them dependent on outside caregivers, family members, or friends and neighbors (BCM & AMA, 2006; Krousel-Wood, et al., 2008; Rothman & Brown). In a disaster, the effects of these disabilities are exacerbated. An older person who has lost the sensory functions of hearing or eyesight may misinterpret emergency announcements or miss them altogether, while in the case of a sensory loss related to smell the older person may be unable to distinguish spoiled foods (Oriol, 1999).

Moreover, limited mobility is especially devastating as it potentially leads to delays in evacuation, lack of access to services, dependence on transportation assistance that may or may not be available, and even abandonment (HelpAge International, 2006; Lamb, O'Brien, & Fenza, 2008; Oriol, 1999). Carballo, Heal, and Horbaty (2006) wrote that older persons with physical disabilities oftentimes are dependent on physical prostheses, which are frequently lost or damaged during disasters and are very difficult to replace. During disasters, the support systems that the vulnerable or disabled older person has come to rely on are often lost, leaving them abandoned unless aid workers make concerted efforts to identify and help these vulnerable people.

Older persons with chronic medical conditions, such as hypertension, heart disease, and arthritis, also are vulnerable to mistreatment (Lamb, et al., 2008). In addition to potentially limiting a person's physical function, chronic medical conditions require constant care, either through a regimen of medications or the attention of doctors and other health professionals. However, in a disaster, medications can often be lost with no recourse for replacement. Obtaining appropriate health care becomes difficult as health resources are scarce or disorganized. Emergent issues often are seen as more important than chronic conditions (Lamb, et al.). In addition, disasters can often exacerbate debilitating chronic conditions by disrupting the food and water supply and the provision of appropriate shelter, increasing stress and exposing residents to infection (Mokdad, et al., 2005). Such disruptions are especially worrisome for older persons with altered immune function who are at an increased risk of infectious disease (AARP, 2006). According to Greenough and Kirsch (2005, p. 1546), the major health issue of Hurricane Katrina "was and will continue to be the inability of the displaced population to manage their chronic diseases."

Psychosocial Characteristics

In addition to the physical issues associated with the aging process, there are also covert psychosocial changes that can make the older person vulnerable to DREM. Specifically, these include cognitive impairments such as dementia and delirium as well as emotional problems such as depression. These cognitive problems are generally more prevalent in older as opposed to younger adults (Oriol, 1999). Dementia manifests itself via impairments in memory, judgment, abstract thinking, language, and, at times, mood, personality, and behavior. Older persons with dementia may be prone to getting lost, unable to control their impulses, or resistant to medical care (BCM & AMA, 2006). In contrast to dementia, delirium is sudden and temporary, revealing itself through confusion and delusional moments. Both dementia and delirium in the older population are problematic in normal daily life and are made much worse in disaster situations. Associated Press news reports of Hurricane Katrina brought attention to the plight of older persons with dementia who went missing during the storm (Huus, 2005).

While cognitive impairments associated with old age are well documented, the emotional problems may be unknown or overlooked by aid workers. Oriol (1999) asserts that old age can be a difficult developmental stage. He suggests that older populations may face numerous emotional life crises: fears of impairment; the death of friends, families, and spouses; financial worries related to retirement; and new social roles and living arrangements. Older persons who have become disabled due to a disaster may fear losing their independence by being sheltered in places such as nursing homes, experience "transfer trauma" associated with moving, or fear being invisible to aid and health care workers (AARP, 2006, p. 20). The latter anxiety can be seen clearly in the aftermath of the Southeast Asia tsunami; aid workers during that disaster did not tailor support specifically to the older population, in effect shutting them out from the help they needed (Mudur, 2005). This is another form of mistreatment that potentially could be avoided with adequate planning and contingency-based protocols. It is possible that these emotional disturbances could have long-lasting effects leading to a diagnosis of PTSD. However, the research regarding this issue is still unclear. Ehrenreich and McQuaide (2001, p. 29) echoed this uncertainty but noted that while research does not show any definitive long-lasting effects, the emotional vulnerability of the older person is often overlooked, partly because these forms of distress "may not take on exactly the same symptom pattern as among younger people."

Sociodemographic Characteristics

While it is important to recognize the changes the older person deals with during his or her individual aging process, it is also important to realize there are inherent cultural and sociodemographic characteristics that affect this perception and response. According to AARP (2006), older persons are more likely to have lower literacy levels when compared to younger adults, be non-English speakers, be unable to drive, or live alone in isolated rural areas. Oftentimes, when older persons are separated from or lose spouses or family, they become isolated (Centers for Disease Control and Prevention, 2003; U.S. Administration on Aging & Kansas Department of Aging, 2003). This isolation can be seen as a measure to protect themselves from theft or abuse (Weems, et al., 2007). However, during disasters this isolation will prevent older persons from obtaining essential services (HelpAge International, 2006). During the New York City blackout, hurricanes, wildfires, and also during terrorist attacks, isolated older people who had not received services were found by relief or rescue workers or neighbors long after the disaster. The literature provides additional examples of older persons who remained in their apartments during disasters, unaware of what had transpired beyond their private space. Sometimes this isolation effect is the result of cultural parochialism. Whatever the reason, the result is socially debilitating to an older population that generally lacks a real support system. Relief agencies and local communities are potential sources of service for isolated older persons during disasters.

FROM VULNERABILITY TO RISK OF MISTREATMENT

It is clear that older persons are a vulnerable population, particularly during disasters. Geroff and Olshaker (2006) reviewed the literature concerning how certain risk factors made older persons more likely to be mistreated. While most research indicates a significant relationship between mistreatment and both older age and poor mental health (National Center on Elder Abuse, 1998), the relationship is not as clear when dealing with other variables such as gender or infirmity (Charatan, 2006; Cherniack, 2008; Cherniack, Sandals, Brooks, & Mintzer, 2008; Geroff & Olshaker, 2006).

Moreover, Ehrenreich and McQuaide (2001) noted how during disasters there is a larger chance of older persons being victimized (Hyer, Polivka-West, & Brown, 2007; Jones, Walker, & Krohmer, 1995), and, as previously stated, relief response tends to be inconsistent with the actual need of the older population. Within the context of the impact of a disaster on the overall community, meeting the needs of older people may take on a lower priority from a responder's or community's perspective (Ehrenreich & McQuaide). Additionally, stress from a disaster can lead to physical or other forms of abuse (Oriol, 1999). The literature on older persons who live with extended family (Oriol) shows a resulting stressful impact on the existing social support structure of the host family. It may lead to extensive stress on the family breadwinner with a subsequent ripple effect of abuse and mistreatment (Kar, 2006; Lach, Langan, & James, 2005). On the other hand, some cultures seem to be supportive of such interfamilial relocation (HelpAge International, 2006) as long as there are not any direct repercussions on the older person.

Common Risk Factors

Isolation, drug and alcohol addiction, psychiatric problems, dependence, and familial stress are identified as the most critical among the high-risk factors in the geriatric literature (Torgusen & Kosberg, 2006).

Elmore and Brown (2007) and Ehrenreich and McQuaide (2001) described how the lack of a rigorous support structure necessary to deter the isolation effect of a disaster might lead to heightened vulnerabilities (Maeda, 2007). This has been confirmed in postassessment analysis of evacuations (Laska & Morrow, 2006; McGuire, Ford, & Okoro, 2007) and the subsequent relocation of older persons to government or community shelters (Chaffee, 2005). Vulnerable people are susceptible to fraudulent contractors and con artists (AARP, 2006; Oriol, 1999). Older populations in shelters can become easy prey and targets for scammers and thieves and even sexual assault (Ehrenreich & McQuaide; Elmore & Brown; U.S. Department of Justice, 2002). Older persons who are dropped off at shelters without care instructions or medical records (Lamb, et al., 2008) and who may be disorientated or demented commonly receive inappropriate medical treatment (Okumura, Nishita, & Kimura, 2008). There seems to be no known pattern of neglect in the older community during disasters (Bolin & Klenow, 1983, 1988). This leads to an increased potential of prolonged isolation and invisibility to aid workers (Brown, 2007) during the most needed time after a disaster (AARP, 2006).

Moreover, these risk indicators may be markers of unmeasured and unobserved confounders as they can be the source of the relationship between causal factors and elder mistreatment (Morrow, 1999). For example, depression in a caregiver may be a causal risk factor in that a depressed caregiver may be more likely to neglect the care of an elder by virtue of the fatigue (O'Brien, 2003), social withdrawal, and lack of interest associated with depression. Living with others has been associated with an increased probability of mistreatment (Elmore & Brown, 2007). However, this may not be a direct causal relationship because living with others is a contextual factor in which mistreatment is more likely to occur (Ehrenreich & McQuaide, 2001). It may be possible to reduce the risk of mistreatment by modifying other factors associated with living with others (Pattillo, 2005; Pekovic, Seff, & Rothman, 2007) rather than changing the living circumstances of the older person. Changes in living arrangements are often difficult and disruptive for older persons (Elmore & Brown).

PTSD is the most prevalent postdisaster psychiatric ailment and in older persons may be an indicator of negligence or mistreatment. Clinicians should be aware that PTSD can be seen in subjects directly exposed to the disaster (Schinka, Brown, Borenstein, & Mortimer, 2007) as well as in older persons for whom the disaster triggers memories of past trauma (Cook, 2002; Cook, Arean, Schnurr, & Sheikh, 2001) that can lead to disabling anxiety (Lantz & Buchalter, 2003).

Portelli and Fulmer (2006) described how debilitating depression after mistreatment could be another serious sequelae after a disaster. Feelings of depression may be even stronger if the older person feels isolated or that no one understands him or her (Somasundaram & van de Put, 2006). The clinician should be aware of symptoms of depression (Rao, 2006), which may include (1) suicidal ideation, (2) isolation, (3) sudden changes in weight, (4) insomnia, and (5) alcohol or drug abuse, including prescription drugs (Cook, et al., 2001). As a consequence of the aging process but also a side effect of mistreatment, older persons may experience multiple losses; transfer trauma, for example, may result in serious psychological ailments and sometimes even death. The psychological task associated with adjusting to new surroundings and routines can lead to aggravation (Torgusen, Kosberg, & Lowenstein, 2004), depression, increased irritability, and serious illness and can sometimes make frail older persons more susceptible to mistreatment (Ridenour, Cummings, Sinclair, & Bixler, 2007).

Older persons are not a homogenous group. Sociocultural and religious factors play roles in determining the vulnerability and neglect of the older population (Rosenkoetter, Covan, Bunting, Cobb, & Fugate-Whitlock, 2007; Rosenkoetter, Covan, Cobb, Bunting, & Weinrich, 2007). What might be acceptable to an 85 year-old person may not be suitable for a person 65 years of age. Individualized care is necessary, and the diversity of the older population must be kept in mind. Neglect is commonly presumed if the health care provider does not apply an optimal level of health care delivery (Rhoads & Clayman, 2008). The older population presents unique features and challenges to disaster clinicians or relief workers that might result in mistreatment. Therefore, it is suggested that clinicians should exercise special sensitivity toward this reality (Saliba, Buchanan, & Kington, 2004).

There may also be mediating factors that allow for a supporting structure for an older person in need during a disaster (Tumosa, 2007). This may not be the sole responsibility of a familial support structure, such as where an extended family takes in or fosters an older person; it also can be a community-oriented mediating factor. Lamb and colleagues (2008) described how having social contacts, group activities, and a friend living nearby lead to the empowerment of the older person. Religion can play a similar role. When examining the spiritual coping and resiliency mechanisms of older Black hurricane survivors, Lawson and Thomas (2007, p. 34) found that they placed "extensive reliance on a Higher Power to cope with the hurricane and its aftermath."

Older persons are commonly stereotyped and portrayed as generally ill or frail, especially in the case of a disaster. However, the literature increasingly portrays older persons as resilient and experiencing successful aging (Rowe & Kahn, 1997). This positive portrayal of older persons may reduce the exposure of older persons to mistreatment (Drew & Dewan, 2006). Rowe and Kahn (p. 443) described this as "multidimensional, encompassing three distinct domains: avoidance of disease and disability, maintenance of high physical and cognitive functions, and sustained engagement in social and productive activities." Thus, it is erroneous to categorize all older adults as frail when studies show that the older population in most developed countries is developing in healthy strata. This same healthy strata has a strong support system and will be less exposed to mistreatment.

ELDER MISTREATMENT NEEDS ASSESSMENT

Given the vulnerability of older persons and the possibility for mistreatment, aid workers and caretakers must be aware of the presence of older persons during disasters and the special requirements of this population (HelpAge International, 2006). During the aftermath of Hurricane Katrina, approximately 23,000 individuals, many of whom were older persons without family support, found shelter in the Reliant Astrodome

Complex (RAC). To address the needs of this population, geriatric specialists within the RAC developed a triage tool called Seniors Without Families Triage, or SWiFT (BCM & AMA, 2006; Burnett, Dyer, & Pickins, 2007). The purpose of this tool was to "screen for the most in need of help by assessing the issues of cognition, medical and social services needs, and the ability to perform activities of daily living" (BCM & AMA, p. 8). SWiFT was categorized according to three levels, noting appropriate actions given each level of severity (BCM & AMA). During the course of 2 weeks, over 300 SWiFT assessments were completed, with 68%, 18%, and 4% placed in Levels I, II, and III respectively (Burnett, et al.). These results show the utility of the SWiFT tool in postdisaster situations (Dyer, Regev, Burnett, Festa, & Cloyd, 2008). The developers of the tool also noted it can be used prior to the occurrence of a disaster as it provides a hierarchy of disability to allow seniors to prepare for an impending disaster (BCM & AMA).

While the SWiFT tool is designed to ensure the critical and immediate needs of older persons are cared for during disasters, there also can be long-term consequences from disasters, specifically in terms of long-term mental health and psychological effects (Elmore & Brown, 2007). Norris, Friedman, and Watson (2002, p. 70) indicated "disasters do have significant implications for mental health for a significant proportion of persons who experience them." However, it is not clear from the research how older persons are specifically affected. Regardless of the conflicting research, caregivers must be aware of issues such as PTSD, ASD, and depression as well as the impact of both personal and material losses (Elmore & Brown).

An accurate assessment should include stress factors that could highlight the vulnerability and possibility for mistreatment in older persons (Bloodworth, Kevorkian, Rumbaut, & Chiou-Tan, 2007). During massive disasters survivors who have been directly impacted may be exposed to or witness events that may make them extremely vulnerable to serious stress reactions. Being aware of these risk factors is important and could ease the assessment process. Emphasis on postassessment maintenance or re-establishment of communication with family, peers, and counselors in order to talk about the experiences is crucial for the older person's well-being and as a contingency plan to avoid mistreatment (Dosa, Grossman, Wetle, & Mor, 2007; Dosa, et al., 2008). It is also a prerequisite, incumbent upon the professional, to identify key resources such as FEMA, the Red Cross, the Salvation Army, and local and state health departments (Elmore & Brown, 2007) for health, housing, and basic emergency assistance (Barratt, 2007). Identifying local cultural or community supports helps maintain or reestablish normal activities such as attending religious services.

Mental health screening for older persons (Elmore & Brown, 2007) has been shown to be critical since the most common psychosocial symptoms distinguished in diagnosis and treatment in cases of disaster are ASDs and acute and chronic PTSD. The main criteria/symptoms to look for in an assessment, as described by the *DSM-IV* (American Psychiatric Association, 2000), should include the exposure to the traumatic event, persistent re-experiencing of the event, avoidance of stimuli associated with the trauma (Fujita, et al., 2008; Portelli & Fulmer, 2006), and reduced responsiveness to the environment as well as increased arousal not present before the trauma, including mistreatment events (Grady, 2006). Symptoms must be present for at least 1 month and must have caused significant impairment in social, occupational, and other areas of function (Bolin & Klenow, 1983, 1988). Due to the fact that PTSD is often complicated by underlying neurological and physical disorders, a differential diagnosis could document depression, adjustment disorders, obsessive-compulsive disorders, schizophrenia, anxiety, alcohol or substance abuse, or any combination of these (Bonnie & Wallace, 2002). A full assessment would include the examination of symptoms such as re-experiencing, emotional numbing, autonomic arousal, and avoidance. The clinician's main role is to differentiate between normal and abnormal responses to the disaster (Bonder & Wagner, 2001; Goldstein, 1996; Portelli & Fulmer), provide the support and comfort needed, and effectively diagnose the underlying stressors leading to the illness (Andresen, Rothenberg, & Zimmer, 1997). At the same time, the clinician must identify high-risk individuals and follow up with proper referral or treatment and care.

The International Society for Traumatic Stress Studies (ISTSS) explains how some older persons are more vulnerable than others, especially individuals with prior or other underlying traumatic events in life, such as accidents, abuse, assault, combat, emargination, or chronic medial illnesses (Portelli & Fulmer, 2006). With such clients, the clinician needs to encourage discussion and provide constant orienting information and assurances regarding the situation. The clinician needs to engage with the older person and assist in building a support structure around the patient while assessing the reliability of the family or client support group. "Victims are forever changed by the experience of disaster" (U.S. Department of Justice, 2002, p. 456). Facing life with a new experience in the background and trying to understand its meaning doesn't always help overcome tragedy since the feeling of loss may remain for a long time. Therefore, during assessments it is important to offer practical suggestions. A good assessment, including observation by mental health specialists, could result in an intervention to reduce stress symptoms and promote postdisaster adjustment (Fulmer, Guadagno, Bitondo Dyer, & Connolly, 2004), especially after potential mistreatment. Addressing the basic needs of shelter and finding a safe haven that provides food and water, sanitation, privacy, and opportunities to sit quietly, relax, and sleep, at least briefly, improves the clinician-patient alliance and prevents mistreatment (Portelli & Fulmer, 2006). It is essential that older persons be encouraged to avoid alcohol and other drugs since these substances interfere with healing (Polivka-West & Berman, 2008). Re-establishing old routines is a practical way to decrease tension; staying busy with work or hobbies can provide a distraction to occupy the mind. Seeking information, advice, and help from others such as family, clergy, and support workers provides support and eases the negative effects of painful memories. However, it must be remembered that although most people are honest and trustworthy, some unscrupulous individuals try to take advantage of victims in the aftermath of a disaster (Acierno, Ruggiero, Kilpatrick, Resnick, & Galea, 2006).

DREM PREVENTION STRATEGIES AND MANAGEMENT

Since Hurricane Katrina, a number of agencies have created guidelines for caring for older persons during disasters, although few have addressed the specifics of DREM. Baylor College of Medicine and the AMA (2006) created a set of recommendations for managing older disaster victims that include the following strategies:

1. Develop a tracking system for the elderly.
2. Provide separate shelters for the elderly.
3. Involve aging specialists in planning for care and training aid workers.
4. Involve local social services and community organizations.
5. Use a triage system to ensure that the most critical victims are cared for.
6. Establish a means for shelter personnel to remain in touch with central administration.
7. Provide protection from abuse and fraud.

8. Plan for evacuation of residents of long-term-care facilities.
9. Prepare disaster plans and conduct readiness drills.

While the authors do specifically mention that abuse and fraud are possibilities that need to be prevented, they do not provide specific recommendations. Similarly, research on elderly mistreatment has provided guidelines for identifying and treating abuse but not specifically with regard to disasters (BCM & AMA, 2006).

HelpAge International (2006), an organization dedicated to caring and advocating for older persons, has developed guidelines that specifically address DREM that include these recommendations:

1. Be aware of the possibility of elder abuse and provide protection (Aldrich & Benson, 2008). This applies not only to caregivers and aid workers but also to members of the community (Andresen, et al., 1997) who can help reduce the possibility of intimidation, exploitation, and theft of older persons.
2. Be knowledgeable about the power dynamic between men and women, especially in shelters, where a need to fill quotas may create a gender imbalance. The authors stress that the risk of sexual abuse of older women increases when shelters have mixed genders without the informed consent of women.
3. Avoid the presence of large cohorts of older people without families, either due to loss, abandonment, or isolation (Weinstein, Fletcher, & Stover, 2007). Steps should be taken to find support for these people either through community organizations, foster families, or extended family via family-tracing services.
4. Be sure to account for the sociodemographic and cultural characteristics of older persons when dealing with situations of possible abuse (HelpAge International, 2006).

Medical personnel have an important role to play in the early detection and identification of elder abuse (Geroff & Olshaker, 2006). In the case of DREM, due to the lack of disaster and older persons mistreatment research, medical practitioners follow the AMA's (1992) guidelines, which urge early detection and proper assessment of older persons. The implementation of such a structured protocol to DREM, however well intentioned, could be costly and counterproductive in the absence of careful planning and training for first responders and health care workers. Therefore, appropriate intervention and planning measures are critical

(Geroff & Olshaker). An appropriate planning structure should be the platform for a detail-oriented elder mistreatment assessment. Possible markers of neglect and abuse, including bruises, pressure sores, fractures, burns, and abrasions, are not the only identifiers of abuse (AMA, 1992). It is important to note and document every particular as a key to the interpretation of these markers; identifying their presence as well as their characteristics—such as anatomic location, extent, morphology, severity, and multiplicity—may help differentiate between an intentional injury and an avoidable one (Fernandez, Byard, Lin, Benson, & Barbera, 2002). Therefore, training and educating both health care personnel (clinical, behavioral, and forensic assessors) and older persons would help identify evidence of mistreatment as caused by the conduct (acts or omissions) of an abusing person.

CONCLUSIONS

Disaster preparedness and careful planning for older persons are integral for the prevention of DREM. Referral to experts is important for those who do not feel competent in this new area of practice. For all clinicians, the focus of a health assessment must be on the needs of the older person and may sometimes simply involve asking if the individual feels neglected or inappropriately treated. This may set the stage for the next steps in the DREM-care planning process and provide useful information on appropriate protocol development.

ACKNOWLEDGMENT

Special credit goes to the National Library of Medicine, The Frederick L. Ehrman Medical Library at New York University, and Itty Mathew, disaster informationist for the research and data mining support for this chapter.

REFERENCES

AARP. (2006). *We can do better. Lessons learned for protecting older persons in disasters.* Retrieved May 29, 2009, from http://assets.aarp.org/rgcenter/il/better.pdf

Acierno, R., Ruggiero, K. J., Kilpatrick, D. G., Resnick, H. S., & Galea, S. (2006). Risk and protective factors for psychopathology among older versus younger adults after the 2004 Florida hurricanes. *American Journal of Geriatric Psychiatry, 14*(12), 1051–1059.

Aldrich, N., & Benson, W. F. (2008). Disaster preparedness and the chronic disease needs of vulnerable older adults. *Preventing Chronic Disease, 5*(1), A27.

American Medical Association. (1992). AMA diagnostic and treatment guidelines on domestic violence. *Archives of Family Medicine, 1,* 40–41.

American Psychiatric Association. (2000). *Diagnostic and statistical manual of mental disorders* (4th ed., text revision). Washington, DC: Author.

Andresen, E., Rothenberg, B., & Zimmer, J. G. (1997). *Assessing the health status of older adults.* New York: Springer Publishing.

Barratt, J. (2007). International perspectives on aging and disasters. *Generations: Journal of the American Society on Aging, 31*(4), 57–60.

Baylor College of Medicine, & American Medical Association. (2006). *Recommendation for best practices in the management of elderly disaster victims.* Retrieved May 29, 2009, from http://assets.aarp.org/www.aarp.org_/articles/aboutaarp/baylor_best_practices_guide.pdf

Bloodworth, D. M., Kevorkian, C. G., Rumbaut, E., & Chiou-Tan, F. Y. (2007). Impairment and disability in the Astrodome after Hurricane Katrina: Lessons learned about the needs of the disabled after large population movements. *American Journal of Physical Medicine & Rehabilitation, 86*(9), 770–775.

Bolin, R., & Klenow, D. J. (1983). Response of the elderly to disaster—An age-stratified analysis. *International Journal of Aging and Human Development, 16*(4), 283–296.

Bolin, R., & Klenow, D. J. (1988). Older people in disaster—A comparison of black and white victims. *International Journal of Aging and Human Development, 26*(1), 29–43.

Bonder, B., & Wagner, M. B. (2001). *Functional performance in older adults* (2nd ed.). Philadelphia, PA: F. A. Davis.

Bonnie, R. J., & Wallace, R. B. (2002). *Elder mistreatment: Abuse, neglect, and exploitation in an aging America.* Washington, DC: National Academies Press.

Brown, L. M. (2007). Issues in mental health care for older adults after disasters. *Generations: Journal of the American Society on Aging, 31*(4), 21–26.

Brunkard, J., Namulanda, G., & Ratard, R. (2008). Hurricane Katrina deaths, Louisiana, 2005. *Disaster Medicine & Public Health Preparedness, 2*(4), 215–223.

Burnett, J., Dyer, C. B., & Pickins, S. (2007). Rapid needs assessments for older adults in disasters. *Generations: Journal of the American Society on Aging, 31*(4), 10–15.

Carballo, M., Heal, B., & Horbaty, G. (2006). Impact of the tsunami on psychosocial health and well-being. *International Review of Psychiatry, 18*(3), 217–223.

Castle, N. G. (2008). Nursing home evacuation plans. *American Journal of Public Health, 98*(7), 1235–1240.

Castro, C., Persson, D., Bergstrom, N., & Cron, S. (2008). Surviving the storms: Emergency preparedness in Texas nursing facilities and assisted living facilities. *Journal of Gerontological Nursing, 34*(8), 9–16.

Cefalu, C. A. (2007). Re: To evacuate or not to evacuate: Lessons learned from Louisiana nursing home administrators following hurricanes Katrina and Rita [Letter to the editor]. *Journal of the American Medical Directors Association, 8*(7), 485–486.

Centers for Disease Control and Prevention. (2003). *Disaster preparedness and emergency response.* New York: Department of Health and Mental Hygiene.

Chaffee, M. W. (2005). Hospital response to acute-onset disasters: The state of the science in 2005. *Nursing Clinics of North America, 40*(3), 565.

Charatan, F. (2006). New Orleans doctor is charged with giving lethal injections during floods. *British Medical Journal, 333*(7561), 218.

Cherniack, E. P. (2008). The impact of natural disasters on the elderly. *American Journal of Disaster Medicine, 3*(3), 133–139.

Cherniack, E. P., Sandals, L., Brooks, L., & Mintzer, M. J. (2008). Trial of a survey instrument to establish the hurricane preparedness of and medical impact on a vulnerable, older population. *Prehospital and Disaster Medicine, 23*(3), 242–249.

Cook, J. M. (2002). Traumatic exposure and PTSD in older adults: Introduction to the special issue. *Journal of Clinical Geropsychology, 8,* 149–152.

Cook, J. M., Arean, P. A., Schnurr, P. P., & Sheikh, J. (2001). Symptom differences of older depressed primary care patients with and without history of trauma. *International Journal of Psychiatry in Medicine, 31,* 415–428.

Dosa, D. M., Grossman, N., Wetle, T., & Mor, V. (2007). To evacuate or not to evacuate: Lessons learned from Louisiana nursing home administrators following hurricanes Katrina and Rita. *Journal of the American Medical Directors Association, 8*(3), 142–149.

Dosa, D. M., Hyer, K., Brown, L. M., Artenstein, A. W., Polivka-West, L., & Mor, V. (2008). The controversy inherent in managing frail nursing home residents during complex hurricane emergencies. *Journal of the American Medical Directors Association, 9*(8), 599–604.

Drew, C., & Dewan, S. (2006, July 20). Accused doctor said to have faced chaos at New Orleans hospital. *New York Times,* p. A18.

Dyer, C. B., Regev, M., Burnett, J., Festa, N., & Cloyd, B. (2008). SWiFT: A rapid triage tool for vulnerable older adults in disaster situations. *Disaster Medicine & Public Health Preparedness, 2*(Suppl. 1), S45–50.

Ehrenreich, J. H., & McQuaide, S. (2001). *Coping in disasters: A guidebook to psychosocial intervention.* Retrieved May 29, 2009, from http://www.mhwwb.org/Coping WithDisaster.pdf

Elmore, D. L., & Brown, L. M. (2007). Emergency preparedness and response: Health and social policy implications for older adults. *Generations: Journal of the American Society on Aging, 31*(4), 66–74.

Fernandez, L. S., Byard, D., Lin, C. C., Benson, S., & Barbera, J. A. (2002). Frail elderly as disaster victims: Emergency management strategies. *Prehospital and Disaster Medicine, 17*(2), 67–74.

Fujita, Y., Inoue, K., Seki, N., Inoue, T., Sakuta, A., Miyazawa, T., et al. (2008). The need for measures to prevent "solitary deaths" after large earthquakes—Based on current conditions following the great Hanshin-Awaji earthquake. *Journal of Forensic & Legal Medicine, 15*(8), 527–528.

Fulmer, T., Guadagno, L., Bitondo Dyer, C., & Connolly, M. T. (2004). Progress in elder abuse screening and assessment instruments. *Journal of the American Geriatrics Society, 52*(2), 297–304.

Geroff, A. J., & Olshaker, J. S. (2006). Elder abuse. *Emergency Medicine Clinics of North America, 24*(2), 491.

Goldstein, M. Z. (1996). Elder maltreatment and posttraumatic stress disorder. In P. E. Ruskin & J. A. Talbott (Eds.), *Aging and posttraumatic stress disorder.* Washington, DC: American Psychiatric Press.

Grady, D. (2006, July 20). Medical and ethical questions raised on deaths of critically ill patients. *New York Times,* p. A18.

Graziano, R. (1997). The challenge of clinical work with survivors of trauma. In J. R. Brandell (Ed.), *Theory and practice in clinical social work.* New York: Free Press.

Graziano, R. (2003). Trauma and aging. *Journal of Gerontological Social Work, 40*(4), 3–21.

Greenough, P. G., & Kirsch, T. D. (2005). Hurricane Katrina. Public health response— Assessing needs. *New England Journal of Medicine, 353*(15), 1544–1546.

HelpAge International. (2006). *Older people in disaster and humanitarian crises: Guidelines for best practice.* Retrieved May 29, 2009, from http://www.reliefweb.int/library/documents/HelpAge_olderpeople.pdf

Huus, K. (2005, Nov 24). Lost in the shuffle: Katrina leaves elderly evacuees displaced, disconnected. *MSNBC.* Retrieved June 26, 2009, from http://www.msnbc.msn.com/id/10180296/

Hyer, K., Polivka-West, L., & Brown, L. M. (2007). Nursing homes and assisted living facilities: Planning and decision making for sheltering in place or evacuation. *Generations: Journal of the American Society on Aging, 31*(4), 29–33.

Islam, T., Muntner, P., Webber, L. S., Morisky, D. E., & Krousel-Wood, M. A. (2008). Cohort study of medication adherence in older adults (CoSMO): Extended effects of Hurricane Katrina on medication adherence among older adults. *American Journal of the Medical Sciences, 336*(2), 105–110.

Jones, J. S., Walker, G., & Krohmer, J. R. (1995). To report or not to report: Emergency services response to elder abuse. *Prehospital and Disaster Medicine, 10*(2), 96–100.

Kar, N. (2006). Psychosocial issues following a natural disaster in a developing country: A qualitative longitudinal observational study. *International Journal of Disaster Medicine, 4,* 169–176.

Kohn, R., Levav, I., Garcia, I. D., Machuca, M. E., & Tamashiro, R. (2005). Prevalence, risk factors, and aging vulnerability for psychopathology following a natural disaster in a developing country. *International Journal of Geriatric Psychiatry, 20*(9), 835–841.

Krousel-Wood, M. A., Islam, T., Muntner, P., Stanley, E., Phillips, A., Webber, L. S., et al. (2008). Medication adherence in older clinic patients with hypertension after hurricane Katrina: Implications for clinical practice and disaster management. *American Journal of the Medical Sciences, 336*(2), 99–104.

Lach, H. W., Langan, J. C., & James, D. C. (2005). Disaster planning: Are gerontological nurses prepared? *Journal of Gerontological Nursing, 31*(11), 21–27.

Lamb, K. V., O'Brien, C., & Fenza, P. J. (2008). Elders at risk during disasters. *Home Healthcare Nurse, 26*(1), 30–38.

Lantz, M. S., & Buchalter, E. N. (2003). Posttraumatic stress disorder: When older adults are victims of severe trauma. *Clinical Geriatrics, 11*(04), 122–131.

Laska, S., & Morrow, B. H. (2006). Social vulnerabilities and Hurricane Katrina: An unnatural disaster in New Orleans. *Marine Technology Society Journal, 40*(4), 16–26.

Lawson, E. J., & Thomas, C. (2007). Wading in the waters: Spirituality and older Black Katrina survivors. *Journal of Health Care for the Poor & Underserved, 18*(2), 341–354.

Maeda, K. (2007). Twelve years since the great Hanshin Awaji earthquake, a disaster in an aged society. *Psychogeriatrics, 7*(2), 41–43.

McGuire, L. C., Ford, E. S., & Okoro, C. A. (2007). Natural disasters and older U.S. adults with disabilities: Implications for evacuation. *Disasters, 31*(1), 49–56.

Mokdad, A. H., Mensah, G. A., Posner, S. F., Reed, E., Simoes, E. J., Engelgau, M. M., et al. (2005). When chronic conditions become acute: Prevention and control of chronic diseases and adverse health outcomes during natural disasters. *Preventing Chronic Disease, 2*(Special issue A04), 23.

Morrow, B. H. (1999). Identifying and mapping community vulnerability. *Disasters, 23*(1), 1–18.

Mudur, G. (2005). Aid agencies ignored special needs of elderly people after tsunami. *British Medical Journal, 331*(7514), 422.

National Center on Elder Abuse. (1998). *The national elder abuse incidence study: Final report.* Retrieved May 28, 2009, from http://www.aoa.gov/AoARoot/AoA_Programs/ Elder_Rights/Elder_Abuse/docs/ABuseReport_Full.pdf

Norris, F. H., Friedman, M. J., & Watson, P. J. (2002). 60,000 disaster victims speak: Part II. Summary and implications of the disaster mental health research. *Psychiatry, 65*(3), 240–260.

O'Brien, N (2003, January–February). *Emergency preparedness for older people* (Issue Brief). New York: International Longevity Center-USA.

Okumura, J., Nishita, Y., & Kimura, K. (2008). Pharmaceutical supply for disaster victims who need chronic disease management in region with aging population based on lessons learned from the Noto peninsula earthquake in 2007. *Yakugaku Zasshi—Journal of the Pharmaceutical Society of Japan, 128*(9), 1275–1283.

Oriol, W. E. (1999). *Psychosocial issues for older adults in disasters* (DHHS Pub. No. ESDRB SMA 99-3323). Retrieved May 29, 2009, from http://download.ncadi.samhsa. gov/ken/pdf/SMA99-3323/99-821.pdf

Pattillo, M. (2005). City-wide efforts to provide shelter and care to elderly evacuees. *Journal of Gerontological Nursing, 31*(11), 62–64.

Pekovic, V., Seff, L., & Rothman, M. B. (2007). Planning for and responding to special needs of elders in natural disasters. *Generations: Journal of the American Society on Aging, 31*(4), 37–41.

Polivka-West, L., & Berman, A. (2008). Safeguarding seniors during hurricanes. *American Journal of Nursing, 108*(1), 28.

Portelli, I., & Fulmer, T. (2006). *Assessing disaster preparedness and response.* In J. Gallo, T. Fulmer, G. Paveza, & H. R. Bogner (Eds.), *Handbook of geriatric assessment* (4th ed.). Sudbury, MA: Jones and Bartlett Publishers.

Rao, K. (2006). Psychosocial support in disaster-affected communities. *International Review of Psychiatry, 18*(6), 501–505.

Rhoads, J., & Clayman, A. (2008). Learning from Katrina: Preparing long-term care facilities for disasters. *Geriatric Nursing, 29*(4), 253–258.

Ridenour, M. L., Cummings, K. J., Sinclair, J. R., & Bixler, D. (2007). Displacement of the underserved: Medical needs of hurricane Katrina evacuees in West Virginia. *Journal of Health Care for the Poor & Underserved, 18*(2), 369–381.

Rosenkoetter, M. M., Covan, E. K., Bunting, S., Cobb, B. K., & Fugate-Whitlock, E. (2007). Disaster evacuation: An exploratory study of older men and women in Georgia and North Carolina. *Journal of Gerontological Nursing, 33*(12), 46–54.

Rosenkoetter, M. M., Covan, E. K., Cobb, B. K., Bunting, S., & Weinrich, M. (2007). Perceptions of older adults regarding evacuation in the event of a natural disaster. *Public Health Nursing, 24*(2), 160–168.

Rothman, M., & Brown, L. M. (2007). The vulnerable geriatric casualty: Medical needs of frail older adults during disasters. *Generations: Journal of the American Society on Aging, 31*(4), 16–20.

Rowe, J. W., & Kahn, R. L. (1997). Successful aging. *The Gerontologist, 37*(4), 433–440.

Saliba, D., Buchanan, J., & Kington, R. S. (2004). Function and response of nursing facilities during community disaster. *American Journal of Public Health, 94*(8), 1436–1441.

Schinka, J. A., Brown, L. M., Borenstein, A. R., & Mortimer, J. A. (2007). Confirmatory factor analysis of the PTSD checklist in the elderly. *Journal of Traumatic Stress, 20*(3), 281–289.

Somasundaram, D. J., & van de Put, W.A.C.M. (2006). Management of trauma in special populations after a disaster. *Journal of Clinical Psychiatry, 67*, 64–73.

Torgusen, B. L., & Kosberg, J. I. (2006). Assisting older victims of disasters: Roles and responsibilities for social workers. *Journal of Gerontological Social Work, 47*(1–2), 27–44.

Torgusen, B. L., Kosberg, J. I., & Lowenstein, A. (2004). The impact of disasters on the lives of older persons: Applied implications. *Gerontologist, 44*(Special Issue 1), 242.

Tumosa, N. (2007). Disaster: Nursing homes need to be prepared. *Journal of the American Medical Directors Association, 8*(3), 135–137.

U.S. Administration on Aging, & Kansas Department on Aging. (2003). *The disaster preparedness manual: Impact of disaster on older adults*. Retrieved December 29, 2008, from http://www.dmhas.state.ct.us/trauma/olderadults.pdf

U.S. Department of Justice, Office for Victims of Crime, Victims and Family Assistance. (2002). *OVC handbook for coping after terrorism: A guide to healing and recovery*. Retrieved December 29, 2008, from http://www.ojp.usdoj.gov/ovc/publications

Weems, C. F., Watts, S. E., Marsee, M. A., Taylor, L. K., Costa, N. M., Cannon, M. F., et al. (2007). The psychosocial impact of Hurricane Katrina: Contextual differences in psychological symptoms, social support, and discrimination. *Behaviour Research & Therapy, 45*(10), 2295–2306.

Weinstein, H. M., Fletcher, L. E., & Stover, E. (2007). Human rights and mass disaster: Lessons from the 2004 tsunami. *Asia-Pacific Journal of Public Health, 19*(Spec. No.), 52–59.

A Guide to Developing Training Programs for Disaster Preparedness for Older Persons

JUDITH L. HOWE, ANNETTE M. ATANOUS, AND JOHN A.TONER

Since 2003, the GEPR Collaborative of the federal HRSA-funded GECs has addressed the needs of older persons in emergencies through the development, dissemination, and evaluation of education and training programs. Six GECs, located in California, New York, Kentucky, Texas, Missouri, and Ohio, and Mathers LifeWays in Illinois form this successful collaborative. Specifically, the CNYGEC received funding in 2005 to develop a curriculum on the mental health effects of disasters on older adults as discussed in Chapter 3. The CNYGEC curriculum was intended for distribution throughout the GEC network, area health education centers, area agencies on aging, health professional schools, local and state public health agencies, and community agencies serving older people and their families.

This book was conceptualized by the editors to serve as an evidence-based guide for professionals working with older adults at risk for suffering mental health issues in the face of emergencies and disasters. These events include earthquakes, floods, tornadoes, heat waves, flu outbreaks, and fires in addition to man-made disasters such as terrorist attacks. Training on preparedness, and specifically the mental health effects of these events, increases the chance of survival among older persons and makes communities more resilient. The editors also hope this book provides a framework for the development of training programs in disaster preparedness. Training programs can vary and may include face-to-face, Web-based, and self-study modalities, among others. It is crucial that health care agencies throughout the country begin creating and implementing training programs in geriatric emergency preparedness in an effort to meet the special needs of a growing older population. According to the U.S. Department of Health and Human Services Administration on Aging, the population of individuals 65 and older will increase from 35 million in 2000 to 40 million in 2010, a 15% increase, and then to 55 million in 2020, a 36% increase for that decade. By 2030, there will be about 72.1 million older persons, almost twice as many as in 2007. People 65 years old and older made up 12.6% of the population in 2007 but are projected to be 19.3% of the population by 2030. The 85-and-older population is expected to increase from 5.5 million in 2007 to 5.8 million in 2010 and then to 6.6 million in 2020 (Administration on Aging, 2008).

All health care professionals need to be prepared in the event they are called upon to assist older persons during or after an emergency. Historically, older people have been overlooked in emergencies and disasters as many of this book's chapters have underscored. Disasters in the United States such as September 11, 2001, Hurricane Katrina, and Hurricane Rita are just a few examples of major emergencies both unforeseen and extremely difficult to control afterward. Older persons and other vulnerable groups, such as the disabled, often fell between the cracks during and after these disasters in part because health care providers and other emergency responders were not prepared to address their unique needs.

STEPS IN SETTING UP A TRAINING PROGRAM

Several important steps will help assure success when setting up a training program in geriatric emergency preparedness. While there may be variations to procedures due to the size and purpose of a particular program, certain measures should be followed by any organization. If a training program already is developed and in place, it is vital that the agency review how it is currently managed and evaluated. If no programs are in place, the following suggestions may be useful when setting up a training program within your organization (Versitas Corporation, 2006).

Management Approval

One of the first steps in creating an emergency preparedness training program is to receive proper management approval. Permission to create and implement a program is at the discretion of the management. Please follow your agency guidelines and go through the proper channels.

Establish a Budget

After approval has been granted, an internal budget should be created to determine the cost of implementing an emergency training program within an organization's infrastructure. Budget constraints may influence the length of training offered. The organization's fiscal department will be able to assist in short-term and long-term budget planning.

Needs Assessment

One of the most critical steps in developing geriatric emergency preparedness training is to conduct a needs assessment of the organization. This will determine where the agency lacks disaster preparedness knowledge, prevention, and intervention. A thorough needs assessment will aid tremendously in planning and implementing a training program.

Implementing the Training

After designing a tailored geriatric emergency preparedness program specific to the needs of the organization, the next step is to actually implement the training program. The administrator or director should determine any applicable mandates, such as whether the agency's entire staff is required to participate, the length and frequency of the training, and any post-training certifications offered for training participants.

Post-Training Assessment and Evaluation

The final step in implementing a geriatric emergency preparedness program at a particular agency or organization is to properly assess the program. Participants of the training should complete an itemized questionnaire or other applicable tool to evaluate the program. Findings should be written up, evaluated, and submitted to organizational leadership for future planning.

Principles of Adult Learning

Since the trainees will generally be adults with varied backgrounds and experiences, it is imperative that the curriculum be geared toward meeting the needs of adult learners. In the mid-20th century, American adult educator Malcolm Knowles adapted the concept of *andragogy*— the art and science of helping adults learn—and forever influenced the way adults learn and retain information. This principle of adult learning theory states that the relationship between teacher and student is one of mutual respect, that the student's experience counts as much as the teacher's knowledge, and that learning is student centered rather than teacher centered. In Knowles's model of learning, the adult learner has a problem-centered orientation to learning, an accumulation of life experiences upon which new learning experiences can be built, an intrinsic motivation to learn, and a need to be self-directed (Slusarski, 1994). Knowles's model of adult learning promotes a climate of openness, collaboration, competence, creativity, and success. When developing training programs, the principles of adult learning may be incorporated through understanding and application, self-direction, collaboration, and critical thinking.

Target Audience for the Training Program

Training programs in geriatric emergency preparedness are beneficial at all levels of organization and government. Funding, training guidelines, and certifications will vary depending on the level of training. A list of potential government funders of training programs is provided in Table Appendix I.1. Ideally, experts in the field of geriatric emergency training should facilitate such programs, although there are currently no formal teaching certifications implemented in this area. Officials, directors, and administrators at all levels are highly encouraged to sponsor training programs in geriatric emergency preparedness.

All health care workers will benefit from participating in these training programs given their likely involvement in emergencies that impact on older persons. These include medical doctors, registered nurses, licensed practical nurses, social workers, pharmacists, audiologists, psychologists, home health attendants/aides, mental health counselors, and so forth. In addition, staff of long-term-care institutions, acute care facilities, rehabilitation hospitals, community mental health clinics, and emerging first responders are all appropriate audiences. Furthermore, academic and public disaster preparedness centers, health associations, and foundations specializing in geriatric issues can use this manual for identifying educational programs in geriatric mental health and disaster preparedness and for developing their own in-service training.

Table Appendix I.1

GOVERNMENTAL SPONSORS OF TRAINING PROGRAMS

GOVERNMENT LEVEL	AGENCY TYPES
Federal	■ Federal Emergency Management Agency (FEMA) ■ Administration on Aging (AoA) ■ Centers for Disease Control and Prevention (CDC)
State	■ State offices for the aging ■ State health departments ■ Regional and state agency disaster officers ■ Eldercare locator
Municipal	■ Departments for the aging ■ Health care institutions (hospitals, nursing homes, walk-in health centers) ■ Housing sites (senior housing, assisted living facilities, subsidized housing) ■ Other sponsors (senior centers, churches, food banks, Salvation Army)

Learning Modalities

When designing geriatric emergency preparedness training, several learning modalities are most effective, including the following:

Tabletop Exercises

Conducting tabletop exercises is an excellent way to present a group of trainees with simulated emergency situations and allow for concrete discussion. Tabletop exercises do not have any time restraints, thus enabling trainees to closely examine a hypothetical emergency situation, discuss ways in which the situation may be resolved, and plan for rescue and follow-up interventions. Tabletop exercises work best with groups. They promote open dialogue and team approaches to disaster preparedness. For this reason, the level of discussion will inevitably affect the success of tabletop exercises.

Cases

Incorporating case examples into geriatric emergency preparedness training gives trainees the opportunity to discuss real-life situations or cases that may have occurred in their settings. Case examples are generally detailed and serve as instructive examples of the topic at hand. Case examples enable the trainees to put their gathered information in context. Case examples on emergency preparedness may also illustrate any shortcomings during and after a crisis.

Role-Plays

In emergency preparedness training, role-playing is an excellent way for trainees to practice simulated emergency situations and attempt rescue efforts. Role-plays are often used in group learning so the learners may play the roles of particular characters. This type of learning modality is extremely challenging for participants because it offers a practical, firsthand way to perform emergency response methods and identifies any inadequacies throughout the process.

Trigger Tapes

Trigger tapes may be used in both one-on-one and group learning. Trigger tapes are excellent tools whereby trainees watch short films that depict emergency situations and then trigger discussions about the topics. Trigger tapes related to emergency preparedness often illustrate both good and bad emergency preparedness interventions. They are a useful resource for training participants and trainers alike.

Exemplar Models for Training Programs

There are currently several exemplar models developed by GECs for geriatric emergency preparedness in the United States (Johnson, et al., 2006).

GEPR Collaborative

Composed of HRSA-funded GECs in California, New York, Kentucky, Texas, Missouri, Ohio, and Mathers LifeWays in Illinois, this group was created to help increase national awareness of the issues of emergency preparedness for aging, advocacy for older persons, and funding to educate faculty, students, and health care providers who work with older persons. The work of this collaborative has been nationally and internationally recognized and replicated.

Consortium of New York Geriatric Education Centers

This GEC offers a 3-day emergency preparedness certificate program for health care professionals working with the older population.[1]

Ohio Valley Appalachia Regional Geriatric Education Center

Numerous portable tools for long-distance learning are offered by this organization including emergency planning tools,[2] distance learning modules and interactive videos,[3] and e-newsletters on emergency preparedness.[4]

Texas Consortium of Geriatric Education Centers

This consortium is responsible for designing a comprehensive curriculum on bioterrorism and emergency preparedness in aging that is being taught throughout the state of Texas.[5]

SAMPLE TRAINING PLAN

Depending on time and budget constraints, training programs vary dramatically in format. An ideal geriatric emergency preparedness training is 1 day. Table Appendix I.2 provides a sample 1-day training for use in all facilities. It may be shortened or extended to meet specific agency needs. In addition, all training programs, regardless of length, should have designated learning objectives for all learners. Table Appendix I.3 lists sample learning objectives that may be applied to various training programs (Howe, Sherman, & Toner, 2006).

CONCLUSION

There is no question that our country is aging rapidly. It is vital that all health care professionals become better equipped to meet the needs of an aging population. Having knowledge and proper training in geriatric emergency preparedness is one of many ways in which we are best able to serve our elders. Individuals interested in this very important task are strongly urged to speak with their agency administrators and directors to implement an emergency preparedness curriculum within their

Table Appendix I.2

SAMPLE 1-DAY TRAINING

8:00–8:30 AM: Check-in; light refreshments

8:30–9:00 AM: Introduction

- Purpose of training
- Goals and objectives for the day
- Pre-test

9:00–10:00 AM: Overview of Disaster Preparedness Mental Health Effects of Disasters on Older Persons

One or two speakers should cover the following topics:

- Demographics of aging population
- Major disasters in recent years (Katrina, Rita, 9/11, Thailand tsunami)
- Displacement of elderly
- Overall impact of disasters on the elderly (individual and public outcomes)

10:00–10:10 AM: Break

10:10–11:00 AM: Mental Disorders Common in Older Persons

11:00–11:10 AM: Break

11:10 AM–12:00 PM: Assessment and Screening Tools

- Mini-Mental State Exam (MMSE)
- Post traumatic Stress Disorder (PTSD) Checklist
- Patient Health Questionnaire (PHQ)

12:00–12:30 PM: Lunch

12:30–2:00 PM: Interactive Exercise(s) Focused on Interventions

Choose from the following modalities:

- Tabletop exercises
- Cases
- Role-plays
- Trigger tapes
- FEMA Emergency Preparedness Checklist http://www.fema.gov/pdf/library/epc.pdf

2:00–2:10 PM: Break

2:10–3:00 PM: Special Considerations/Populations

- Tabletop exercises
- Diverse cultures
- Veterans: PTSD, TBI, Pre-existing psychological conditions, etc.

3:00–3:10 PM: Break

3:10–4:00 PM: Policy Implications

- Government involvement
- Educational program development throughout the country

4:00–4:30 PM: Wrap-up

- Q & A
- Post-Test

4:30–5:00 PM: Evaluations, Networking

Table Appendix I.3

LEARNING OBJECTIVES

AT THE CONCLUSION OF THE INTRODUCTORY SESSION, LEARNERS WILL:

Knowledge

- Articulate the rationale for this training
- Describe the importance of a structured curriculum in geriatric mental health and emergency disaster preparedness and response
- Describe the overall goals and objectives of the training plan
- Assess their current knowledge of geriatric mental health and disaster preparedness and response through a pre-test

Attitudes

- Realize that older adults require special consideration—for both mental and physical health needs—during and after disasters
- Understand the importance of training health care professionals to integrate this material into their practice
- Appreciate the importance of the interdisciplinary team approach, which is a key aspect of this curriculum

Skills

- Be able to implement the training plan
- Know how to use the available resource material to augment their knowledge before teaching this curriculum
- Be able to select and effectively employ interactive teaching methods appropriate for the level and type of learner they will be training.

organization. Agencies may get more information on developing training programs for their staff by contacting city and state officials. Policy makers at the state and federal levels must also allot funding sources for such training programs as they will become increasingly significant in future years. While much research needs to be conducted to show the mental health effects of disasters on older persons, prevention and education will continue to be the most effective ways of minimizing adverse mental health effects caused by disasters and meeting the special needs of this vulnerable and ever-growing population.

NOTES

1. Detailed information can be found on their Web site at http://www.nygec.org/.

2. Further information about emergency planning tools can be found at http://www.mc.uky.edu/aging//gec.html.

3. Distance training models and interactive videos can be reviewed at http://ky.train.org.

4. The link for e-newsletters is http://cwte.louisville.edu/ovar/emergency/winter 2009.htm.

5. For curriculum details, log onto http://www.hcoa.org/tcgec/tcgec.htm.

REFERENCES

Administration on Aging. (2008). *Profiles of older Americans.* Retrieved August 10, 2009, from http://www.aoa.gov/AoAroot/Aging_Statistics/Profile/2008/docs/2008profile.pdf

Howe, J., Sherman, A., & Toner, J. (Eds.). (2007). Geriatric mental health disaster and emergency preparedness curriculum. *Portal of Geriatric Online Education (POGOe),* Product Number 18848. Retrieved from http://www.pogoe.com

Johnson, A., Howe, J. L., McBride, M., Palmisano, B., Perweiler, E. A., Roush, R. E., et al. (2006). Bioterrorism and emergency preparedness in aging (BTEPA): HRSA-funded GEC collaboration for curricula and training. *Gerontology and Geriatrics Education, 26*(4), 63–86.

Slusarski, S. B. (1994). Enhancing self-direction in the adult learner: Instructional techniques for teachers and trainers. *New Directions for Adult and Continuing Education, 64,* 71–79.

Versitas Corporation. (2006). *Setting up a training program for your company.* Retrieved August 10, 2009, from http://www.versotas.com/setting-up-training-program.php

APPENDIX II

Glossary of Terms Commonly Used in Geriatric Mental Health and Disaster Preparedness

Those items marked with an asterisk are from Tener Goodwin Veenema (Ed.), *Disaster Nursing and Emergency Preparedness*. Copyright © 2007 Springer Publishing Company, LLC. Reproduced with the permission of Springer Publishing Company, LLC, New York, NY 10036.

Acute Stress Disorder. Acute stress disorder is an anxiety disorder characterized by symptoms of motor tension, hypervigilance, and autonomic hyperarousal. Acute stress disorder is symptomatically similar to PTSD but is distinguished by a duration of a minimum of 2 days to a maximum of 4 weeks with the onset of symptoms within 4 weeks of the traumatic stimulus event.

Anxiety Disorders. Anxiety disorders are characterized by excessive, uncontrollable worries with accompanying symptoms of motor tension, hypervigilance, and autonomic hyperarousal such as palpitations, dry mouth, dizziness, hot flashes, and gastrointestinal distress. Anxiety disorders include phobic disorder, panic disorder, generalized anxiety disorder, obsessive-compulsive disorder, and PTSD.

Activities of Daily Living (ADLs). Self-maintenance skills such as dressing, bathing, toileting, grooming, eating, and ambulating.

Acute Treatment. Formally defined procedures used to reduce and remove the signs and symptoms of depression and to restore psychosocial function.

Adequate Treatment Analysis. Analysis of data in terms of the relationship between the number of patients who received a predetermined minimum amount of treatment and the number who responded.

*Advanced Life Support. A medical procedure performed by paramedics that includes the advanced diagnosis and protocol-driven treatment of a patient in the field.

Affective Lability. Rapidly changing or unstable expressions of emotion or mood.

Agnosia. Loss or impairment of the ability to recognize, understand, or interpret sensory stimuli or features of the outside world such as shapes or symbols.

Agoraphobia. A disorder characterized by a fear of open, public places or crowded situations.

Anhedonia. An absence of or the inability to experience a sense of pleasure from any activity.

Aphasia. Prominent language dysfunction affecting an individual's ability to articulate ideas or comprehend spoken or written language.

Apraxia. Loss or impairment of the ability to perform a learned motor act in the absence of sensory or motor impairment (e.g., paralysis or paresis).

*Basic Life Support. Noninvasive measures used to treat unstable patients, such as extraction of airway obstructions, cardiopulmonary resuscitation, care of wounds and hemorrhages, and immobilization of fractures.

Behavioral Therapy. A form of psychotherapy focused on modifying observable problematic behaviors by systematic manipulation of the environment.

*Bioterrorism. The unlawful release of biologic agents or toxins with the intent to intimidate or coerce a government or civilian population to further political or social objectives; humans, animals, and plants are often targets.

Bipolar Disorder. A major mood disorder characterized by episodes of major depression and mania or hypomania, formerly called manic-depressive psychosis, circular type. The diagnosis of bipolar I disorder requires one or more episodes of mania. The diagnosis of bipolar II disorder requires one or more episodes of hypomania and is excluded by the history or presence of a manic episode. Current episode may be manic, depressed, hypomanic, or mixed manic.

*Case Definition. Standardized criteria for deciding whether a person has a particular disease or health-related condition; often used in investigations and for comparing potential cases; case definitions help decide which disaster-specific conditions should be monitored with emergency information surveillance systems.

*Case Management. The collaborative process that assesses, plans, implements, coordinates, monitors, and evaluates the options and services required to meet an individual's health needs.

*Casualty. Any person suffering physical and/or psychological damage that leads to death, injury, or material loss.

Clinical Management. Education of and discussion with patients and, when appropriate, their families about the nature of depression, its course, and the relative costs and benefits of treatment options. It also includes assessment and management of the patient while in treatment along with resolution of obstacles to treatment adherence, monitoring and management of treatment side effects, and assessment of outcome.

Cognition. The conscious faculty or process of knowing, including all aspects of awareness, perception, reasoning, thinking, and remembering.

Cognitive Functions. Mental processes, including memory, language skills, attention, and judgment.

Cognitive Therapy. A treatment method that focuses on revising a person's maladaptive processes of thinking, perceptions, attitudes, and beliefs. Cognitive therapy has been developed for different disorders, including depression.

*Community Profile. The characteristics of the local environment that are prone to a chemical or nuclear accident [these characteristics can include population density; age distribution; number of road-ways, railways, and waterways; type of buildings; and local relief agencies].

*Comprehensive Emergency Management. A broad style of emergency management, encompassing prevention, preparedness, response, and recovery.

Comprehensive Mental Status Examination. Assessment of multiple cognitive functions that provides a detailed cognitive profile of the patient.

Confrontation Naming. The ability to name an object when shown a picture of it.

Continuation Treatment. Treatment designed to prevent the return of the most recent mood episode.

*Crisis Management. Administrative measures that identify, acquire, and plan the use of resources needed to anticipate, prevent, and/or resolve a threat to public health and safety.

Cyclothymic Disorder. A mood disorder of at least 2 years' duration characterized by numerous periods of mild depressive symptoms not sufficient in duration or severity to meet the criteria for major depressive episodes interspersed with periods of hypomania. Some view this condition as a mild variant of bipolar disorder.

Delirium. A temporary disordered mental state characterized by the acute and sudden onset of cognitive impairment, disorientation, disturbances in attention, decline in level of consciousness, or perceptual disturbances.

Dementia. A syndrome of progressive decline in multiple areas (domains) of cognitive function eventually leading to a significant inability to maintain occupational and social performance. This group of mental disorders involves a general loss of intellectual abilities, including memory, judgment, and abstract thinking. There may be associated poor impulse control and/or personality change. Dementias may be progressive, reversible, or static and have a variety of causes.

Direct Costs. The expense of diagnostic, treatment, and care services.

*Disaster. Any event, typically occurring suddenly, that causes damage, ecological disruption, loss of human life, deterioration of health and health services, and which exceeds the capacity of the affected community on a scale sufficient to require outside assistance. These events can be caused by nature, equipment malfunction, human error, or biological hazards and disease [e.g., earthquake, flood, fire, hurricane, cyclone, typhoon, significant storms, volcanic eruptions, spills, air crashes, drought, epidemic, food shortages, civil strife].

*Disaster Field Office (DFO). The office established in or near the disaster area that supports federal and state response as well as recovery operations. The Disaster Field Office houses the Federal Coordinating Officer (FCO), the Emergency Response Team (ERT), the State Coordinating Officer (SCO), and support staff.

*Disaster Severity Scale. A scale that classifies disasters by the following parameters: the radius of the disaster site, the number of dead, the number of wounded, the average severity of the injuries sustained, the impact time, and the rescue time.

Dysthymia. A mood disorder characterized by depressed mood and loss of interest or pleasure in customary activities, with some additional signs and symptoms of depression, that is present most of the time for at least 2 years. Many patients with dysthymia go on to develop major depressive episodes.

Effect Size. A summary statistic that provides an index of the ability of a screening or test instrument to discriminate between persons with and without a particular symptom, cluster of symptoms, or disease.

Electroconvulsive Therapy. A treatment method usually reserved for very severe or psychotic depressions or manic states that are not responsive to medication treatment. A low-voltage alternating current is sent to the brain to induce a convulsion or seizure, which induces the therapeutic effect.

*Emergency. Any natural or man-made situation that results in severe injury, harm, or loss of humans or property.

*Emergency Management Agency (EMA). (Also referred to as the Office of Emergency Preparedness (OEP).) The EMA, under the authority of the governor's office, coordinates the efforts of the state's health department, housing and social service agencies, and public safety agencies during an emergency or disaster. The EMA also coordinates federal resources made available to the states, such as the National

Guard, the Centers for Disease Control, and the Public Health Service [e.g., Agency for Toxic Substances Disease Registry (ATSDR)].

*Emergency Medical Services (EMS) System. The coordination of the prehospital system [e.g., public access, dispatch, EMTs/and medics, ambulance services] and the in-hospital system [e.g., emergency departments, hospitals, and other definitive care facilities and personnel] to provide emergency medical care.

*Emergency Medical Technicians (EMTs) and Paramedics (EMT-Ps). Trained emergency medical responders, paramedics and EMTs, are trained to diagnose and treat the most common medical emergencies in the field and to provide medical treatment while en route to the hospital. Paramedics are more highly trained than EMTs.

*Emergency Operations Center (EOC). The location where department heads, government officials, and volunteer agencies coordinate the response to an emergency.

*Emergency Response Team. A team of federal personnel and support staff that is deployed by FEMA during a major disaster or emergency; the duty of the team is to assist the Federal Coordinating Officer (FCO) in carrying out his or her responsibilities under the Stafford Act; team members consist of representatives from each federal department or agency that has been assigned primary responsibility for an emergency support function as well as key members of the FCO's staff.

*Epidemic. The occurrence of any known or suspected contagion that occurs in clear excess of normal expectancy. [A threatened epidemic occurs when the circumstances are such that a disease may reasonably be anticipated to occur in excess of normal expectancy.]

Episodic Memory. Memory of one's own experiences that is unique and localizable in time and space.

*Evacuation. An organized removal of civilians from a dangerous or potentially dangerous area.

Executive Functions. Goal formulation, planning, and execution of plans.

*Exposure Surveillance. To look for risk exposure in a disaster setting. Exposure may be based on the physical or environmental properties of the disaster event and may also be known as a risk factor variable, predictor variable, or independent variable.

Factor Analysis. A statistical procedure designed to determine if variability in scores can be related to one or more factors that are reliably influencing performance.

False Negative. Erroneous finding that a patient does not have a particular medical condition (e.g. dementia) when the person does have it.

False Positive. Erroneous finding that a patient does have a particular medical condition (e.g., dementia) when the person does not have it.

***Federal Coordinating Officer (FCO).** The person appointed by FEMA following a presidential declaration of a severe disaster or of an emergency to coordinate federal assistance. The FCO initiates immediate action to assure that federal assistance is provided in accordance with the disaster declaration, any applicable laws or regulations, and the FEMA-state agreement.

***Federal On-Scene Commander (OSC).** The official that ensures appropriate coordination of the United States government's overall response with federal, state, and local authorities; the OSC maintains this role until the United States Attorney General transfers the Lead Federal Agency (LFA) role to FEMA.

***First Responder.** Local police, fire, and emergency medical personnel who arrive first on the scene of an incident and take action to save lives, protect property, and meet basic human needs.

Focused History. A patient history confined to questions designed to elicit information related to cognitive impairment or a decline in function consistent with dementia and to document the chronology of the problems.

Focused Physical Examination. A physical examination that seeks to identify life-threatening or rapidly progressing illness while paying special attention to conditions that might cause delirium. The examination typically includes a brief neurological evaluation as well as assessment of mobility and cardiac, respiratory, and sensory functions.

Further Assessment. An additional evaluation concluded after the initial assessment and intended to clarify information gleaned from that assessment to make a decision about the presence of a dementing disorder.

Generalized Anxiety Disorder. Generalized anxiety disorder is a chronic mental health condition that involves excessive, uncontrollable worries accompanied by motor tension (shakiness, muscle tension, restlessness, fatigue) and hypervigilance (difficulty concentrating, insomnia, irritability, and heightened startle response). Symptoms occur most days for a minimum of 6 months.

Hypomania. An episode of illness that resembles mania, but is less intense and less disabling. The state is characterized by a euphoric mood, unrealistic optimism, increased speech and activity, and a decreased need for sleep. For some, there is increased creativity, while others evidence poor judgment and impaired function.

Incremental Validity. The notion that information from multiple, reliable sources enhances the validity of the assessment.

Indigenous Workers. Crisis counselors who come from within the local community, cultural, or ethnic group targeted for crisis counseling services. They are members of, familiar to, and recognized by their own communities. They may be spouses of community leaders, natural leaders in their own right, or have nurturing roles in their communities. Examples of indigenous workers may also include retired persons, students, active community volunteers, and so forth. Indigenous workers may or may not have formal training in counseling or related professions; they may be paraprofessionals or professionals.

Indirect Costs. The expense of morbidity (the value of lost or reduced productivity of a patient, an unpaid caretaker, or both) caused by illness and mortality (the present value of future earnings lost because of premature death from disease).

Initial Assessment (for Dementia). An evaluation conducted when the patient, clinician, or someone close to the patient first notices or mentions symptoms that suggest the presence of a dementing disorder. This evaluation includes a focused history, a focused physical examination of mental status and function, and consideration of confounding and comorbid conditions.

Instrumental Activities of Daily Living (IADLs). Complex, higher order skills such as managing finances, using the telephone, driving a car, taking medications, planning a meal, shopping, and working in an occupation.

Intent-to-Treat Analysis. Analysis of data in terms of the relationship between the number of patients randomized to treatment and the number whose condition improved.

Interpersonal Psychotherapy. A time-limited psychotherapeutic approach that aims to clarify and resolve one or more of the following interpersonal difficulties: role disputes, social isolation, prolonged grief reaction, or role transition. The patient and therapist define the nature of the difficulty and work to its resolution.

*Man-Made or Human-Generated Disasters; Complex Emergencies. Technological events that are caused by humans and occur in human settlements [for example, fire, chemical spills and explosions, and armed conflict].

Maintenance Treatment. Treatment designed to prevent a new mood episode (e.g. depression, mania, or hypomania).

Major Depressive Disorder. A major mood disorder characterized by one (single) or more (recurrent) episodes of major depression, with or without full recovery between episodes.

Major Disaster. A major disaster refers to any natural or man-made catastrophe (including any hurricane, tornado, storm, high water, wind-driven water, tidal wave, tsunami, earthquake, volcanic eruption, landslide, mudslide, snowstorm, drought, or terrorist activity) that by the determination of the president causes damage of sufficient severity and magnitude to warrant major disaster assistance to supplement the efforts and available resources of states, local governments, and disaster relief organizations in alleviating the damage, loss, hardship, or suffering .

Mania. An episode of illness usually seen in the course of bipolar I disorder and characterized by hyperexcitability, euphoria, and hyperactivity. Rapid thinking and speaking, agitation, a decreased need for sleep, and a marked increase in energy are nearly always present. During manic episodes, some patients also experience hallucinations or delusions. Manic episodes can also be caused by selected general medical disorders.

*Maslow's Theory of Human Motivation and Hierarchy of Basic Needs. This theory of human development proposes a hierarchical structure for human needs—from physiological drives to needs for safety, belonging, love, esteem, and self-actualization at the top of the pyramid.

Melancholic Features. Symptoms usually found in severe major depressive episodes, including marked loss of pleasure, psychomotor retardation or agitation, weight loss, and insomnia.

*Medical Coordination. The coordination between health care providers during the transition from the prehospital to the hospital phase of patient care; simplification and standardization of materials and methods are a prerequisite.

Meta-Analysis. Any systematic method that uses statistical analysis to integrate data from a number of independent studies.

*Mitigation. Measures taken to reduce the harmful effects of a disaster by attempting to limit the disaster's impact on human health and economic infrastructure.

Mood Disorders. A grouping of psychiatric conditions that have as a central feature a disturbance in mood usually manifest as profound sadness or apathy, euphoria, or irritability. These disorders may be episodic or chronic.

*Natural Disasters. Natural phenomena with acute onset and profound effects [e.g., earthquakes, floods, cyclones, tornadoes] that causes damage, ecological disruption, loss of human life, deterioration of health and human services, and which exceeds the capacity of the affected community on a scale sufficient to require outside assistance.

Nonreversible Dementias. Term used to distinguish cognitive disorders that cannot be treated effectively to restore normal or nearly normal intellectual function, such as Alzheimer's disease, from those that can.

Obsessive-Compulsive Disorder. A condition characterized by the presence of obsessions and/or compulsions. Obsessions are recurrent, intrusive thoughts—usually irrational worries—that often necessitate behaviors to prevent untoward consequences (e.g., fears of contamination from dirt requiring the individual to wear gloves at all times). Compulsions are recurrent behaviors beyond the normal range that the individual feels compelled to undertake, usually to preserve personal safety, to avoid embarrassment, or to perform adequately (e.g., checking multiple times to see that the gas is turned off before leaving home). This disorder affects 1% to 2% of the population.

Open Trial. A trial of a treatment in which both patient and practitioner are aware of the treatment being used.

Outreach. Outreach is a method for delivering crisis counseling services to disaster survivors and victims. It consists primarily of face-to-face contact with survivors in their natural environments in order to provide disaster related crisis counseling services. Outreach is the means by which crisis counseling services are made available.

Panic Disorder. An anxiety disorder characterized by discrete intense periods of fear and associated symptoms. Panic disorder may be accompanied by agoraphobia.

Phobias. Phobias are recurring, persistent, irrational fears of situations, objects, or activities that result in a change of lifestyle characterized by avoidance of the phobic stimulus.

Polypharmacy. The administration of many drugs together.

Posttraumatic Stress Disorder (PTSD). PTSD is characterized by a re-experiencing of the symptoms related to a previous trauma, including but not limited to distressing recollections, dreams, or flashbacks. Symptoms of PTSD include persistent avoidance of stimuli associated with the original trauma, numbing of general responsiveness (such as feelings of detachment, restricted range of affect, loss of interest in activities), and symptoms of hyperarousal.

Praxis. The performance of an action, movement, or series of movements.

*Preparedness. All measures and policies taken before an event occurs that allow for prevention, mitigation, and readiness. [Preparedness includes designing educational programs and resources, warning systems, planning for evacuation and relocation storing food and water, building temporary shelter, devising management strategies, and holding disaster drills and exercises.] Contingency planning is also included in preparedness as well as planning for post-impact response and recovery.

*Prevention. Primary, secondary, and tertiary efforts that help avert an emergency; these activities are commonly referred to as "mitigation" in the emergency management model [for example, in public health terms, prevention refers to actions that prevent the onset or deterioration of mental health and other diseases, disability, and injury].

*Primary Prevention. Preventing the occurrence of death, injury, or illness in a disaster [e.g., evacuation of a community in a flood-prone area, sensitizing warning systems for tornadoes and severe storms].

Procedural memory. Memory for certain ways of doing things or for certain movements.

Psychometric. Relating to the systematic measurement of mental processes; psychological variables such as intelligence, aptitude, and personality traits; and behavioral acts.

*Readiness. Links preparedness to relief; an assessment of readiness reflects the current capacity and capabilities of the organizations involved in relief activities.

Remission. A return to the asymptomatic state usually accompanied by a return to the usual level of psychosocial functioning.

*Recovery. Actions of responders, government, and the victims that help return an affected community to normal by stimulating community cohesiveness and government involvement. [One type of recovery involves repairing infrastructure, damaged buildings, and critical facilities. The recovery period falls between the onset of the emergency and the reconstruction period.]

*Recovery Plan. A plan to restore areas affected by disaster; developed on a state-by-state basis with assistance from responding federal agencies.

*Response. The phase in a disaster when relief, recovery, and rehabilitation occur; also includes the delivery of services, the management of activities and programs designed to address the immediate and short-term effects of an emergency or disaster.

Reversible Dementias. Term used to distinguish cognitive disorders that can be treated effectively to restore normal or nearly normal intellectual function from those that cannot.

*Risk Assessment. A systematic process that determines the likelihood of adverse health effects to a population after exposure to a hazard; health consequences may depend on the type of hazard and damage to infrastructure, loss of economic value, loss of function, loss of natural resources, loss of ecological systems, and environmental impacts and deterioration of health, mortality, and morbidity. [The major components of a risk assessment include a hazard identification analysis and a vulnerability analysis that answer the following questions: What are the hazards that could affect a community? What can happen as a result of those hazards? How likely is each of the possible outcomes? When the possible outcomes occur, what are the likely consequences and losses?] Risk assessment is a fundamental planning tool for disaster management, especially during prevention and mitigation activities.

*Secondary Prevention. Mitigates the health consequences of disasters. [Examples include the use of carbon monoxide detectors when operating gasoline-powered generators after the loss of electric power, employing appropriate occupant behavior in multi-story structures during earthquakes, and building "safe rooms" in dwellings located in tornado-prone areas.] Secondary prevention may be instituted when disasters are imminent.

Semantic Memory. What is learned as knowledge; it is timeless and spaceless (e.g., the alphabet or historical data unrelated to a person's life).

Sensitivity (of a Test Instrument). Ability to identify cases of a particular medical condition (e.g., dementia) in a population that includes persons who do not have it. Also called diagnostic sensitivity.

Somatization Disorder. A disorder characterized by multiple, often long-standing somatic complaints of bodily dysfunction (e.g., pain complaints and gastrointestinal disturbances). The disorder usually begins before the age of 30 and has a chronic, fluctuating course.

Specificity (of a Test Instrument). Ability to identify those who do not have a particular medical condition (e.g., dementia) in a population that includes persons who do have it. Also called diagnostic specificity.

*State Coordinating Officer. An official designated by the governor of an affected state upon the declaration of a major disaster or emergency to coordinate state and local disaster assistance efforts with those of the federal government and to act in cooperation with the FCO to administer disaster recovery efforts.

Supportive Therapy. Psychotherapy that focuses on the management and resolution of current difficulties and life decisions using the patient's strengths and available resources.

Symptom Breakthrough. The return of symptoms in the course of either continuation or maintenance treatment.

*Tertiary Prevention. The minimization of the effects of disease and disability among those with preexisting health conditions. Tertiary prevention shields persons with health conditions from negative health effects relating to a disaster. [Examples of tertiary prevention include protecting persons with respiratory illnesses and those prone to respiratory conditions from haze and smoke byproducts of forest fires and sheltering elderly who are prone to heat illnesses during episodes of extreme ambient temperatures.]

Vascular Dementia. Dementia with a stepwise progression of symptoms, each with an abrupt onset, often in association with a neurologic incident. Also called multi-infarct dementia.

Visuospatial Ability. Capacity to produce and recognize three-dimensional or two-dimensional figures and objects.

Vegetative Symptoms. A group of symptoms that refer to sleep, appetite, and/or weight regulation.

*Voluntary Agency (VOLAG). A nonprofit, nongovernmental, private association maintained and supported by voluntary contributions that provides assistance in emergencies and disasters.

Vulnerability. The susceptibility of a population to a specific type of event; it is also associated with the degree of possible or potential loss from a risk that results from a hazard at a given intensity. The factors that influence vulnerability include demographics, the age and resilience of the environment, technology, social differentiation, and diversity as well as regional and global economics and politics.

Vulnerability Analysis. The assessment of an exposed population's susceptibility to the adverse health effects of a particular hazard.

*Weapons of Mass Destruction (WMD). Any device, material, or substance used in a manner, in a quantity or type, or under circumstances evidencing an intent to cause death or serious injury to persons or significant damage to property.

Word Fluency. Ability to generate quickly a list of words that all belong to a common category or begin with a specific letter.

Index